URINARY INCONTINENCE

Edited by **Ammar Alhasso**
and **Ashani Fernando**

Urinary Incontinence
Edited by Ammar Alhasso and Ashani Fernando

Published by InTech

Janeza Trdine 9, 51000 Rijeka, Croatia

Publishing Process Manager Danijela Duric

Technical Editor Teodora Smiljanic

Cover Designer InTech Design Team

Additional hard copies can be obtained from orders@intechopen.com

Urinary Incontinence, Edited by Ammar Alhasso and Ashani Fernando
p. cm.
ISBN 978-953-51-0484-1

For EU product safety concerns:
IN TECH d.o.o., Prolaz Marije Krucifikse Kozulić 3, 51000 Rijeka, Croatia,
info@intechopen.com or visit our website at intechopen.com.

Meet the editors

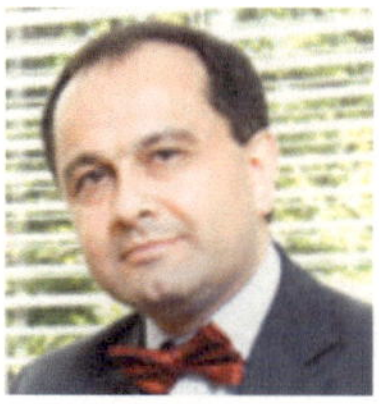

Dr Ammar Alhasso is a Consultant Urological Surgeon at the University of Edinburgh Teaching Hospitals. Providing both general urology expertise and subspecialisation in female urology, urodynamics and reconstructive urology. He was a research fellow at Imperial College School of Medicine, University of London studying bladder cancer and achieved a Masters degree in Surgical Sciences in 2000. He is also a reviewer for the Cochrane Collaboration/Incontinence group and has published systematic reviews and meta-analyses on urinary incontinence in men and women. With commitment to training and education, Ammar is the urology module organiser for undergraduates at Edinburgh University Medical School, Faculty member of the core skills for urologist course at the Royal College of Surgeons of Edinburgh, a member of the local scientific committee for ICS- 2011 and recently took up role of module leader for the Master of Surgery (ChM) in Urology course at University of Edinburgh.

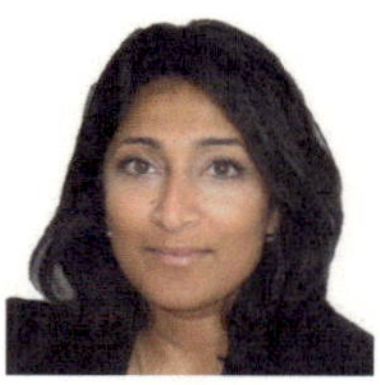

Ms Ashani Fernando graduated from Auckland University, New Zealand with a degree in medicine in 2004. Her Urological training was undertaken in New Zealand culminating in attaining her FRACS(urol) in 2011. Working as a fellow in reconstructive urology at the Western General Hospital in Edinburgh, UK, a center of excellence, she is focusing on urodynamics, voiding dysfunction and urethral and bladder reconstruction. She has published on stone disease and is a reviewer for the Cochrane collaboration/Incontinence group. She is also an organiser for post-graduate training modules in reconstructive urology.

Contents

Preface

Urinary incontinence is a condition that affects a significant proportion of the population. The prevalence increases with age and there is a female preponderance. With the advent of more aggressive management strategies for prostate cancer, there is an increase in the proportion of men struggling with incontinence as well. Incontinence has social, physical, psychological and economic implications for the individual as well as society as a whole. This book attempts to look at the aetiology, investigation and current management of urinary incontinence along with setting it within the framework of clinical practice.

Management strategies are framed within a multidisciplinary team structure and as such a range of specialists ranging from psychologists, specialist nurses, gynaecologists and urologists author the chapters. There are some novel methods outlined by the authors with their clinical application and utility described in detail, along with exhaustive research on epidemiology, which is particularly relevant in planning for the future. We would like to acknowledge all the authors for all the hard work and dedication to excellence in completing this book.

Mr Ammar Alhasso
Consultant Urological Surgeon
and Honorary Clinical Senior Lecturer
at University of Edinburgh,
UK

Ms Ashani Fernando
Fellow in Urologic Reconstructive Surgery
Western General Hospital, Edinburgh,
UK

Part 1

The Basics

1

The Role of Altered Connective Tissue in the Causation of Pelvic Floor Symptoms

B. Liedl[1,*], O. Markovsky[1], F. Wagenlehner[2] and A. Gunnemann[3]
[1]*Pelvic Floor Centre Munich,*
[2]*Urological Clinic of the University of Giessen,*
[3]*Urological Department Klinikum Detmold,*
Germany

1. Introduction

The pelvic floor consists of muscles and connective tissue. In the past, the components' relative contribution to the structural support of the pelvic floor and its functions has been a subject of controversy (Corton 2009). With increasing age women can develop vaginal and pelvic organ prolapse as well as symptoms such as stress urinary incontinence, voiding dysfunction, urgency and frequency and nocturia, and may also develop fecal incontinence, obstructive defecation and pelvic pain (Petros 2010). All of these symptoms can be associated - to a greater or lesser extent - with pelvic floor defects.

What events are responsible for these defects? One theory says that an important cause of prolapse and pelvic floor dysfunction is likely to be partial denervation (Swash et al 1985, Smith et al. 1989). But Pierce et al. (2008) demonstrated in nulliparous monkeys that bilateral transection of the levator ani nerve resulted in atrophy of denervated levator ani muscles but not in failure of pelvic support. This indicates that connective tissue components could compensate for weakened pelvic floor muscles. According to South et al. (2009), in up to 30 percent of all vaginal childbirths, pelvic floor muscles are partially denervated. However, such functions are known to recover and reinnervate often within months (Snooks et al 1984, Lin et al. 2010) .

In a direct test of the question, "connective tissue or muscle damage?", Petros et al 2008 performed a blinded prospective study with muscle biopsies of m.pubococcygeus taken at the same time as a midurethral sling operation for urinary stress incontinence (USI) was done, an operation which works by creating an artificial collagenous neoligament (Petros PE, Ulmsten U, Papadimitriou 1990). Out of 39 patients with histological evidence of muscle damage, 33 (85%) were cured immediately after surgery, indicating that connective tissue, not muscle damage was most likely the major cause of the USI.

Further, the muscle itself can change. It is known that the number and density of urethral striated muscle fibers declines with age (Huisman 1983, Perucchini et al. 2002), an idea that has been confirmed in studies about the vastus lateralis muscle (Lexell et al. 1988). Muscle

---

*Corresponding Author

avulsions have been reported at the pelvic floor (Dietz and Lanzarone 2005, Dietz et al. 2007), but it is more likely that the insertion areas of muscles are dislocated by connective tissue alterations than muscle tears (Petros 2008).

From a mechanical point of view, the pelvic floor is composed of both muscles and connective tissue. The muscles are the active components that are - through their contractions - responsible for all functions of the pelvic floor. The connective tissues, with their elastic and collagen fibres and their extracellular matrices, provide structural support for the vagina and other organs such as uterus, urethra, bladder and rectum (Abramowitch 2009). It has been shown, that connective tissue changes occur during pregnancy (Rechberger et al. 1988, Harkness 1959). Weakening of collagen cross bonding (Rechberger et al. 1988) added to dilatation of the vaginal canal at childbirth can lead to overdistension or rupture of connective tissue. Extracellular matrix proteases contribute to progression of pelvic organ prolapse in mice and humans (Budatha et al. 2011, Connell 2011). The first vaginal birth is especially associated with the development of a prolapse, whereas additional vaginal births do not show significant increases in the odds of prolapse (Quiroz et al. 2011). Aging is characterized by a loss of collagen, degeneration of the elastic fibre network and a loss of hydration as a result of imbalance between biosynthesis and degradation (Uitto und Bernstein 1998, Campisi 1998)

In addition to that, there is a significant variability of tissue due to inborn variations (Dietz et al 2004) and collagen-associated disorders (Lammers et al. 2011, Campeau et al. 2011).

Surgical procedures can reduce structural support of the organs, especially those which cut or displace the uterosacral and cardinal ligaments during hysterectomy or which partially resect vaginal tissue or perineal body during colporrhaphy.

Petros and Ulmsten (1993) stated that looseness or laxity of the vagina and its supporting ligaments can cause stress incontinence as well as urge. Since then the theory has been expanded to include other symptoms such as pelvic pain, voiding dysfunction and more recently, fecal incontinence and constipation (Petros & Swash 2008). In order to fix such loose ligaments Petros et al. (1990) have introduced alloplastic material for planned formation of an artificial neo-ligament. From this rather basic research, new surgical techniques have been developed, such as tapes for midurethral slings (TVT, TOT) and for repair of other pelvic floor ligaments (Petros and Ulmsten 1990, 1993). The new developments and the recent focus on connective tissue are important, not least because looseness of tissues can be repaired surgically..

2. Basic effect of altered connective tissues (looseness) on muscle function

Gordon (1966) studied the relation between muscle force and sarcomere length (figure 1). As a muscle fiber consists of a distinct number of sarcomeres, the determined relation can be leveraged for the full length of the muscle, for which the same relation can be assumed.

This implies that a muscle has a special range of lengths, in which it can perform its peak force. If the muscle is shortened, its force decreases and goes down towards zero. If a muscle is overlengthened, its force goes down, too, sometimes even all the way to zero, at a length half of the one that gives optimal force. This means that a fully innervated muscle with normal morphology can have very low or even no force when it is over-stretched. The same process occurs in women with descending or prolapsing vaginal wall and pelvic organs. The muscles which attaches directly or indirectly to the vagina or the pelvic organs change their length and their direction of action. This alters muscle force and function according to the relation shown in Figure 1. After re-positioning of the prolapsed organs, the muscle can reach its normal length and function. Hence, atrophy of muscle by immobilization (Hvid et al. 2011) can be avoided at least with some patients.

A prime example of this principle is restoration of urethral closure by a midurethral sling which restores the integrity of the pubourethral ligament. In the original description of the „tension-free" sling (Ulmsten et al 1996), the operation was performed under local anesthesia and the tape was lifted upwards while the patient was coughing, until the urine leakage ceased.

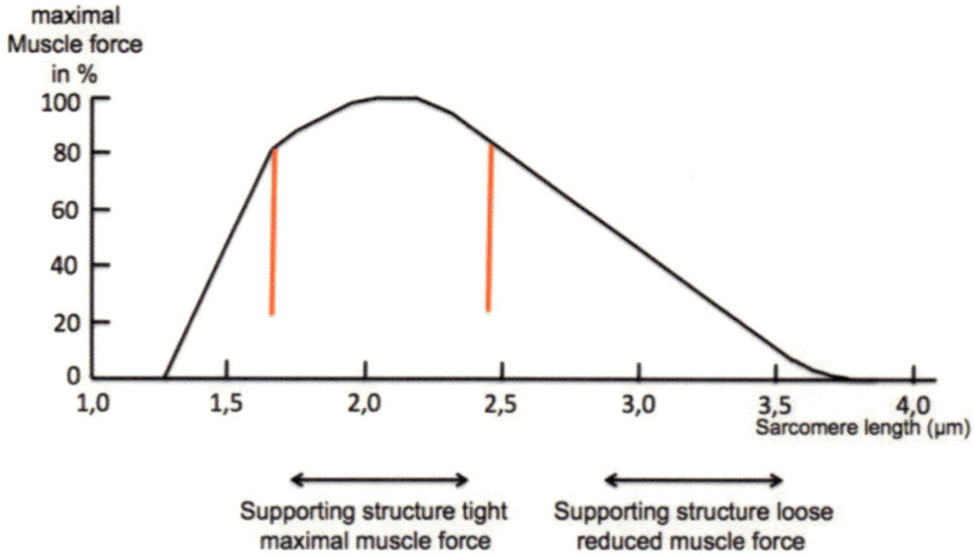

Fig. 1. Relationship of maximal muscle force to muscle (sarcomere)length (modified after Gordon 1966). Maximal muscle strength is exerted over a very short length (between red lines). Contractile strength falls rapidly with muscle lengthening and shortening, for example, due to lax connective tissue attachments.

3. Pelvic floor muscles and their functions (figure 2)

In many studies morphology of pelvic floor muscles has been explained with only few limited reference to muscle action. There is no doubt that the pelvic floor muscles and ligaments have immense importance for stress incontinence, micturition and anorectal functions. It was P. Petros who explained the directional muscle forces (Petros and Ulmsten 1993, Petros and Ulmsten 1997) and their significant role in pelvic floor dysfunctions.

From a functional and clinical aspect, it is important to consider 4 major muscle groups of the pelvic floor which are able to move the vaginal wall and pelvic floor organs (Petros 2010):

1. The anterior and medial portions of the pubococcygeus muscle (PCM) arise on either side from the inner surface of the pubic bone and attach to the lateral walls of the distal vagina (Zacharin 1963, Petros und Ulmsten 1997, Corton 2009). This muscle portion, called pubococcygeus muscle (PCM) by Petros and Ulmsten (1993) and pubovaginal muscle by Corton (2009) can pull the distal vagina forward to close the distal urethra during effort (coughing or straining). This muscle needs intact pubourethral ligaments for optimal action.
2. The levator plate in the upper layer runs horizontally, goes into the posterior wall of the rectum, and thus plays a major role in any backward movement of this organ. This muscle needs intact pubourethral and uterosacral ligaments and an intact perineal body to optimize its various actions.
3. The conjoint longitudinal muscle of the anus (LMA) is a striated muscle which constitutes the middle layer. It is vertically oriented, creates the downward force for bladder neck closure during effort and stretches open the outflow tract during micturition. It takes fibers superiorly from the levator plate (LP), the lateral part of the pubococcygeus and puborectalis muscle. It is well anchored by extra-anal sphincter (Courtney 1950). This muscle needs intact uterosacral ligaments for optimal action.
4. The puborectalis muscle (PRM) originates just medially to PCM and traverses all three muscle layers. It is orientated vertically and runs forward medially below PCM. It is closely applied to the lateral walls of the rectum and surrounds them (Courtney 1950).

The lower layer of pelvic floor muscles is an important anchoring layer. It consists of perineal membranes and component muscles - bulbocavernosus, ischiocavernosus and the deep and superficial transverse perinei muscles. The deep transverse perinei muscle anchors the upper part of the perineal body to the descending pubic ramus. It is a strong muscle and it stabilizes the perineal body laterally. The external anal sphincter acts as a tensor of the perineal body and represents the principal insertion point of the LMA. The bulbocavernosus muscle stretches and anchors the distal part of the urethra. The ischiocavernosus muscle helps stabilize the perineal membrane and may act to stretch the external urethral meatus laterally via its effect of the bulbocavernosus. Between the extra-anal sphincter and the coccyx lies the postanal plate, a tendinous structure which also contains striated muscles inserting into the extra-anal sphincter (Petros 2010).

The striated rhabdosphincter of the urethra surrounds the urethra in the middle third of its length for approximatly 1,5 cm (Oelrich 1983).

4. Important connective tissue structures at the pelvic floor (figures 2 and 8)

At the pelvic floor at least 9 sites of connective tissue can be defined as loose. With regard to its function, P. Petros (2010) divides the connective tissue defects in three zones (figure 2).

The **anterior zone**, which reaches from the external meatus of the urethra to the bladder neck, embraces three important structures:

The extraurethral ligament runs from the pubis anteriorly to the meatus urethrae anterior to the perineal membrane.

The pubourethral ligament, a ligament with key relevance for stress urinary continence, originates from the lower end of the posterior surface of the pubic symphysis and descends like a fan to insert into the pubococcygeus muscle and lateral part of the mid urethra (Zacharin 1963, Petros 1998).

The suburethral vagina acts as a hammock for the urethra. The antero-medial portion of the pubococcygeus muscles is attached laterally on each side of the hammock

In the **middle zone**, which reaches from the bladder neck to the cervix, three further structures are important:

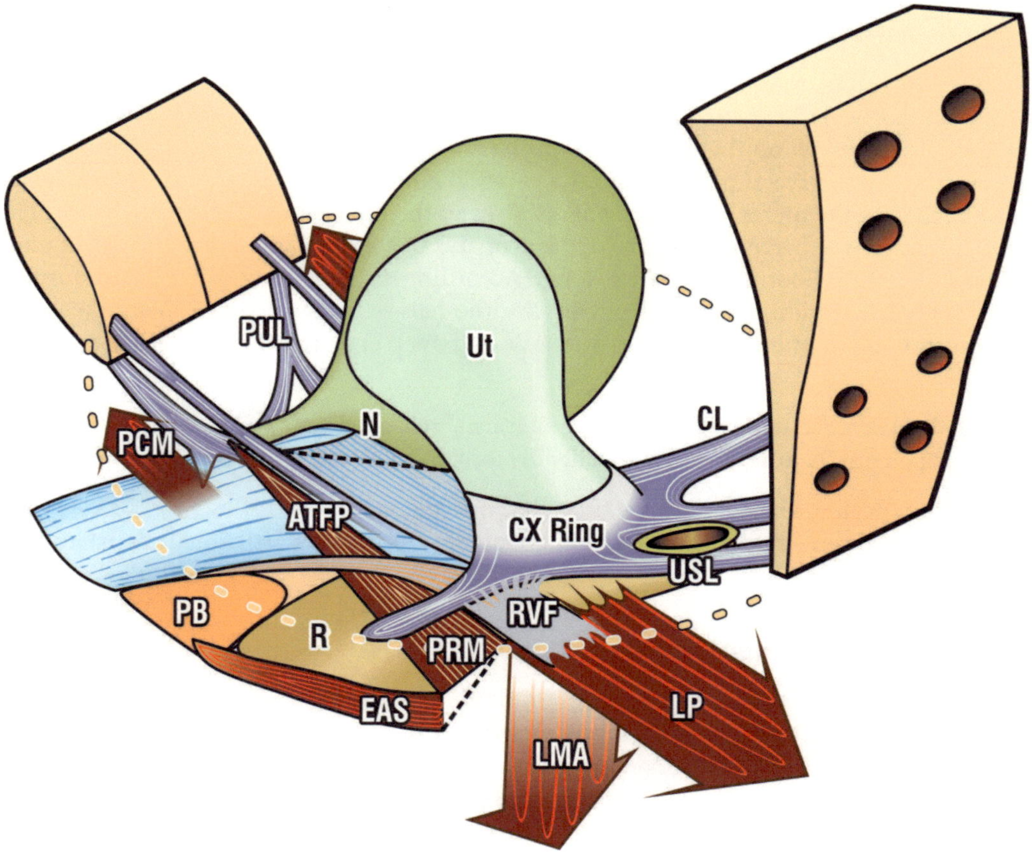

PCM: pubococcygeus muscle, LP: levator plate, LMA: longitudinal muscle of the anus
PRM: puborectalis muscle, EAS: extraanal sphincter
PUL: pubourethral ligament, ATFP: Arcus tendineus fasciae pelvis, CL: cardinal ligament
CX-Ring: cervical ring, USL: uterosacral ligament, RVF: rectovaginal fascia
PB: perineal body, B: bladder, Ut: uterus, R: rectum
N: stretch receptor at bladder base

Fig. 2. Important muscles and connective tissue structure at the pelvic floor (from P. Petros 2010, by permission)

The arcus tendineus fascia pelvis (ATFP) are horizontal ligaments which arise just superior to the pubourethral ligaments at the pubis symphysis and insert into the ischial spine. The vagina is suspended from the ATFP by its fascia, much like a sheet slung across two washing lines (Nichols 1989). The cardinal ligaments are attached to the cervical ring and pubocervical fascia and extend laterally towards and above the ischial spine. The cervical ring surrounds the cervix and acts as an attachment point for the cardinal and uterosacral ligaments as well as the pubocervical and rectovaginal fascia. It consists mainly of collagen. The "pubocervical fascia" – a term still used by surgeons - stretches from the lateral sulci of the vagina to the anterior part of the cervical ring, it is a vaginal muscularis and fibromuscular wall (Corton 2009).

In the **posterior zone**, which reaches from the cervix to the anal canal, the following 3 structures can be loose.

The uterosacral ligaments arise from the sacral vertebrate S2,3,4 and attach to the cervical ring posteriorly. It is an effective insertion point of the downward muscle force, the longitudinal muscle of the anus (LMA). The rectovaginal fascia extends as a sheet between the lateral rectal pillars, from the perineal body below to the levator plate above. It is attached to the uterosacral ligaments (USL) and the fascia surrounding the cervix. The perineal body lies between the distal third of the posterior vaginal wall and the anus below the pelvic floor. It is 3-4 cm long. According to DeLancey (1999), it is formed primarily by the midline connection between the halves of the perineal membrane. It is the insertion point of bulbocavernosus muscle and deep and superficial transverse perinei muscles.

Micturition Broken line below bladder signifies relaxation of PCM; LP/LMA vectors actively open out the urethra exponentially decreasing frictional resistance to micturition

Defecation Broken line behind rectum signifies relaxation of PRM; LP/LMA vectors actively open out the anorectum, exponentially decreasing frictional resistance to defecation

5. Stress urinary continence and incontinence

During stress (coughing or straining) the intraurethral pressure rises in normal patients. The rise in pressure within the urethra precedes the rise in pressure in the bladder by 160-240 milliseconds (Enhorning 1961, Constantinou and Govan 1982, van der Kooi et al. 1984, Pieber et al. 1998). This means, that the increased pressure within the urethra during stress must be due to an active muscle contraction and cannot be a passive transmission of the abdominal pressure.

In addition to the contraction of the rhabdosphincter at midurethra, the PCM pulls the distal vagina forward to close the distal urethra (figure 3). Furthermore, the bladder and posterior vaginal wall is pulled backwards (by levator plate) and downwards (by LMA). With intact pubourethral ligament the urethra is stretched and angulated to "kink" the proximal urethra (Petros and Ulmsten 1995). This action is an important closing mechanism, which, as known, helps many patients maintain continence after excision of the distal urethra.

The Integral Theory (1990, 1993) states that „stress urinary incontinence ... derives mainly from laxity in the vagina or its supporting ligaments, a result of altered collagen/elastin". A hypermobile urethra results from loose connective tissue. In stress situations, abdominal forces stretch loose tissues in the anterior zone (pubourethral ligament, extraurethral ligament, hammock), leading to overlengthening of the rhabdosphincter. According to Gordon`s relation between muscle length and muscle force, as soon as the muscle force diminishes … (by half/etc), the patient is stress incontinent. Overstretched connective tissue leads also to an increased radius within the rhabdosphincter and the urethra. According to Laplace's law, the pressure within the urethra correlates inversely to the radius within the rhabdosphincter. In loose connective tissue, the pressure within the urethra thus diminishes in line with the increasing radius. The Hagen-Poiseuille`s law is also helpful in describing continence. The resistance to flow within the urethra in stress situations correlates directly to the length of the urethra and indirectly to the radius within the urethra in the 4th power (Bush et al. 1997). Stress in patients with loose connective tissue will open the urethra. The stress flow then correlates to the radius of the urethra in 4th power.

In other words, loose connective tissue can lead to reduced muscle force by overstretching the muscle, reduced urethral pressure by increasing the radius within the rhabdosphincter, and reduced resistance to flow by widening the urethral radius.

These correlations have a major impact on interpretation of urodynamic results and should be considered in the future.

Petros has been developing the midurethral sling since 1986 based on research on the laxities of the vagina and supporting ligaments and loose connective tissue. (Petros and Ulmsten 1990, 1993)

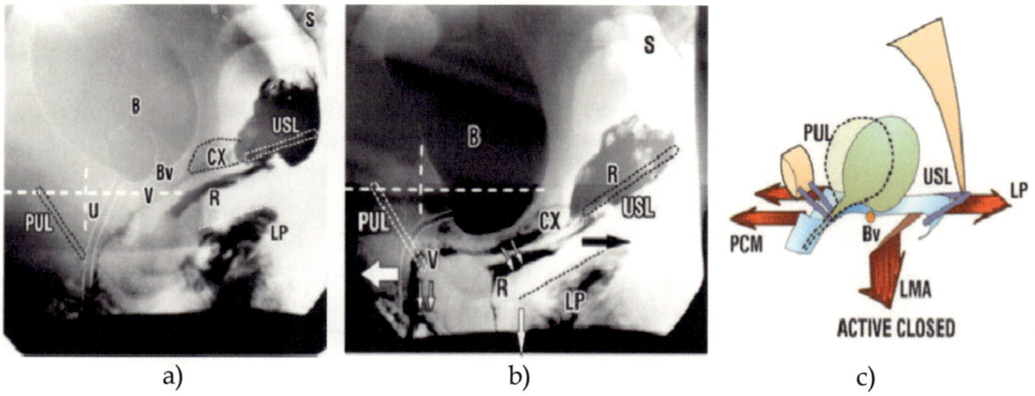

a) b) c)

B=bladder; U=urethra; V=vagina; CX=cervix; R=rectum; PUL=pubourethral ligament; Bv=attachment of bladder base to vagina; LMA= conjoint longitudinal muscle of the anus; LP=levator plate; USL=uterosacral ligament.

Fig. 3. Directional movements of bladder and urethra during effort. a) Lateral xray in resting position, sitting. b) Lateral xray during straining, same patient, shows forward movement of distal vagina and urethra and backward/downward rotation of proximal vagina and urethra ,around the pubourethral ligament (PUL) at the midurethral point. c) Muscle actions during effort- schematic view. PCM pulls the distal vagina forwards to close the distal urethra; LP/LMA stretch the proximal vagina and urethra backwards/downwards to close off the proximal urethra. (From PPetros 2010, by permission).

6. Normal micturition and abnormal emptying of the bladder

Micturition is another complex mechanism that has to be understood when performing pelvic floor surgery. Thus, not only sphincter relaxation and detrusor contraction have to be taken into consideration. EMG-measurements in the posterior fornix have demonstrated commencement of muscle contraction prior to commencement of voiding (Petros 2010). Radiologically, it was shown that the anterior vaginal wall is stretched and moved backward and downward during micturition (figures 4b). The bladder also moves backward and downward and the proximal urethra funnels (figure 4a). This can only be explained by active muscle contractions of levator plate (LP) and longitudinal muscle of anus (LMA). Relaxation of the forward force (PCM) and relaxation of urethral sphincter allows the backward and downward forces to open up the outflow tract (figure 4c)

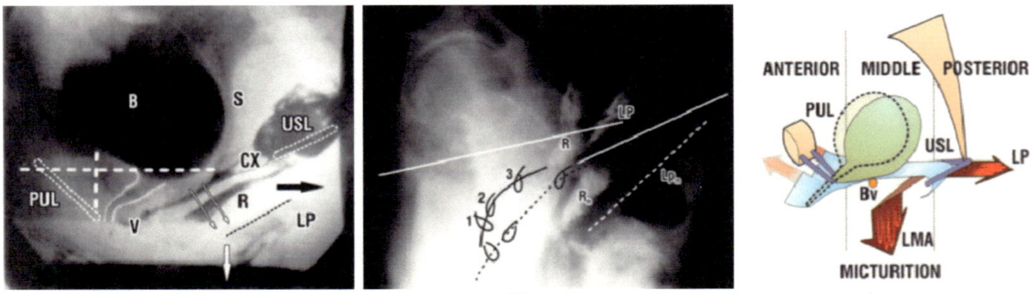

a) b) c)

Fig. 4. Normal micturition. a) Lateral xray, same patient as fig. 3. During micturition, the bladder and vagina move backwards and downward, opening out the posterior urethral wall. b) Superimposed lateral xray.s At rest (unbroken lines) and micturition (broken lines) vascular clips placed at midurethra "1", bladder neck "2" and bladder base "3". c) Muscle actions during micturition . PCM relaxes. This allows the posterior muscle forces LP/LMA (red arrows) to stretch vagina and posterior urethral wall backwards/downwards to open out the outflow tract. Same labelling as fig. 3. (From P Petros 2010, by permission).

The posterior muscles (LP and LMA) only contribute in opening the bladder neck and urethra when the connective tissue architecture and its insertion points are intact in a way that they can pull normally (see figure 1). If the uterosacral ligaments are loose (insertion points of the LMA) or a cystocele is present the posterior forces cannot pull normally, the muscles are shortened or overstretched and have reduced force. Even a minor degree of prolapse can be the cause of defective micturition. Kinking of the urethra by prolapse can also be a cause of abnormal emptying of the bladder. A location of the tape too high up the bladder neck or proximal urethra as well as anterior fixation of the bladder neck after colposuspension can disturb funnelling of the urethra.

7. Stability at the bladder base by a tensioned vaginal wall, urgency and frequency

In their first publication of the "Integral theory" Petros and Ulmsten (1990) stated that "symptoms of stress and urge derive mainly from laxity in the vagina or its supporting ligaments, a result of altered collagen/elastin". Following their publication, evidence was increasingly found that supported their claim that a correlation between the prolapse and an overactive bladder exists (de Boer et al. 2010).

Figures 2, 3b and 5 show that the bladder lies on the vaginal wall. With effort the posterior vaginal wall is orientated horizontally and the bladder lies on this part of tensioned vaginal wall (figure 3b), which acts as a "trampoline". The vagina is attached to the pelvic rim by the uterosacral ligaments posteriorly, the arcus tendineus and the cardinal ligaments laterally as well as the pubourethral ligament anteriorly. Anterior and posterior muscle forces (red arrows in figure 5) add to tension the vaginal wall. While the slow twitch fibres are active when at rest, the fast twitch fibres are active during effort. At the bladder base stretch receptors are present which are connected by afferent nerves to the cortex (Wyndaele et al. 2008, Everaerts et al. 2008, Petros & Ulmsten 1990). Efferent nerves can activate the pelvic floor musculature (figure 5).

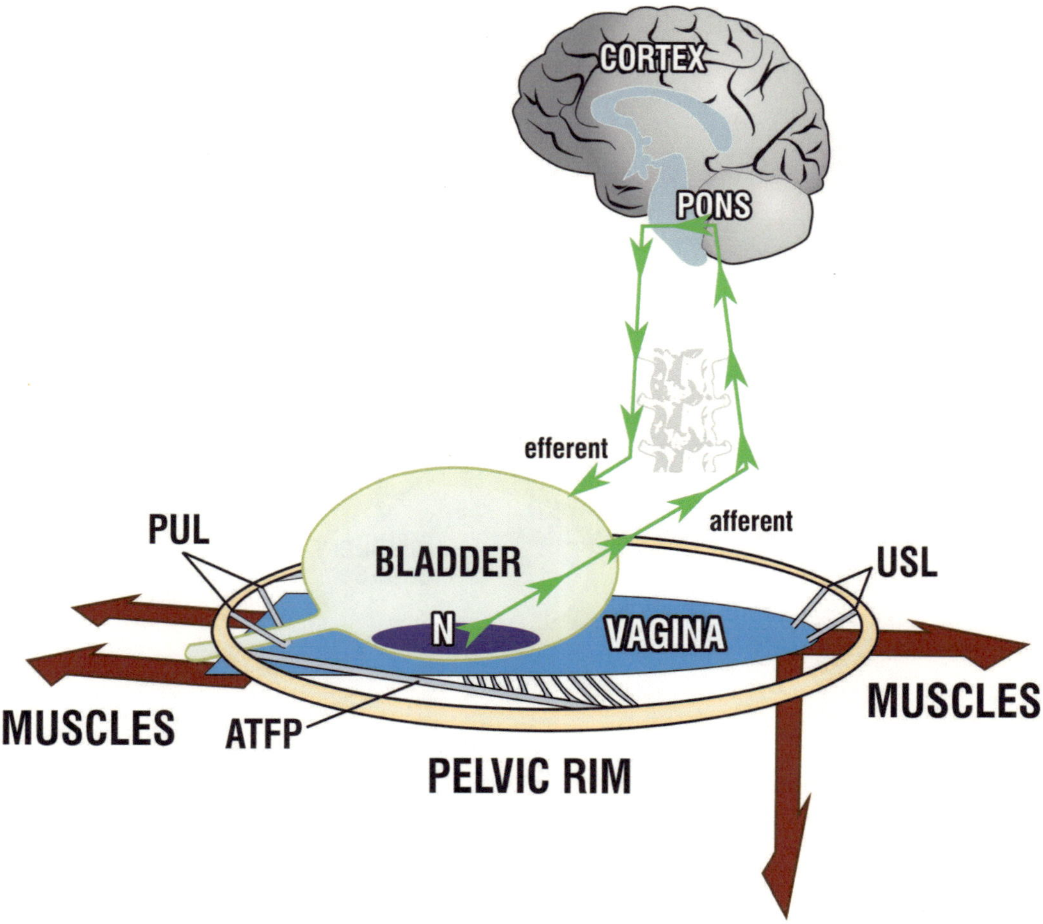

Fig. 5. Stability at the bladder base by a tensioned vaginal wall "Trampoline Analogy". (From P Petros 2010, by permission).

Petros and Ulmsten (1993) postulated that urgency could lead to a premature activation of the micturition reflex. A lax vagina at the anterior, middle or posterior zone reduces the tension of the vagina below the bladder base, the stretch receptors can be activated by afferent nerves, the cortex gets the information of full bladder and this creates the sensation of urge. Prematurely the micturition reflex can be activated and even urge incontinence can occur.

8. Nocturia

Many patients with vaginal vault or uterine prolapse - even if of a minor degree - complain about nocturia. Figure 6 explains the mechanism that leads to nocturia.. When the patient is asleep, the force of gravity pulls down the bladder base. Normally, with firm uterosacral ligaments, the bladder is held high (dotted line in Figure 6). When the patient is asleep and the uterosacral ligaments are loose, the pelvic floor muscles are relaxed, the bladder descends posteriorly, the bladder base is stretched and the stretch receptors "N" are stimulated.

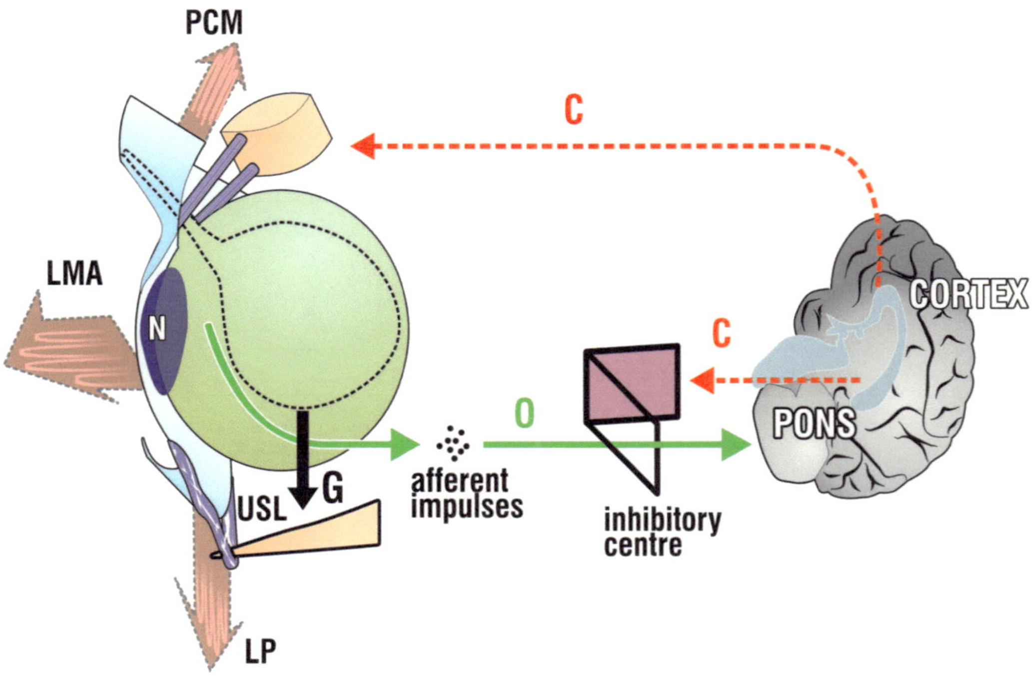

Fig. 6. Mechanism of nocturia- schematic view- patient asleep. The pelvic muscles (arrows) are relaxed. As the bladder fills, it is pulled downwards by the force of gravity 'G'. In the normal patient, bladder descent is limited by the uterosacral ligaments "USL". If "USLs" are loose, the bladder descends more, the stretch receptors "N" are stimulated, the micturition reflex is activated at a low bladder volume, "nocturia". (from P Petros 2010, by permission)

9. Anorectal function, fecal incontinence and obstructive defecation

The anecdotal observation that midurethral slings and repair of loose uterosacral ligaments can cure fecal incontinence has led Petros and Swash (2008) to establish a new theory of anorectal function. A new complex musculo-elastic sphincter mechanism was detected. Its mechanism is similar to that of bladder neck closure. Directional muscle forces stretch the rectum backwards and downwards around an anus firmly anchored by the puborectalis muscle. Anorectal closure occurs when the backward muscle forces of LP and LMA stretch the rectum around the anus, which is anchored by PRM-contraction. Upon comparing Figure 3b with Figure 3a, the rectum above the anal canal has been markedly angulated (and closed) by muscle actions during effort. Upon relaxation of PRM, LP/LMA vectors open out the anal canal for evacuation (broken lines, Fig2)

Fecal incontinence can occur when connective tissue at the anterior zone is loose. Then the insertion points of the puborectalis muscle are dislocated and the muscle is weak. Furthermore, the anterior insertion points of the levator plate are loose and the muscle is weak and the anorectal closure is weak, also.

When connective tissue at the posterior zone is loose, the muscles also cannot act optimally and fecal incontinence can occur. Lax uterosacral ligaments can explain rectal intussusception and obstructive defecation. The levator plate cannot tension the rectovaginal fascia. The perineal body is an important anchoring point and, if loose, it can contribute to fecal incontinence and obstructive defecation (Petros 2010, Abendstein and Petros 2008).

10. Pelvic pain

Many patients with vaginal vault prolapse or uterus prolapse report pelvic pain, a low abdominal dragging pain which occurs mainly in an upright position and is generally relieved in a lying position. This pain may be associated with vulvodynia. Both types of pain have been temporarily relieved by injection of local anaesthetic into the uterosacral ligaments (Bornstein et al 2005, Petros et al 2004), supporting the hypothesis that this pain is a referred pain arising from the inability of lax uterosacral ligaments to support the nerves running along the ligament (figure 7). These nerves are stretched by gravity or during intercourse to cause pain. This pain is almost invariably associated with other symptoms deriving from posterior zone laxity, Figure 8. In a recent study, restoration of uterosacral ligament tension using a posterior tensioned sling showed improvement in posterior zone symptoms as follows: nocturia >2/night 83%; urge-incontinence >2/day 78%; abnormal emptying, 73% ; pelvic pain, 86% fecal incontinence, 87% (Petros PEP, Richardson PA, 2010)

11. The association of pelvic floor dysfunctions and different zones of connective tissue looseness at the pelvic floor (figure 8)

The three zones of connective tissue looseness (see above) are associated with different symptoms. Petros (2010) developed the diagnostic algorithm (Figure 8) through considering the pathophysiology of dysfunctions and through practical experiences with the patients that had different forms and degrees of descensus/prolapse of the vaginal wall.

Many symptoms are associated with these different forms of descensus/prolapse: stress urinary incontinence, abnormal emptying of the bladder, urgency and frequency, nocturia, faecal incontinence, obstructed defecation and pelvic pain.

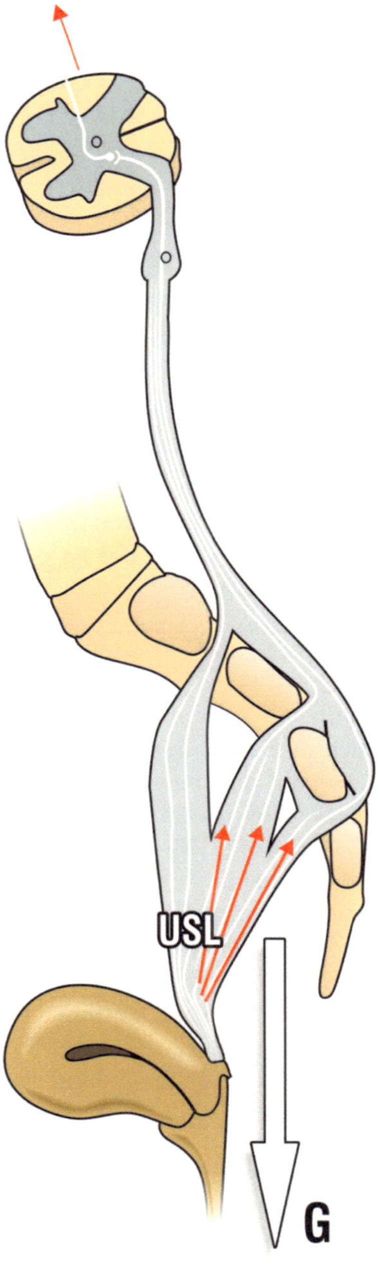

Fig. 7. Pelvic pain caused by loose uterosacral ligaments (USL). Especially in the standing position, the uterus or vaginal vault prolapses under the influence of gravity 'G'. The unmyelinated nerves which run along the USLs are stretched by 'G', causing pain. (from P Petros 2010, by permission)

This algorithm summarizes the relationship between structural damage (prolapse) in the three zones and the respective functions (symptoms). The size of the bar gives an approximate indication of the prevalence (probability) of the symptom. Stress urinary incontinence is mainly caused by anterior defects. Defects in the posterior zone cause different dysfunctions like abnormal emptying of the bladder, frequency and urgency, nocturia, fecal incontinence, obstructed defecation, pelvic pain known as the "posterior fornix syndrome" (Petros & Ulmsten 1993). Nocturia and pelvic pain are specific for posterior zone. Cystoceles mainly are associated with symptoms of abnormal emptying of the bladder and frequency and urgency. The significance of the association between zones and the respective symptoms has been shown by Hunt et al. (2000) using Bayesian networks and decision trees.

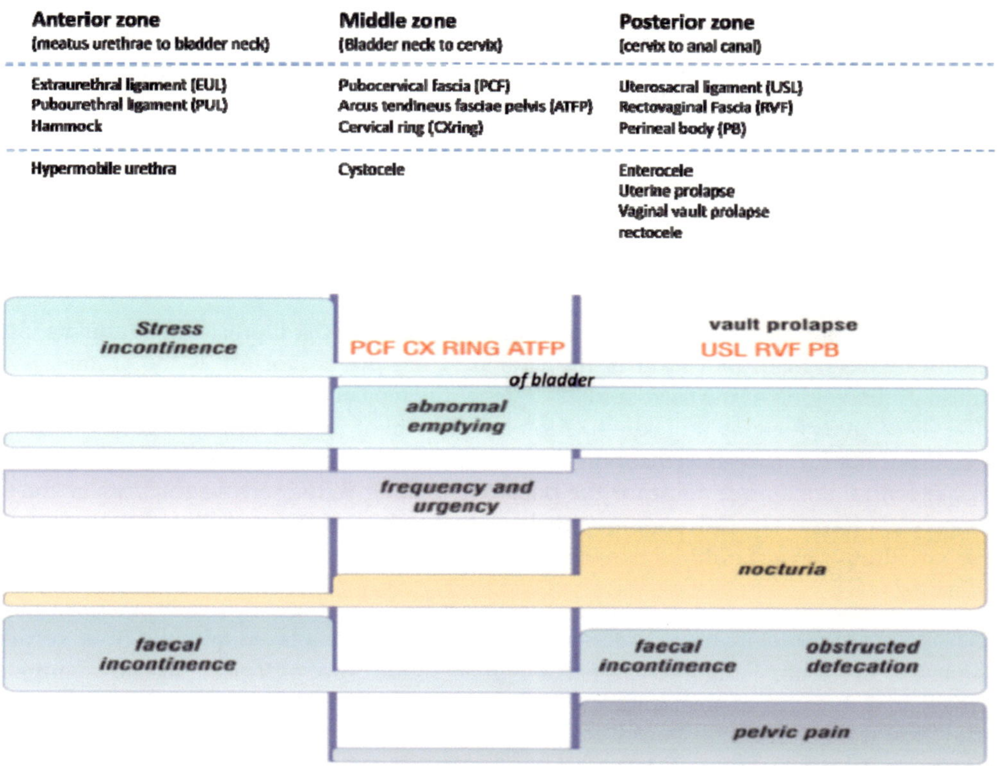

Fig. 8. Diagnostic algorithm. Pictorially elaborates the association between connective tissue looseness at different zones, their relationship with specific prolapses and symptoms, and how repair of the ligaments/fascia in each zone may cure or improve both the prolapse and the symptom(s). The size of the bars gives an approximate indication of the prevalence (probability) of the symptom. (modified after Petros 2010, by permission)

12. Consequences of the diagnostic algorithm for surgical treatments

In the past surgery has only been performed for prolapse and stress incontinence. We now recognise that symptoms of different degrees and combinations can be present in different forms and degrees of prolapse, as seen in Figure 8. Because of the peripheral neurological origin of some symptoms such as urgency and pain, major symptoms may occur with only minimal prolapse. Therefore the new anatomical and functional findings, as summarized in Figure 8 have to be considered in modern pelvic floor surgery.

In daily practice, first, the different symptoms have to be identified with the help of a standardized questionnaire, for instance using Petros`s questionnaire (Petros 2010, pages 270-273). Then the existing pelvic floor defects are assessed. Very helpful are the diagnostic algorithm (Figure 8) and "simulated operations" (Petros 2010) to indicate the appropriate surgery. An example of a "simulated operation" is the controlled urine loss on coughing by applying unilateral digital pressure at midurethra (Pinch-Test). Another is exposure of latent stress incontinence by pushing the prolapse back into the vagina, and asking the patient to cough.

"Restoration of form (structure) leads to restoration of function" (Petros 2010). This principle directly applies Gordon's Law: exact restoration of the insertion points of the pelvic floor muscles allows the muscles to act optimally. The function - even if complex - should thus have the optimal chance to recover.

When repair of weak tissues by conventional techniques such as suturing is not possible (for example repair of a pubourethral ligament for cure of USI), or the recurrence rate is too high, the use of alloplastic materials is an option. Because normal function requires a neurologically complex co-ordination of smooth and striated muscle, any surgery must mimic the natural anatomy as closely as possible if it is to restore function.

The axis of the posterior vagina is nearly horizontal because the uterosacral ligaments insert dorsally between S2-4. Elevation of the vagina to the promontorium is too cranial, while fixation of the vagina to the sacrospinous ligament is too caudal. It is a surgical compromise to use these areas for easy and safe fixation but the site of the uterosacral ligament remains the optimal site for its reconstruction. The uterus needs to be conserved whenever possible. It is the central anchoring point for the posterior ligaments, the rectovaginal fascia and the pubocervical fascia. The descending branch of the uterine artery is a major blood supply for these structures, and should be conserved where possible even if subtotal hysterectomy is performed.

It is important to understand that tissue structure is often displaced laterally (e. g. cardinal ligaments, uterosacral ligaments, rectovaginal fascia, pubocervical fascia, hammock, perineal body). Surgical techniques, which bring the tissues together in the midline or bridge it with alloplastic tapes at the anatomically correct position, should be applied and further developed. Simply applying a large mesh provides a barrier to the prolapse and does not restore the damaged anatomy or function. Instead, such meshes have the tendency to shrink and reduce elasticity of tissues. Furthermore, they obliterate the organ spaces. This may cause pain, dyspareunia, and erosions and may negatively affect the dissection required in cases where the patient develops rectal or bladder carcinoma. The use of alloplastic materials has to be reduced to the necessary amount and their application sites carefully considered. The conventional techniques have to be evaluated following these fundamental principles (Liedl 2010, Wagenlehner et al. 2010)

In order to minimize pain, surgery to the perineal skin and tension when suturing the vagina should be avoided. Vaginal excision should be avoided even in patients with large bulging prolapse. After repair of underlying ligamentous fascial defects, the vaginal wall contracts and will be more elastic than after excision. Tightness or elevation of the bladder neck area of the vagina as well as indentation of the urethra with a midurethral sling should be avoided in order to avoid urinary retention.

Looking at the bladder neck closure mechanism the midurethral tape should be positioned along the pubourethral ligament, which inserts retropubically. This seems especially important in patients with severe stress urinary incontinence or recurrence.

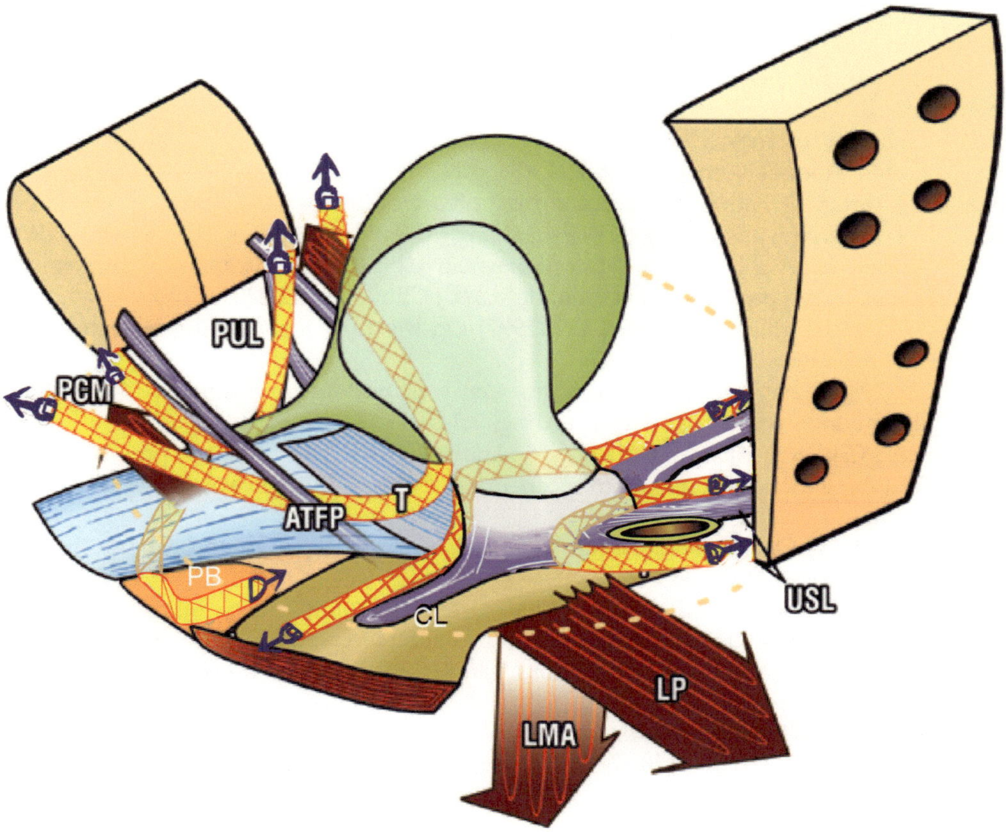

Fig. 9. The use of tensioned tapes to strengthen the principal connective tissue structures which support the vagina, bladder, uterus and rectum: pubourethral ligament (PUL), arcus tendineus fascia pelvis (ATFP), cardinal ligament (CL), uterosacral ligaments (USL), perineal body (PB). These 5 structures are the effective insertion points of the directional muscle forces (arrows) which support the organs, and which open and close the urethra and anorectum, anteromedial part of pubococcygeus muscle (PCM), levator plate (LP) and longitudinal muscle of the anus (LMA). (from P Petros 2010, by permission)

The transobturatoric approach for tape insertion may be an option for mild and moderate cases. New techniques using mini tissue anchors are promising. The TFS (Tissue Fixation System) tensioned tapes (Petros 2010) accurately reinforce the main suspensory ligaments - pubourethral (PUL), uterosacral (USL), cardinal (CL), arcus tendineus fascia pelvis (ATFP) and perineal body (PB) while bringing the laterally displaced tissues towards the midline (figure 9). This action more precisely restores the musculoelastic tension required to also restore function. The meshes with sling fixation transobturatorially or at the sacrospinous ligaments only produces long lasting barriers. At the moment the pelvic floor surgery is in a fundamental development to a minimal invasive surgery. It should be the aim to restore the defects in a way which optimizes the pelvic floor muscles and the functions.

13. References

Abramowitch SD (2009) Tissue mechanics, animal models, and pelvic organ prolapse: A review. Eur J Obstet Gynecol Reprod Biol 144S: S146-S156

Abendstein B, Petros PE, Richardson PA, Goeschen K, Dodero D (2008) The surgical anatomy of rectocele and anterior rectal wall intussusception. Int Urogynecol J Pelvic Floor Dysfunct 19: 705-710

Bornstein J, Zarfati, D, Petros PEP, Causation of vulvar vestibulitis ANZJOG 2005, 45: 538–541

Budatha M, Roshanrava S, Zheng Q, Weislander c, Chapman SL, Davis EC, Starcher B, Word A, Yanagisawa H (2011) Extracellular matrix proteases contribute to progression of pelvic organ prolapse in mice and humans. J Clin Invest 121:2048-2059

Bush MB, Petros P, Barrett-Lennard BR (1997) On the flow through the human urethra. Biomechanics 30: 967-969

Campisi J (1998) The Role of Cellular Senescence in Sin Aging. Journal of Investigative Dermatology Symposium Proceedings 3:1-5

Campeau L, Gorbachinsky I, Badlani GH, Andersson KE (2011) Pelvic florr diesorders: linking genetic risk factors to biochemical changes. BJU Int Aug 26 (Epub ahead of print)

Connell KA (2011) Elastogenesis in the Vaginal Wall and Pelvic-Organ Prolapse. N Engl J Med 364 (24):2356-2358

Constantinou CE, Govan DE (1982) Spatial distribution and timing of transmitted and reflexly generated urethral pressures in healthy women. J Urol 127:964-969

Corton MM (2009) Anatomy of Pelvic Floor Dysfunction. Obstet Gynecol Clin N Am 36:401-319

Courtney H (1950) Anatomy of the pelvic diaphragm and ano-rectal musculature related to sphincter preservation in ano-rectal surgery. American Journal Surgery 79:155-173

De Boer TA, Salvatore S, Cardozo L, Chapple C et al. (2010) Pelvic Organ Prolapse and Overactive Bladder. Neurourol Urodynam 29: 30-39

DeLancey JOL (1999) Structural anatomy of the posterior pelvic compartment as it relates to rectocele. Am J Obstet Gynecol 180:815-823

Dietz HP, Eldridge A, Grace M, Clarke B (2004) Pelvic organ descent in yound nulligravid women. Am J Obstet Gynecol 191:95-99

Dietz HP, Lanzarone V (2005) Levator trauma after vaginal delivery. Obstet Gynecol 106:707-712

Dietz HP, Gillespie AV, Phadke P (2007) Avulsion of the pubovisceral muscle associated with large vaginal tear after normal delivery at term. Aus N Z J Obstet Gynaecol 47: 341-344

Enhorning G. Simultaneous recording of intravesical and intraurethral pressure. Acta Chir Scandinavica, (1961), (Supplement) Vol. 27:61-68.

Everaerts W, Gevaert T, Nilius B, De Ridder D (2008) On the origin of bladder sensing: Tr(i)ps in urology. Neururol Urodyn 27:264-273

Gordon AM, Huxley AF, Julian FJ (1966) The variation in isometric tension with sarcomere length in vertebrate muscle fibers. J Physiol 184: 170-192

Harkness MLR, Harkness RD (1959) Changes in the Physical Properties of the Uterine Cervix of the Rat during Pregnancy. J Physiol 148:524-547

Hunt M, von Konsky B, Venkatesh S, Petros P (2000) Bayesian Networks and Decision Trees in the Diagnosis of Female Urinary Incontinence. Engineering in Medicine and Biology Society 2000. Proceedings of the 22nd Annual International Conference of the IEEE. Volume 1 Issue: 551-554

Huisman AB. Aspects on the anatomy of the female urethra with special relation to urinary continence. Contr Gynecol & Obstets., (1983), Karger Basel, Vol.10:1-31.

Hvid LG, Ortenblad N, Aagaard P, Kjaer M, Suetta C (2011) Effects of aging on single muscle fibre contractile function following short-term immobilisation. J Physiol 2011 Aug 8 (Epub ahead of print)

Lammers K, Lince SL, Spath MA, van Kempen LC, Hendriks JC, Vierhout ME, Kluivers KB (2011) Pelvic organ prolapse and collagen-associated disorders. Int Urogynecol J Aug 3 (Epub ahead of print)

Lexell J, Taylor C., Sjostrom M (1988) What ist the cause of the ageing atrophy? Total number, size and proportion of different fiber types studied in whole vastus lateralis muscle from 15- to 83-year-old men. J Neurol Sci 84:275-294

Liedl B (2010) Male and female urinary incontinence from the viewpoint of the pelvic floor surgeon. Urologe A 49:289-303

Lin YH, Liu M, Xiao N, Daneshgari F (2010) Recovery of continence function following simulated birth trauma involves repair of muscle and nerves in the urethra in the female mouse. Eur Urol 57:506-512

Nichols DH & Randall CL (1989) Vaginal Surgery, 3rd Ed, Williams Wilkins, Baltimore. 1-46

Oelrich TM (1983) The strited urogenital sphincter muscle in the female. The Anatomical Record 205:223-232

Perucchini D, DeLancey JO, Asthon-Miller JA, Peschers U, Kataria T (2002) Age effects on urethral striated muscle. I. Changes in number and diameter of striated muscle fibers in the ventral urethra. Am J Obstet Gynecol 186:351-355

Petros PE and Bornstein J Vulvar vestibulitis may be a referred pain arising from laxity in the uterosacral ligaments- a hypothesis based on 3 prospective case reports , ANZJO&G (2004) 44: 483–486

Petros PEP, Richardson PA, TFS posterior sling improves overactive bladder, pelvic pain and abnormal emptying, even with minor prolapse –a prospective urodynamic study, (2010) Pelviperineology 29: 52-55

Petros PE, Ulmsten U (1990) An Integral Theory of female incontinence. Acta Obstetrica et Gynecologica Scandinavia, Supplement 153, Vol 69: 1-79

Petros PE, Ulmsten U (1993) An Integral Theory and its Method for the Diagnosis and Management of Female Urinary Incontinence. Part II. The biomechanics of vaginal tissue, and supporting ligaments with special relevance to the pathogenesis of female urinary incontinence. Scand J Urol Nephrol Supp. 153: 29-40

Petros PE, Ulmsten U, Papadimitriou J (1990) The Autogenic Neoligament procedure: A technique for planned formation of an artificial neo-ligament. Acta Obstetrica et Gynecologica Scandinavia, 69 (Suppl. 153) 43-51

Petros PE, Ulmsten U (1993) An Integral Theory and its Method for the Diagnosis and Management of Female Urinary Incontinence. Part I. Theory, morphology, radiographic correlations and clinical perspective. Scand J Urol Nephrol Supp. 153: 5-28

Petros P, Ulmsten U (1993) Bladder instability in women: A premature activation of the micturition reflex. Neurourol Urodynam 12:235-239

Petros PE, Ulmsten U (1995) Urethral and bladder neck closure mechanisms. Am J Obstet Gynecol 173: 346-347

Petros PE, Ulmsten U (1997) Role of the Pelvic Floor in Bladder Neck Opening and Closure I: Muscle Forces. Int Urogynecol J 8:74-80

Petros PE (1998) The pubourethral ligament - an anatomical and histological study in the live patient. Int J Urogynecology 9:154-157

Petros PE (2010) The Female Pelvic Floor. Function, Dysfunction and Management According to the Integral Theory. Springerverlag, Berlin-Heidelberg

Petros PE (2008) Pubovisceral muscle avulsion. Aust N Z J Gynaecol 48:124

Petros PE, Swash M (2008) The Musculoelastic Theory of anorectal function and dysfunction. J Pelviperineology 27:89-93

Petros P, Swash M, Kakulas B The Musculo-Elastic Theory of anorectal function and dysfunction, Experimental Study No. 8: Stress urinary incontinence results from muscle weakness and ligamentous laxity in the pelvic floor Pelviperineology 2008; 27: 106 -109

Pierce LM, Coates KW, Kramer LA, Bradford JC, Thor KB, Kuehl TJ (2008) Effects of bilateral levator ani nerve injury on pelvic support in the female squirrel monkey. Am J Obstet Gynecol 198: 585.e1-585.e8

Pieber D, Zivkovic F, Tamussino K (1998) Timing of urethral pressure pulses before and after continence surgery. Neururol Urodyn 17:9-23

Quiroz LH, Munoz A, Shippey SH, Gutman RE, Handa VL (2010) Vaginal parity and pelvic organ prolapse. J Reprod Med 55:93-98

Rechberger T, Uldbjerg N, Oxlund H. (1988) Connective tissue Changes in the Cervix Curing Normal Pregnancy and Pregnancy Complicated by Cervical Incompetence. Obstet Gynecol 71:563-567

Smith ARB, Hoskel GL, Warrel DW (1989) The role of partial denervation of the pelvic floor in the etiology of genitourinary prolapse and stress incontinence of urine: a neurophysiologic study. Br J Obstet Gynaecol 96:24-28

South MM, Stinnett SS, Sanders DB, Weidner AC (2009) Levator ani denervation and reinnervation 6 months after childbirth. Am J Obstet Gynecol 200:519.e1-7

Snooks S J, Swash M, Setchell M and Henry M M. Injury to innervation of pelvic floor sphincter musculature in childbirth. LANCET 1984 2 546-550.

Swash M, Henry MM, Snooks SJ Unifying concept of pelvic floor disorders and incontinence. *Journal of the Royal Society of Medicine*, (1985),78: 906-911.

Ulmsten U, Henriksson L, Johnson P, and Varhos G An ambulatory surgical procedure under local anesthesia for treatment of female urinary incontinence, Int Urogynecol J (1996); 7: 81-86.

Uitto J, Bernstein EF (1998) Molecular Mechanisms of Cutaneous Aging: Connective Tissue Alterations in the Dermis. Journal of Investigative Dermatology Symposium Proceedings 3:41-44

Van der Kooi JB, van Wanroy PJ, De Jonge MC, Kornelis JA (1984) Time separation between cough pulses in bladder, rectum and urethra in women. J Urol 132: 1275-1278

Wagenlehner F, Bschleipfer T, Liedl B, Gunnemann A, Petros P, Weidner W. (2010) Surgical reconstruction of pelvic floor descent: Anatomic and functional aspects. Urologia internationalis 84: 1-9.

Wyndaele JJ, De Wachter S (2008). The sensory bladder (1): an update on the different sensations described in the lower urinary tract and the physiological mechanisms behind them. Neurourol Urodyn 27: 274-278

Zacharin RF (1963) A suspensory mechanism of the female urethra. Journal of Anatomy 97:423-427

2

Epidemiology of Urinary Incontinence in Pregnancy and Postpartum

Stian Langeland Wesnes,
Steinar Hunskaar and Guri Rortveit
Department of Public Health and Primary Health Care,
University of Bergen,
Norway

1. Introduction

Urinary incontinence is a common condition in pregnancy and postpartum. There are published more than a thousand articles on urinary incontinence (UI) in pregnancy. Incidence and prevalence figures of UI in association with pregnancy vary substantially.

Not many reviews have focused solely on incidence and prevalence of UI in association with pregnancy. One report gives a range of prevalence of UI in pregnancy from 32 to 64 % (Milsom et al., 2009). There are published few reviews on incident UI postpartum, most of them are based on a small number of studies. However, one systematically review (Thom & Rortveit, 2010) and several traditional reviews have been published on prevalence of UI postpartum.

This chapter on epidemiology of urinary incontinence in pregnancy and postpartum reviews the incidence and prevalence of UI in pregnancy and postpartum on the basis of a non-systematic PubMed search. The selected articles are chosen due to relevance, quality, citation and sample size.

Published articles will be listed in tables. Tables will contain data on author and article, country of origin of the study, type of study, number of participants, time point in pregnancy and postpartum of information gathering, means of information gathering (questionnaire, interview, objective testing), and prevalence and incidence figures. Parity is an established risk factor for UI. Tables will therefore be stratified for primiparous and parous women. Large studies of good quality are referred to in the text. We will summarize incidence and prevalence figures from single papers; both range of all figures and a more narrow range of figures without the two highest and lowest outliers will be given. We will also give estimates from former reviews.

Prevalence and incidence estimates of UI in association with pregnancy vary very much and with a factor of 7 - 10. We will discuss study design, characteristics of the study population, biases, definitions and other methodological reasons for the diverging estimates, and try to help the reader understand why estimates differ. Hopefully this will give a better understanding of incidence and prevalence estimates of urinary incontinence in association with pregnancy.

2. Urinary incontinence in pregnancy

2.1 Incidence of urinary incontinence in pregnancy

Urinary incontinence (UI) is common also among women who have not given birth (nulliparous women). A Norwegian study found prevalence of UI among nulliparous women aged 20 - 34 and 35 - 44 to be 8 % and 15 %, respectively (Rortveit et al., 2001). Other studies have found that 11 % (Brown et al., 2010, MacLennan et al., 2000) of nulliparous women had UI before pregnancy. Prevalence of UI increases considerably in pregnancy due to increased incidence of stress and mixed UI (Solans-Domenech et al., 2010).

Incidence of UI is low in 1. trimester, rising rapidly in 2. trimester and continues to rise, though more slowly, in 3. trimester (Marshall et al., 1998, Morkved & Bo, 1999, Solans-Domenech et al., 2010).

The nulliparous continent pelvis represents the best available clinical model of the unexposed pelvis, thereby the best study-population to assess incident UI in pregnancy.

Among published cross-sectional studies, Glazener et al published in 2006 data on incident UI in pregnancy among 3,405 nulliparous women with mean age of 25 years (Glazener et al., 2006). They found an incidence of UI in pregnancy of 11 %. A cross sectional study of 7,771 women from UK used questionnaire data collected postpartum (Marshall et al., 1998). They found an incidence of UI in pregnancy of 50 % and 45 % among nulliparous and parous women, respectively.

Several large population-based cohorts have been published during the recent years. A large Spanish cohort study from 2010 consisting of 1,128 nulliparous women who were continent before pregnancy had questionnaire data from each trimester. The article reported a cumulative incidence of UI in pregnancy of 39 % (Solans-Domenech et al., 2010). An Australian cohort study from 2009 consisting of 1,507 nulliparous women had interview data from early and late pregnancy. The authors found an incidence of any UI of 45 % in pregnancy (Brown et al., 2010). Results from 43,279 pregnant women in the Norwegian mother and child cohort study show a cumulative incidence of any UI in week 30 of pregnancy among nulliparous and parous women of 39 % and 49 %, respectively (Wesnes et al., 2007). Stress UI was the most common type of UI.

Several studies on incident UI in pregnancy are cross sectional. The lowest incidence estimates are reported in the cross sectional studies and in studies with focus on stress UI only. Some studies use questionnaire data while others use interview and objective testing. This might explain the diverging estimates.

No systematic review has presented pooled incidence of UI in pregnancy. Epidemiologic data are somewhat scarce and differ substantially for cumulative incidence of UI in pregnancy; from 8 - 57 % in different studies (Table 1). The majority of studies report incidence estimate of any UI in pregnancy between 28 - 45 % among primiparous, and 45 - 54 % among parous women.

Authors, year	Origin	Design	N	Data collection	Time of UI	Nulli-parous	Parous
(Al-Mehaisen et al., 2009)	Jordan	Cohort	181	Interv.	3. trimester	45 %	54 %
(Arrue et al., 2010)	Spain	Cohort	396	Ex., interv.	Delivery	31 %	
(Brown et al., 2010)	Australia	Cohort	1,507	Quest., interv.	3. trimester	45 %	
(Chiarelli & Campbell, 1997)	New - Zealand	Cross-S	304	Interv.	During pregn.		57 %
(Dimpfl et al., 1992)	Germany	Cross-S	180	Interv.	During pregn.		54 %
(Eliasson et al., 2005)	Sweden	Cohort	665	Quest.	3. trimester	45 %	
(Glazener et al., 2006)	UK, N.Z.	Cross-S	3,405	Quest.	During pregn.	11 %	
(Groutz et al., 1999)	Israel	Cross-S	300	Interv.	3 days PP	28 %	49-50%
(Hvidman et al., 2002)	Denmark	Cross-S	642	Quest.		17 %	8 %
(Iosif, 1981)	Sweden	Cohort	1,411	Ex, interv.	1-2 weeks PP		5 %(s)
(King & Freeman, 1998)	UK	Cohort	103	Ex, interv.	During pregn.	48 %	
(Kristiansson et al., 2001)	Sweden	Cohort	200	Quest.	3. trimester		14 % (s)
(Marshall et al., 1998)	UK	Cross-S	7,771	Quest.	3 days PP	50 %	45 %
(Morkved & Bo, 1999)	Norway	Cross-S	144	Ex., interv.	During pregn.		38 %(s)
(Sharma et al., 2009)	India	Cohort	240	Quest.	3. trimester		18 %
(Solans-Domenech et al., 2010)	Spain	Cohort	1,128	Quest.	During pregn.	39 %	
(Thomason et al., 2007)	USA	Cross-S	121	Ex., interv.	During pregn.	16 %	
(Viktrup et al., 1992)	Denmark	Cohort	305	Interv.	1 week PP	10 % (s)	
(Wesnes et al., 2007)	Norway	Cohort	43,279	Quest.	3. trimester	39 %	49 %

cross-s = cross sectional study, Quest. = Questionnaire, Interv. = interview, Ex. = examination, PP = postpartum, (s) = stress UI

Table 1. Incidence of urinary incontinence in pregnancy by parity.

2.2 Prevalence of urinary incontinence in pregnancy

Data from a large number of cross-sectional studies and cohort studies indicate that UI in women is highly prevalent in pregnancy. More than 50 % of all pregnant women experience UI. UI when running, jumping, coughing or laughing (stress UI) is the most common symptom of UI in association with pregnancy.

In a cross-sectional study from Ireland 7,771 women received a questionnaire on UI 2-3 days postpartum (Marshall et al., 1998). Prevalence of UI was 55 % and 66 % among primiparous and parous women, respectively. The study has somewhat insufficient descriptive data which makes it difficult to evaluate the external validity. In 1999 Hojberg et al found a prevalence of UI of 4 % and 14 % among 7,794 Danish nulliparous and parous women, respectively (Hojberg et al., 1999). The low prevalence might be due to UI was reported in early in pregnancy (week 16).

Several cohorts have investigated prevalence of UI during pregnancy. One of the first studies to put focus on UI in pregnancy was done by Francis in 1960 (Francis, 1960). In this cohort he found the prevalence of UI to be 52 % and 85 % among nulliparous and parous women, respectively. Similar results were found in an Australian cohort study that used a validated questionnaire on UI on 1,507 nulliparous women (Brown et al., 2010). Prevalence of UI at least once a month was found to be 56 % in week 31 of pregnancy. New cases of stress UI accounted for more than two thirds of the reported UI prevalence in pregnancy. A study from USA found by structured questionnaire interview on 553 women a prevalence 60 % for UI during pregnancy (Burgio et al., 2003). In the large Norwegian mother and child cohort the prevalence of any UI in third trimester was 48 % among nulliparous and 67 % among parous women (Wesnes et al., 2007). Stress UI was the most common type of UI, affecting 31 % and 41 % of all nulliparous and parous women. The majority of women leaked only small amounts.

Lower prevalence estimates are reported in other cohorts; Dolan et al investigated prevalence of any UI in week 32 to term in a cohort of 492 nulliparous women in England (Dolan et al., 2004). Prevalence of UI was 36 % in pregnancy. However, prevalence of UI before pregnancy was only 2.6 %, which might explain a somewhat low UI prevalence in pregnancy. The majority of the women reported little impact on quality of life. The highest prevalence estimates were reported from a very small cohort recruiting 113 women from an American tertiary care hospital (Raza-Khan et al., 2006). A prevalence of 70 % and 75 % were found among nulliparous and parous women, respectively.

Prevalence estimates for UI in pregnancy among nulliparous women vary from 4 - 70 %, while estimates for parous women vary from 14 - 85 % (Table 2). However, the majority of studies appear to report prevalence estimates between 35 - 55 % among primiparous women, and somewhat higher figures for parous women. No systematic review on UI in pregnancy has been published. The International consultation on incontinence published in 2009 their latest report "Epidemiology of Urinary (UI) and Faecal (FI) Incontinence and Pelvic Organ Prolapse (POP)" (Milsom et al., 2009). It describes period prevalence of any UI in pregnancy of 32 - 64% among all women.

Author, year	Origin	Design	N	Data collection	Time of UI	Nulli-parous	Parous
(Burgio et al., 2003)	USA	Cohort	523	Interv.	2 days PP		60 %
(Brown et al., 2010)	Australia	Cohort	1,507	Quest, interv.	3. trimester	56 %	
(Chaliha et al., 1999)	UK	Cohort	549	Interv.	3. trimester	44 %	
(Dimpfl et al., 1992)	Germany	Cross-s	350	Interv	During pregn.		55 %
(Dolan et al., 2004)	UK	Cohort	492	Quest.	3. trimester	36 %	
(Francis, 1960)	England	Cohort	400	Ex, interv.	During pregn.	53 %	85 %
(Groutz et al., 1999)	Israel	Cross-s	300	Interv.	3 days PP	49 %	50 %
(Hojberg et al., 1999)	Denmark	Cross-s	7,795	Quest.	2. trimestr	4 %	14–16%
(Hvidman et al., 2003)	Denmark	Cross-s	376	Quest.			18 %
(Hvidman et al., 2002)	Denmark	Cross-s	642	Quest.		20 %	24 %
(Iosif, 1981)	Sweden	Cohort	1,411	Quest.	1-2 weeks PP		22 % (s)
(Kristiansson et al., 2001)	Sweden	Cohort	200	Quest.	3. trimester		26 % (s)
(Marshall et al., 1998)	Irland	Cross-s	7,771	Quest.	3 days PP	55 %	66 %
(Mason et al., 1999)	England	Cohort	717	Quest.	3. trimester	32 % (s)	59 % (s)
(Morkved & Bo, 1999)	Norway	Cross-s	144	Ex., interv.	8 weeks PP	35 %	37–70%
(Raza-Khan et al., 2006)	USA	Cohort	113	Quest.	3. trimester	70 %	75 %
(Scarpa et al., 2006)	Brasil	Cross-s	340	Interv.	3. trimester	46 % (s)	55–64%
(Thomason et al., 2007)	USA	Cross-s	121	Ex., interv.	During pregn.	55 %	
(van Brummen et al., 2006)	Netherland	Cohort	515	Quest.	2. trimester	42 % (s)	
(Viktrup et al., 1992)	Denmark	Cohort	305	Interv.	1 week PP	32 % (s)	
(Wesnes et al., 2007)	Norway	Cohort	43,279	Quest.	3. trimester	48 %	67 %

cross-s = cross sectional study, Ex. = examination, Quest. = questionnaire, Interv. = interview, PP = postpartum, (s) = stress UI.

Table 2. Prevalence of urinary incontinence in pregnancy by parity.

3. Urinary incontinence postpartum

3.1 Incidence of urinary incontinence postpartum

Prevalence of UI postpartum is a so called "mixed bag" of incident UI before pregnancy, incident UI in pregnancy and incident UI postpartum (Iosif, 1981, Nygaard, 2006). Risk factors for incident UI at the different time points vary. Mode of delivery; vaginal delivery, vacuum and forceps, are risk factors for incident UI postpartum compared to cesarean section (Glazener et al., 2006). Incident UI is also called *de novo UI* or *new onset UI*.

Cross-sectional studies on incident UI postpartum must rely on maternal recall of UI status during pregnancy. Several large cross-sectional studies have data on incident UI postpartum. A large population-based cross-sectional study from USA investigated incidence of UI postpartum among 5,599 primiparous women (Boyles et al., 2009). The incidence of UI 6 months postpartum was 10 %. About 25 % of the study population had delivered by cesarean section, which might explain the low incidence. Glazener et al published in 2006 cross-sectional data on incident UI in pregnancy among 3,405 primiparous women with mean age of 25 years (Glazener et al., 2006). They found an incidence of UI 3 months postpartum of 15 %. Wilson used questionnaires to investigate incident UI postpartum among 1,505 women who were resident in the Dunedin area, New Zealand (Wilson et al., 1996). The incidence of UI 3 months postpartum was 12 % and 21 % among primiparous and parous women, respectively.

Prospective data on incident UI among 595 primiparous Canadian women 6 months postpartum by a validated questionnaire showed an incidence of any UI of 26 % (Farrell et al., 2001). The use of a research nurse to clarify and complete the questionnaire with each participant might explain the high incidence. Several Scandinavian cohort studies have reported incidence of UI postpartum; in the 30 year old Swedish cohort of 1,411 primiparous women, 19 % reported incident stress UI 6 months post partum (Iosif, 1981). Wesnes et al found a similar incidence of any UI 6 months postpartum (21 %) among 12,679 primiparous women who were continent before pregnancy (Wesnes et al., 2009). Eliasson found an identical incidence of UI 12 months postpartum among 665 Swedish primiparous women (Eliasson et al., 2005). In a smaller Danish cohort of 305 primiparous women Viktrup et al found an incidence of stress UI of 7 % 3 months after vaginal delivery (Viktrup et al., 1992).

Mode of delivery affects the incidence estimates, as study populations with high CS rate is likely to report lower incidence of UI postpartum. Prolonged pressure from baby's head and trauma as baby passes through the vaginal canal may affect the pelvic floor and urethral support. These mechanisms are likely to be involved in incident UI postpartum. The reported incidence of UI among primiparous and parous women postpartum varies between 0 - 26 % and 4 - 21 %, respectively (Table 3). The majority of reported incident UI postpartum are in the range of 5 - 21 % among primiparous women, and 8 - 15 % among parous women. No systematic review on incident UI postpartum has been identified. In a review on the association between CS on UI postpartum Nygaard reported the range of incident UI postpartum to be 7 - 15 % among all women (Nygaard, 2006). For women who become incontinent postpartum, not many women achieve spontaneous continence during the first postpartum year (Thom & Rortveit, 2010)

Author, year	Origin	Design	N	Data collection	Time of UI PP	Primi-parous	Parous
(Arya et al., 2001)	USA	Cohort	315	Interv.	3 mth.	10 % (s)	
(Boyles et al., 2009)	USA	Cross-s	5,599	Quest.	6 mth	10 %	
(Burgio et al., 2003)	USA	Cohort	523	Interv.	3 mth		10 %
(Chaliha et al., 1999)	England	Cohort	549	Interv.	3 mth	6 %	
(Dimpfl et al., 1992)	Germany	Cross-s	350	Interv.	3 mth	4 % (s)	4 %
(Eliasson et al., 2005)	Sweden	Cohort	665	Quest.	12 mth	21 %	
(Farrell et al., 2001)	Canada	Cohort	595	Quest.	6 mth	26 %	
(Foldspang et al., 2004)	Denmark	cross-s	1,232	Quest.	> 12 mth		14 %
(Francis, 1960)	England	Cohort	400	Ex., interv.	3 mth	0 %	
(Glazener et al., 2006)	UK, N.Z.	Cross-S	3,405	Quest.	3 mth	15 %	
(Hvidman et al., 2003)	Denmark	Cross-S	642	Quest.	3 mth		8 %
(Iosif, 1981)	Sweden	Cohort	1,411	Quest.	6-12 mth		19 % (s)
(King & Freeman, 1998)	UK	Cohort	103	Ex, interv.	3 mth	4 %	
(Mason et al., 1999)	England	Cohort	717	Quest.	3 mth		15 %
(Morkved & Bo, 1999)	Norway	Cross-S	144	Ex., interv.	2 mth		19 %
(Raza-Khan et al., 2006)	USA	Cohort	113	Quest.	Postpartum		4 %
(Solans-Domenech et al., 2010)	Spain	Cohort	1,128	Quest.	2 mth	5 %	
(Thomason et al., 2007)	USA	Cross-S	121	Ex., interv.	6 mth	16 %	
(Stanton et al., 1980)	UK	Cohort	189	Interv.	Postpartum	6% (s), 9% (u)	11% (s), 7% (u)
(Viktrup et al., 1992)	Denmark	Cohort	305	Interv.	3 mth	7% (s), 4% (u)	
(Wesnes et al., 2009)	Norway	Cohort	12,679	Quest.	6 mth	21 %	
(Wilson et al., 1996)	New Zealand	Cross-S	1,505	Quest.	3 mth	12 %	21 %

Cross-s = cross sectional study, Ex. = examination, Quest. = questionnaire, Interv. = interview, PP = postpartum, (s) = stress UI, (u) = urgency UI, mth = month.

Table 3. Incidence of urinary incontinence postpartum by parity.

3.2 Prevalence of urinary incontinence postpartum

Vaginal delivery is an important and well documented risk factor for UI postpartum, also when compared with cesarean section. If a woman delivers by caesarean section only, a protective effect on UI compared with vaginal delivery is documented 12 years after delivery (MacArthur et al., 2011). The population based cross sectional EPINCONT study found that women aged 50- 64 years who had delivered by cesarean section or vaginal only had similar UI prevalence, suggesting that any protection from caesarean section might be lost with advancing age (Rortveit et al., 2003).

UI after delivery may affect women for the rest of their lives. Several studies have presented data on the long term prognoses of UI postpartum. Farrell found that prevalence of UI did not change from 6 weeks postpartum to 6 months postpartum (Farrell et al., 2001). A six year follow up study concluded that 24 % of the women had persisting UI from 3 months postpartum to 6 years postpartum (MacArthur et al., 2006). A 12 year prospective study indicates that onset of UI in pregnancy or postpartum increased the risk for UI 12 years later (Viktrup et al., 2006). A systematic review found only small changes in prevalence of UI over the first year postpartum (Thom & Rortveit, 2010). As prevalence figures of UI postpartum appear to be stable, time point of data collection postpartum may be of less importance. We will therefore limit our presentation to studies investigating prevalence of UI during the first year postpartum.

A large questionnaire based cross-sectional study of 5,599 primiparous American women investigated prevalence of UI postpartum (Boyles et al., 2009). The prevalence of any UI was 17 % 6 months postpartum. A similar questionnaire based cross-sectional study was performed in Turkey (Ege et al., 2008). One year postpartum 20 % of the parous women had UI. Stress and mixed UI were most common types of UI.

A large cohort study on 2,390 Swedish women recruited in pregnancy assessed stress UI at 2 and 12 months postpartum by questionnaire (Schytt et al., 2004). UI was defined as any UI last week. Data was linked to the Swedish birth registry. The authors found that 18 % of primiparous women and 24 % of multiparous women had stress UI 12 months postpartum. The largest study (by 2011) on UI during pregnancy and postpartum found a prevalence of UI of 31 % among 12,679 primiparous women 6 months postpartum. All the participants were continent before pregnancy (Wesnes et al., 2009).

There is a wide range of reported prevalences of any UI among primiparous women (6 - 67 %) and parous women (3 - 45 %) (Table 4). The majority of the studies report however estimates 15 - 31 % and 18 - 38 % among primiparous and parous women, respectively. This corresponds well with reports from several reviews on UI postpartum. In a review on UI and its precipitating factors postpartum Herbruck reported prevalences of stress UI of 22 - 33 % postpartum among all women (Herbruck, 2008). The ICI epidemiology report presented prevalence of 15 - 30 % among all women the 1. year postpartum (Milsom et al., 2009). In a review Nygaard reported the prevalence of UI postpartum to be 9 - 31 % among all women (Nygaard, 2006). Authors of a systematic review reported a pooled prevalence of UI of 29 % and 33 % 3 months postpartum among primiparous and parous women, respectively (Thom & Rortveit, 2010).

Author, year	Origin	Design	N	Data collection	Time of UI PP	Primi-parous	Parous
(Altman et al., 2006)	Sweden	Cohort	304	Quest.	5 mth	15 % (s)	
(Arrue et al., 2010)	Spain	Cohort	396	Ex., interv.	6 mth	15 %	
(Baydock et al., 2009)	Canada	Cross-S	632	Interv.	4 mth		23 %
(Bo & Backe-Hansen, 2007)	Norway	Cross-S	40	Quest.	6 weeks		29 %(s)
(Boyles et al., 2009)	USA	Cross-S	5,599	Quest.	6 mth	17 %	
(Burgio et al., 2003)	USA	Cohort	523	Interv.	6 mth		11 %
(Chaliha et al., 2002)	England	Cohort	161	Quest., urodyn	3 mth	30 %	
(Chaliha et al., 1999)	England	Cohort	549	Interv-	3 mth	15 %	
(Diez-Itza et al., 2010)	Spain	Cohort	352	Ex., quest.	12 mth	11 % (s)	
(Dimpfl et al., 1992)	Germany	Cross-S	350	Interv.	3 mth	6 % (s)	
(Dolan et al., 2004)	UK	Cohort	492	Quest.	3 mth	13 %	
(Eason et al., 2004)	Canada	Cohort	949	Quest.	3 mth		31 %
(Ege et al., 2008)	Turkey	Cross-S	1,749	Quest.	12 mth		20 %
(Ekstrom et al., 2008)	Sweden	Cohort	389	Quest.	3 mth	13% (s), 4% (u)	
(Eliasson et al., 2005)	Sweden	Cohort	665	Quest.	12 mth	49 %	
(Ewings et al., 2005)	England	Cohort	723	Quest.	6 mth		45 %
(Farrell et al., 2001)	Canada	Cohort	595	Quest.	6 mth	26 %	
(Foldspang et al., 2004).	Denmark	Cross-S	1,232	Quest.	> 12 mth	26 %	
(Francis, 1960)	England	Cohort	400	Ex, interv.	3 mth	24 %	29 % (s)
(Glazener et al., 2006)	UK, N.Z.	Cross-S	3,405	Quest.	3 mth	29 %	
(Hatem et al., 2005)	Canada	Cross-S	2,492	Quest	6 mth	30 %	
(Hvidman et al., 2003)	Denmark	Cross-S	642	Quest.	3 mth		3 %
(Jundt et al, 2010)	Germany	Cohort	112	Quest, ex.	6 mth	21 %	
(Iosif, 1981)	Sweden	Cohort	1,411	Quest.	6-12 mth		22 % (s)
(King & Freeman, 1998)	UK	Cohort	103	Ex, interv.	3 mth	22 %	
(Mason et al., 1999)	England	Cohort	717	Quest.	3 mth	10 % (s)	31 % (s)
(Morkved & Bo, 1999)	Norway	Cross-S	144	Ex., interv.	2 mth		38 %
(Pregazzi et al., 2002)	Italy	Cross-S	537	Ex., interv.	3 mth	8 %	20 %
(Raza-Khan et al., 2006)	USA	Cohort	113	Quest.	Postpartum	46 %	43 %
(Sampselle et al., 1996)	USA	Cohort	59	Quest., ex.	6 mth	67 % (s)	
(Schytt et al., 2004)	Sweden	Cohort	2,390	Quest.	12 mth	18 % (s)	24 % (s)
(Serati et al., 2008)	Italy	Cohort	336	Interv.	6/12 mth		27/23 %
(Stanton et al., 1980)	UK	Cohort	189	Interv.	3 mth	6 % (s), 8 % (u)	
(Thomason et al., 2007)	USA	Cross-S	121	Ex., interv.	6 mth	45 %	
[Thompson 2002]	Australia	Cohort	1,295	Quest.	6 mth		18 %
(Torrisi et al., 2007)	Italy	Cohort	562	Ex., interv.	3 mth		11 % (s)
(Viktrup et al., 1992)	Denmark	Cohort	305	Interv.	3 mth	7 % (s)	
(Wesnes et al., 2009)	Norway	Cohort	12,679	Quest.	6 mth	31 %	
(Wijma et al., 2003)	Netherland	Cohort	117	Quest., ex.	6 mth	15 %	
(Wilson et al., 1996)	N.Z	Cross-S	1,505	Quest.	3 mth	29 %	34 %
(Yang et al, 2010)	China	cross-s	1,889	Quest.	6 mth	10 %	

cross-s = cross sectional study, Ex. = examination, PP = postpartum, (s) = stress UI, (u) = urgency UI, Urodyn = urodynamic testing, mth = months

Table 4. Prevalence of urinary incontinence postpartum by parity.

4. Why do estimates differ?

A wide range of prevalence estimates of UI in pregnancy and postpartum have been presented. There are several methodological reasons for these diverging incidence and prevalence estimates.

4.1 UI definition

The concept of UI can be based on:

- **symptoms** (a morbid phenomenon or departure from the normal in structure, function, or sensation, experienced by the woman and indicative of disease or a health problem) (Abrams et al., 1988, Abrams et al., 2002, Haylen et al., 2010)
- **signs** (observed by the physician to verify symptoms and quantify them) (Abrams et al., 1988, Abrams et al., 2002, Haylen et al., 2010)
- - **urodynamic findings** (observations made during urodynamic studies) (Abrams et al., 2002)
- **conditions** (the presence of urodynamic observations associated with characteristic symptoms or signs and/or non-urodynamic evidence of relevant pathological processes) (Abrams et al., 2002)

The ICS definitions and terminologies of UI according to the above descriptions have been revised several times (Abrams et al., 1988, Abrams et al., 2002, Haylen et al., 2010). The current definition of UI symptoms is "Complaint of involuntary loss of urine" (Haylen et al., 2010). In the 2002 definition, UI symptoms were not enough to set the UI diagnose; UI signs were needed. Today the majority of studies on UI define UI according to UI symptoms. Studies on UI have used the definitions at the time. As definitions change, prevalence estimates will also change.

4.2 Information gathering

Information on UI in pregnancy and postpartum is often gathered through questionnaires, but objective testing (Morkved & Bo, 1999), personal structured interviews (Chiarelli & Campbell, 1997, Morkved & Bo, 1999) or semi structured interviews (Farrell et al., 2001, Spellacy, 2001) or phone interviews (Baydock et al., 2009) by doctors or assistants, or reviews of existing medical records (Spellacy, 2001) are also used. Information collected by interview makes it possible to clarify and gather more and better information regarding UI. Thom found higher prevalence figures of UI when data was gathered by structured interview compared to questionnaire (Chiarelli & Campbell, 1997, Thom, 1998). Medical records often lack important information, leading to low prevalence estimates. Studies have found low agreement between self reported UI and clinical assessment (Diokno et al., 1988, Milsom et al., 1993). A review on variations in estimates of UI found that objective testing according to the "UI sign" definition led to lower prevalence estimates than questionnaire based studies using the "UI symptom" definition (Thom, 1998).

4.3 Type of study

A large proportion of studies on UI in pregnancy or postpartum are cross sectional (Table 1 - 4) or retrospective. If a woman has UI when answering a retrospective study, this may affect her reporting of UI by improving her memory about earlier UI leading to a recall bias. Cross sectional studies have less valid incidence figures than prospective cohorts. Cross-sectional studies can gather information about the prevalence of UI, but they cannot distinguish between incident and long-established UI. Therefore, cross-sectional studies can usually only measure prevalence of UI. Also, they cannot identify cause-and-effect relationships as exposure and outcome information are gathered at the same time.

4.4 Timing of data collection

Timing of data collection can affect prevalence estimates of UI in pregnancy. Some studies question women about UI during each trimester, but most studies question women at one certain time point in pregnancy (Brown et al., 2010, Lewicky-Gaupp et al., 2008) or just after birth (Sottner et al., 2006). Some studies do not report what time in pregnancy the women reported UI (Sharma et al., 2009). As prevalence of UI increases in pregnancy, the time of information gathering will affect the prevalence estimates of UI during pregnancy. When it comes to data collection postpartum, some studies report on UI at 6 - 9 weeks postpartum (D'Alfonso et al., 2006, Lewicky-Gaupp et al., 2008, Meyer et al., 1998), 3 months (Eason et al., 2004, Hannah et al., 2002), 4 months (Baydock et al., 2009), 6 months (Thomason et al., 2007), 12 months (Serati et al., 2008) or > 12 months (Foldspang et al., 2004, Fritel et al., 2004) postpartum. The time of information gathering postpartum might affect incidence and prevalence estimates of UI. However, a recent review indicates that prevalence of UI is stable first year postpartum (Thom & Rortveit, 2010), and time of data collection postpartum may therefore be of less importance.

4.5 Threshold

Permanence, frequency and volume are used by authors as threshold to define women with UI in association with pregnancy. Permanence or duration can be defined as one or more episodes of UI in the previous month (Brown et al., 2010, Wilson et al., 1996). Some authors use longer periods, like trimesters (Schytt et al., 2004) or the 6 months postpartum period (Schytt et al., 2004). Some authors investigate severe UI defined by weekly or daily leakage (Al-Mehaisen et al., 2009) while others do not report any cut-off (van Brummen et al., 2006). Prevalence estimates are lower for daily UI compared to weekly or monthly UI (Thom, 1998). Some studies have a cut-off for minimum frequency, amount or severity of UI for women to be included in the study as incontinent. A high cut-off decreases the number of women who fulfil the UI criteria in a study. Differing thresholds may explain differing incidence and prevalence estimates of UI.

4.6 Type of UI

Stress UI predominates in young women. Stress UI is more common in pregnancy and postpartum than urgency UI and mixed UI. Also, the incidence of pure urgency UI in pregnancy or postpartum is low compared with incidence of stress UI and mixed UI. The prevalence of pure stress UI is reported to be 2 – 8 times higher than the prevalence of pure urgency UI in pregnancy (Brown et al., 2010, Goldberg et al., 2005, Raza-Khan et al., 2006). Prevalence of mixed UI is reported to be 0.3 – 1.5 times of the prevalence of pure stress UI in pregnancy (Brown et al., 2010, Goldberg et al., 2005, Raza-Khan et al., 2006). The stress/urgency ratio is reduced postpartum as prevalence of stress UI decline. Several studies focus solely on stress UI (Mason et al., 1999, Torrisi et al., 2007, Viktrup et al., 1992). Prevalence figures in these studies are likely to be lower than in studies that include both urgency UI and mixed UI in their analyses (Thom, 1998).

4.7 Characteristics of study population

The study population influences prevalence of UI. Some studies on UI in association with pregnancy use study populations from tertiary care hospitals (Baydock et al., 2009, Raza-Khan et al., 2006), leading to recruitment of highly selected participants. BMI distribution, age distribution, parity distribution, proportion of European or Hispanic population, proportion of women having vaginal delivery all influence prevalence figures of UI. Mothers BMI and age at first delivery have risen the 50 years. These demographic variables might partly explain why studies from 1970-1980 tend to report lower UI estimates compared to recent studies. Some studies include only women having SVD (Altman et al., 2006, Arrue et al., 2010, Baydock et al., 2009), which will give a higher prevalence estimate of UI than if the study also had included CS. Many studies on UI in association with pregnancy either adjust or report stratified analyses for age (Solans-Domenech et al., 2010), BMI (Eason et al., 2004), race (Connolly et al., 2007) and mode of delivery (Eason et al., 2004). Effect estimates are thereby controlled for baseline imbalances in these important patient characteristics. However, dissimilar use of statistical stratification and adjustment makes it difficult to compare findings. Pooled prevalences figures can be misleading and readers should be careful in generalising the findings to a population outside the study population.

4.8 Bias

Many studies on UI in pregnancy try to gather information from all pregnant women in the community; so called population based studies (Boyles et al., 2009, Thompson et al., 2002). Participation rates for epidemiologic studies have been declining during the decades with even steeper declines in recent years (Galea and Tracy, 2007). Several large surveillance surveys in USA report overall decrease in participation rates well below 50 %. Population based studies on UI in association with pregnancy are challenged with the same problems. Boyles reported a response rate of 39 % (Boyles et al., 2009), Wesnes of 45 % (Wesnes et al., 2007). These studies are prone to a biased response rates/selection bias which may invalidate the prevalence estimates. Nulliparous women are more likely to participate and tell their pregnancy stories in studies compared with parous women (Magnus et al., 2006). Declining participation rates and the growing complexity of reasons for study nonparticipation add unpredictability about who is participating in a study and who is not. It challenges the ability of these studies to confidently obtain a population-representative sample (Galea and Tracy, 2007).

Known differences between responders and non-responders may be compensated during analyses. The major problem is unknown response bias, such as the possibility of different response rates between continent and incontinent women (Cartwright, 1983). Due to embarrassment and feeling uncomfortable about reporting UI, incontinent women may deny or not answer questions about UI. Conversely, incontinent women may find the subject particularly relevant, and therefore respond to a greater extent than continent women. At present, we do not know how these factors may affect the response rates. To minimize selection bias one should always aim at the highest possible response rates.

4.9 Questionnaire

It is essential to research on UI that incidence and prevalence estimates can be properly assessed and recorded. As clinicians objective testing and patients' symptoms often differ in their perspective of UI (Milsom et al, 2009), the use of questionnaires to approach patients symptoms are more used recent years. There are an increasing number of questionnaires to assess UI. The Symptom and Quality of Life Committee of the International Consultation on Incontinence performed a systematic review of questionnaires related to urinary incontinence (Avery et al, 2007). They identified 17 questionnaires on UI in women (assessing symptoms, quality of life or both) that were highly recommended; that is questionnaires that were seen as an established measure with documented, rigorous validity, reliability and responsiveness in several clinical studies. However, only 38 % of all clinical trials use these questionnaires (Avery et al, 2007). The proportion in descriptive studies using robust validated questionnaires is likely to be even lower. Some of the variability in UI incidence and prevalence estimates is likely to be related to the range of different questionnaires used.

All the above methodological factors can influence UI estimates in a study. Unfortunately we do not know all factors that influence UI estimates. Some variation in prevalence estimates between studies will always remain.

5. Conclusion

Reported incidence and prevalence estimates in pregnancy and postpartum vary (Table 5). Incidence of UI is high during pregnancy. Close to 50 % of all women experience UI during pregnancy. Delivery is one of many factors that lead to a high incidence of UI postpartum. About 1/3 women experience UI postpartum. This is the first review trying to summarize the UI estimates in association with pregnancy.

Time point	Source of data	Primiparous	Parous
Incidence in pregnancy	Range Table 1	11 - 50 %	8 - 57 %
	Narrow range Table 1	17 - 45 %	45 - 54 %
Prevalence in pregnancy	Range Table 2	4 - 70 %	14 - 85 %
	Narrow range Table 2	35 - 55 %	24 - 67 %
	Report (Milsom et al., 2009)		32 - 64 %
Incidence postpartum	Range Table 3	0 - 26 %	4 - 21 %
	Narrow range Table 3	5 - 21 %	8 - 15 %
	Review (Nygaard, 2006)		7 - 15 %
Prevalence postpartum	Range Table 4	6 - 67 %	3 - 45 %
	Narrow range Table 4	15 - 45 %	18 - 38 %
	Report (Milsom et al., 2009)		15 - 30 %
	Review (Nygaard, 2006)		9 - 31 %
	Systematic review (Thom & Rortveit, 2010)	29 %	33 %

Table 5. Range of incidence and prevalence estimates for any UI by parity.

Many factors contribute to the wide range of incidence and prevalence estimates. The different use of definitions, type of study, methods of data collection, time point of information gathering information gathering, threshold used to define UI, UI type, study population, questionnaire and selection bias are some of the factors that may explain the wide range of estimates.

There is need for systematic reviews giving pooled estimates, preferably for subsets defined by parity, type of delivery and type of incontinence. Future studies ought to follow reporting guidelines for observational studies, like the Strobe criteria (von Elm et al, 2007), as poor reporting hinders the assessment of the strengths and weaknesses of a study and the generalizability of its results.

6. References

Abrams, P.; Blaivas, J.G.; Stanton, S.L. & Andersen, J.T. (1988). The standardisation of terminology of lower urinary tract function. The International Continence Society Committee on Standardisation of Terminology. *Scand J Urol Nephrol,* Vol.114 (suppl), No.5 (Jan 1988), pp. 5-19, ISSN 0300-8886

Abrams, P.; Cardozo, L.; Fall, M.; Griffiths, D.; Rosier, P.; Ulmsten, U.; van Kerrebroeck, P.; Victor, A. & Wein, A. (2002). The standardisation of terminology of lower urinary tract function: report from the Standardisation Sub-committee of the International Continence Society. *Neurourol Urodyn,* Vol.21, No.2 (Feb 2002), pp. 167-178, ISSN 0733-2467

Al-Mehaisen, L.M.; Al-Kuran, O.; Lataifeh, I.M.; Betawie, S.; Sindiyani, A.; Al-ttal, O.F. & Naser, F. (2009). Prevalence and frequency of severity of urinary incontinence symptoms in late pregnancy: a prospective study in the north of Jordan. *Arch Gynecol Obstet,* Vol.279, No.4 (Apr 2009), pp. 499-503, ISSN 1432-0711

Altman, D.; Ekstrom, A.; Gustafsson, C.; Lopez, A.; Falconer, C. & Zetterstrom, J. (2006). Risk of urinary incontinence after childbirth: a 10-year prospective cohort study. *Obstet Gynecol,* Vol.108, No.4 (Oct 2006), pp. 873-878, ISSN 0029-7844

Arrue, M.; Ibanez, L.; Paredes, J.; Murgiondo, A.; Belar, M.; Sarasqueta, C. & Diez-Itza, I. (2010). Stress urinary incontinence six months after first vaginal delivery. *Eur J Obstet Gynecol Reprod Biol,* Vol.(Mar 11 2010), pp. ISSN 1872-7654

Arya, L.A.; Jackson, N.D.; Myers, D.L. & Verma, A. (2001). Risk of new-onset urinary incontinence after forceps and vacuum delivery in primiparous women. *Am J Obstet Gynecol,* Vol.185, No.6 (Dec 2001), pp. 1318-1323; discussion 1323-1314., ISSN 0002-9378

Baydock, S.A.; Flood, C.; Schulz, J.A.; MacDonald, D.; Esau, D.; Jones, S. & Hiltz, C.B. (2009). Prevalence and risk factors for urinary and fecal incontinence four months after vaginal delivery. *J Obstet Gynaecol Can,* Vol.31, No.1 (Jan 2009), pp. 36-41, ISSN 1701-2163

Bo, K. & Backe-Hansen, K. (2007). Do elite athletes experience low back pain, pelvic girdle and pelvic floor complaints during and after pregnancy? *Scand J Med Sci Sports,* Vol.17, No.5 (Oct 2007), pp. 480-487, ISSN 0905-7188

Boyles, S.H.; Li, H.; Mori, T.; Osterweil, P. & Guise, J.M. (2009). Effect of mode of delivery on the incidence of urinary incontinence in primiparous women. *Obstet Gynecol,* Vol.113, No.1 (Jan 2009), pp. 134-141, ISSN 0029-7844

Brown, S.J.; Donath, S.; MacArthur, C.; McDonald, E.A. & Krastev, A.H. (2010). Urinary incontinence in nulliparous women before and during pregnancy: prevalence, incidence, and associated risk factors. *Int Urogynecol J Pelvic Floor Dysfunct,* Vol.21, No.2 (Feb 2010), pp. 193-202, ISSN 1433-3023

Burgio, K.L.; Zyczynski, H.; Locher, J.L.; Richter, H.E.; Redden, D.T. & Wright, K.C. (2003). Urinary incontinence in the 12-month postpartum period. *Obstet Gynecol,* Vol.102, No.6 (Dec 2003), pp. 1291-1298, ISSN 0029-7844

Cartwright, A. 1983. Health surveys in practice and in potential: a critical review of their scope and methods London: King Edward's Hospital Fund for London.

Chaliha, C.; Kalia, V.; Stanton, S.L.; Monga, A. & Sultan, A.H. (1999). Antenatal prediction of postpartum urinary and fecal incontinence. *Obstet Gynecol,* Vol.94, No.5 (Nov 1999), pp. 689-694, ISSN 0029-7844

Chaliha, C.; Khullar, V.; Stanton, S.L.; Monga, A. & Sultan, A.H. (2002). Urinary symptoms in pregnancy: are they useful for diagnosis? *BJOG,* Vol.109, No.10 (Oct 2002), pp. 1181-1183., ISSN 1470-0328

Chiarelli, P. & Campbell, E. (1997). Incontinence during pregnancy. Prevalence and opportunities for continence promotion. *Aust N Z J Obstet Gynaecol,* Vol.37, No.1 (Feb 1997), pp. 66-73, ISSN 0004-8666

Connolly, T.J.; Litman, H.J.; Tennstedt, S.L.; Link, C.L. & McKinlay, J.B. (2007). The effect of mode of delivery, parity, and birth weight on risk of urinary incontinence. *Int Urogynecol J Pelvic Floor Dysfunct,* Vol.18, No.9 (Sep 2007), pp. 1033-1042, ISSN 0937-3462

D'Alfonso, A.; Iovenitti, P. & Carta, G. (2006). Urinary disorders during pregnancy and postpartum: our experience. *Clin Exp Obstet Gynecol,* Vol.33, No.1 (Jun 2006), pp. 23-25, ISSN 0390-6663

Diez-Itza, I.; Arrue, M.; Ibanez, L.; Murgiondo, A.; Paredes, J. & Sarasqueta, C. (2010). Factors involved in stress urinary incontinence 1 year after first delivery. *Int Urogynecol J Pelvic Floor Dysfunct,* Vol.21, No.4 (Apr 2010), pp. 439-445, ISSN 1433-3023

Dimpfl, T.; Hesse, U. & Schussler, B. (1992). Incidence and cause of postpartum urinary stress incontinence. *Eur J Obstet Gynecol Reprod Biol,* Vol.43, No.1 (Jan 1992), pp. 29-33, ISSN 0301-2115

Diokno, A.C.; Brown, M.B.; Brock, B.M.; Herzog, A.R. & Normolle, D.P. (1988). Clinical and cystometric characteristics of continent and incontinent noninstitutionalized elderly. *J Urol,* Vol.140, No.3 (Sep 1988), pp. 567-571, ISSN 0022-5347

Dolan, L.M.; Walsh, D.; Hamilton, S.; Marshall, K.; Thompson, K. & Ashe, R.G. (2004). A study of quality of life in primigravidae with urinary incontinence. *Int Urogynecol J Pelvic Floor Dysfunct,* Vol.15, No.3 (May-Jun 2004), pp. 160-164, ISSN 0937-3462

Eason, E.; Labrecque, M.; Marcoux, S. & Mondor, M. (2004). Effects of carrying a pregnancy and of method of delivery on urinary incontinence: a prospective cohort study. *BMC Pregnancy Childbirth,* Vol.4, No.1 (Feb 2004), pp. 4, ISSN 1471-2393

Ege, E.; Akin, B.; Altuntug, K.; Benli, S. & Arioz, A. (2008). Prevalence of urinary incontinence in the 12-month postpartum period and related risk factors in Turkey. *Urol Int,* Vol.80, No.4 (Jul 2008), pp. 355-361, ISSN 1423-0399

Ekstrom, A.; Altman, D.; Wiklund, I.; Larsson, C. & Andolf, E. (2008). Planned cesarean section versus planned vaginal delivery: comparison of lower urinary tract symptoms. *Int Urogynecol J Pelvic Floor Dysfunct,* Vol.19, No.4 (Apr 2008), pp. 459-465, ISSN 0937-3462

Eliasson, K.; Nordlander, I.; Larson, B.; Hammarstrom, M. & Mattsson, E. (2005). Influence of physical activity on urinary leakage in primiparous women. *Scand J Med Sci Sports,* Vol.15, No.2 (Apr 2005), pp. 87-94, ISSN 0905-7188

Ewings, P.; Spencer, S.; Marsh, H. & O'Sullivan, M. (2005). Obstetric risk factors for urinary incontinence and preventative pelvic floor exercises: cohort study and nested randomized controlled trial. *J Obstet Gynaecol,* Vol.25, No.6 (Aug 2005), pp. 558-564, ISSN 0144-3615

Farrell, S.A.; Allen, V.M. & Baskett, T.F. (2001). Parturition and urinary incontinence in primiparas. *Obstet Gynecol,* Vol.97, No.3 (Mar 2001), pp. 350-356., ISSN 0029-7844

Foldspang, A.; Hvidman, L.; Mommsen, S. & Nielsen, J.B. (2004). Risk of postpartum urinary incontinence associated with pregnancy and mode of delivery. *Acta Obstet Gynecol Scand,* Vol.83, No.10 (Oct 2004), pp. 923-927, ISSN 0001-6349

Francis, W.J.A. (1960). The onset of stress incontinence. *J Obstet Gynaecol Br Empire,* Vol.67, (Dec 1960), pp. 899-903, ISSN 0307-1871

Fritel, X.; Fauconnier, A.; Levet, C. & Benifla, J.L. (2004). Stress urinary incontinence 4 years after the first delivery: a retrospective cohort survey. *Acta Obstet Gynecol Scand,* Vol.83, No.10 (Oct 2004), pp. 941-945, ISSN 0001-6349

Glazener, C.M.; Herbison, G.P.; MacArthur, C.; Lancashire, R.; McGee, M.A.; Grant, A.M. & Wilson, P.D. (2006). New postnatal urinary incontinence: obstetric and other risk factors in primiparae. *BJOG,* Vol.113, No.2 (Feb 2006), pp. 208-217, ISSN 1470-0328

Goldberg, R.P.; Kwon, C.; Gandhi, S.; Atkuru, L.V. & Sand, P.K. (2005). Urinary incontinence after multiple gestation and delivery: impact on quality of life. *Int Urogynecol J Pelvic Floor Dysfunct,* Vol.16, No.5 (Sep-Oct 2005), pp. 334-336, ISSN 0937-3462

Groutz, A.; Gordon, D.; Keidar, R.; Lessing, J.B.; Wolman, I.; David, M.P. & Chen, B. (1999). Stress urinary incontinence: prevalence among nulliparous compared with primiparous and grand multiparous premenopausal women. *Neurourol Urodyn,* Vol.18, No.5 (Jan 1999), pp. 419-425, ISSN 0733-2467

Hannah, M.E.; Hannah, W.J.; Hodnett, E.D.; Chalmers, B.; Kung, R.; Willan, A.; Amankwah, K.; Cheng, M.; Helewa, M.; Hewson, S.; Saigal, S.; Whyte, H. & Gafni, A. (2002). Outcomes at 3 months after planned cesarean vs planned vaginal delivery for breech presentation at term: the international randomized Term Breech Trial. *JAMA,* Vol.287, No.14 (Apr 2002), pp. 1822-1831., ISSN 0098-7484

Hatem, M.; Fraser, W. & Lepire, E. (2005). Postpartum urinary and anal incontinence: a population-based study of quality of life of primiparous women in Quebec. *J Obstet Gynaecol Can,* Vol.27, No.7 (Jul 2005), pp. 682-688, ISSN 1701-2163

Haylen, B.T.; de Ridder, D.; Freeman, R.M.; Swift, S.E.; Berghmans, B.; Lee, J.; Monga, A.; Petri, E.; Rizk, D.E.; Sand, P.K. & Schaer, G.N. (2010). An International Urogynecological Association (IUGA)/International Continence Society (ICS) joint report on the terminology for female pelvic floor dysfunction. *Neurourol Urodyn,* Vol.29, No.1 (Jun 2010), pp. 4-20, ISSN 1520-6777

Herbruck, L.F. (2008). Urinary incontinence in the childbearing woman. *Urol Nurs,* Vol.28, No.3 (Jun 2008), pp. 163-171; quiz 172, ISSN 1053-816X

Hojberg, K.E.; Salvig, J.D.; Winslow, N.A.; Lose, G. & Secher, N.J. (1999). Urinary incontinence: prevalence and risk factors at 16 weeks of gestation. *Br J Obstet Gynaecol,* Vol.106, No.8 (Aug 1999), pp. 842-850, ISSN 0306-5456

Hvidman, L.; Foldspang, A.; Mommsen, S. & Bugge Nielsen, J. (2002). Correlates of urinary incontinence in pregnancy. *Int Urogynecol J Pelvic Floor Dysfunct,* Vol.13, No.5 (Oct 2002), pp. 278-283., ISSN 0937-3462

Hvidman, L.; Foldspang, A.; Mommsen, S. & Nielsen, J.B. (2003). Postpartum urinary incontinence. *Acta Obstet Gynecol Scand,* Vol.82, No.6 (Jun 2003), pp. 556-563, ISSN 0001-6349

Iosif, S. (1981). Stress incontinence during pregnancy and in puerperium. *Int J Gynaecol Obstet,* Vol.19, (Mar 1981), pp. 13-20, ISSN 0020-7292

Jundt K, Scheer I, Schiessl B, Karl K, Friese K & Peschers UM. (2010). Incontinence, bladder neck mobility, and sphincter ruptures in primiparous women. *Eur J Med Res.* Vol.15. No.5 (Aug 2010), pp. 246-252, ISSN 0949-2321.

King, J.K. & Freeman, R.M. (1998). Is antenatal bladder neck mobility a risk factor for postpartum stress incontinence? *BJOG,* Vol.105, No.12 (Dec 1998), pp. 1300-1307, ISSN 0306-5456

Kristiansson, P.; Samuelsson, E.; von Schoultz, B. & Svardsudd, K. (2001). Reproductive hormones and stress urinary incontinence in pregnancy. *Acta Obstet Gynecol Scand,* Vol.80, No.12 (Dec 2001), pp. 1125-1130., ISSN 0001-634

Lewicky-Gaupp, C.; Cao, D.C. & Culbertson, S. (2008). Urinary and anal incontinence in African American teenaged gravidas during pregnancy and the puerperium. *J Pediatr Adolesc Gynecol,* Vol.21, No.1 (Feb 2008), pp. 21-26, ISSN 1083-3188

MacArthur, C.; Glazener, C.; Lancashire, R.; Herbison, P. & Wilson, D. (2011). Exclusive caesarean section delivery and subsequent urinary and faecal incontinence: a 12-year longitudinal study. *BJOG,* Vol.(Apr 8 2011), pp. ISSN 1471-0528

MacArthur, C.; Glazener, C.M.; Wilson, P.D.; Lancashire, R.J.; Herbison, G.P. & Grant, A.M. (2006). Persistent urinary incontinence and delivery mode history: a six-year longitudinal study. *BJOG,* Vol.113, No.2 (Feb 2006), pp. 218-224, ISSN 1470-0328

MacLennan, A.H.; Taylor, A.W.; Wilson, D.H. & Wilson, D. (2000). The prevalence of pelvic floor disorders and their relationship to gender, age, parity and mode of delivery. *BJOG,* Vol.107, No.12 (Dec 2000), pp. 1460-1470, ISSN 1470-0328

Magnus, P.; Irgens, L.M.; Haug, K.; Nystad, W.; Skjaerven, R. & Stoltenberg, C. (2006). Cohort profile: The Norwegian Mother and Child Cohort Study (MoBa). *Int J Epidemiol,* Vol.35, No.5 (Oct 2006), pp. 1146-1150, ISSN 0300-5771

Marshall, K.; Thompson, K.A.; Walsh, D.M. & Baxter, G.D. (1998). Incidence of urinary incontinence and constipation during pregnancy and postpartum: survey of current findings at the Rotunda Lying-In Hospital. *Br J Obstet Gynaecol,* Vol.105, No.4 (Apr 1998), pp. 400-402, ISSN 0306-5456

Mason, L.; Glenn, S.; Walton, I. & Appleton, C. (1999). The prevalence of stress incontinence during pregnancy and following delivery. *Midwifery,* Vol.15, No.2 (Jun 1999), pp. 120-128, ISSN 0266-6138

Meyer, S.; Schreyer, A.; De Grandi, P. & Hohlfeld, P. (1998). The effects of birth on urinary continence mechanisms and other pelvic-floor characteristics. *Obstet Gynecol,* Vol.92, (Oct 1998), pp. 613-618., ISSN 0029-7844

Milsom, I.; Altman, D.; Lapitan, M.; Nelson, R.; Sillèn, U. & Thom, D. 2009. Epidemiology of urinary (UI) and faecal (FI) incontinence and pelvic organ prolapse (POP). p 57.

Milsom, I.; Ekelund, P.; Molander, U.; Arvidsson, L. & Areskoug, B. (1993). The influence of age, parity, oral contraception, hysterectomy and menopause on the prevalence of urinary incontinence in women. *J Urol,* Vol.149, No.6 (Jun 1993), pp. 1459-1462, ISSN 0022-5347

Morkved, S. & Bo, K. (1999). Prevalence of urinary incontinence during pregnancy and postpartum. *Int Urogynecol J Pelvic Floor Dysfunct,* Vol.10, No.6 (Jun 1999), pp. 394-398, ISSN 0937-3462

Nygaard, I. (2006). Urinary incontinence: is cesarean delivery protective? *Semin Perinatol,* Vol.30, No.5 (Oct 2006), pp. 267-271, ISSN 0146-0005

Pregazzi, R.; Sartore, A.; Troiano, L.; Grimaldi, E.; Bortoli, P.; Siracusano, S. & Guaschino, S. (2002). Postpartum urinary symptoms: prevalence and risk factors. *Eur J Obstet Gynecol Reprod Biol,* Vol.103, No.2 (Jun 2002), pp. 179-182., ISSN 0301-2115

Raza-Khan, F.; Graziano, S.; Kenton, K.; Shott, S. & Brubaker, L. (2006). Peripartum urinary incontinence in a racially diverse obstetrical population. *Int Urogynecol J Pelvic Floor Dysfunct,* Vol.17, No.5 (Oct 2006), pp. 525-530, ISSN 0937-3462

Rortveit, G.; Daltveit, A.K.; Hannestad, Y.S. & Hunskaar, S. (2003). Urinary incontinence after vaginal delivery or cesarean section. *N Engl J Med,* Vol.348, No.10 (Mar 2003), pp. 900-907., ISSN 1533-4406

Rortveit, G.; Hannestad, Y.S.; Daltveit, A.K. & Hunskaar, S. (2001). Age- and type-dependent effects of parity on urinary incontinence: the Norwegian EPINCONT study. *Obstet Gynecol,* Vol.98, No.6 (Dec 2001), pp. 1004-1010, ISSN 0029-7844

Sampselle, C.M.; DeLancey, J.O.L. & J., A.-M. (1996). Urinary incontinence in pregnancy and postpartum. *Neurourol Urodyn,* Vol.15, No.4 1996), pp. 329-330,

Scarpa, K.P.; Herrmann, V.; Palma, P.C.; Riccetto, C.L. & Morais, S.S. (2006). Prevalence and correlates of stress urinary incontinence during pregnancy: a survey at UNICAMP Medical School, Sao Paulo, Brazil. *Int Urogynecol J Pelvic Floor Dysfunct,* Vol.17, No.3 (May 2006), pp. 219-223, ISSN 0937-3462

Schytt, E.; Lindmark, G. & Waldenstrom, U. (2004). Symptoms of stress incontinence 1 year after childbirth: prevalence and predictors in a national Swedish sample. *Acta Obstet Gynecol Scand,* Vol.83, No.10 (Oct 2004), pp. 928-936, ISSN 0001-6349

Serati, M.; Salvatore, S.; Khullar, V.; Uccella, S.; Bertelli, E.; Ghezzi, F. & Bolis, P. (2008). Prospective study to assess risk factors for pelvic floor dysfunction after delivery. *Acta Obstet Gynecol Scand,* Vol.87, No.3 (Jun 2008), pp. 313-318, ISSN 1600-0412

Sharma, J.B.; Aggarwal, S.; Singhal, S.; Kumar, S. & Roy, K.K. (2009). Prevalence of urinary incontinence and other urological problems during pregnancy: a questionnaire based study. *Arch Gynecol Obstet,* Vol.279, No.6 (Jun 2009), pp. 845-851, ISSN 1432-0711

Solans-Domenech, M.; Sanchez, E. & Espuna-Pons, M. (2010). Urinary and Anal Incontinence During Pregnancy and Postpartum: Incidence, Severity, and Risk Factors. *Obstet Gynecol,* Vol.115, No.3 (Mar 2010), pp. 618-628, ISSN 1873-233X

Sottner, O.; Zahumensky, J.; Krcmar, M.; Brtnicka, H.; Kolarik, D.; Driak, D. & Halaska, M. (2006). Urinary incontinence in a group of primiparous women in the Czech Republic. *Gynecol Obstet Invest,* Vol.62, No.1 (Oct 2006), pp. 33-37, ISSN 0378-7346

Spellacy, E. (2001). Urinary incontinence in pregnancy and the puerperium. *J Obstet Gynecol Neonatal Nurs,* Vol.30, No.6 (Nov-Dec 2001), pp. 634-641, ISSN 0884-2175

Stanton, S.L.; Kerr, W.R. & Harris, V.G. (1980). The incidence of urological symptoms in normal pregnancy. *Br J Obstet Gynaecol,* Vol.87, No.10 (Oct 1980), pp. 897-900, ISSN 0306-5456

Thom, D.H. & Rortveit, G. (2010). Prevalence of postpartum urinary incontinence: a systematic review. *Acta Obstet Gynecol Scand,* Vol.89, No.12 (Dec 2010), pp. 1511-1522, ISSN 1600-0412

Thomason, A.D.; Miller, J.M. & Delancey, J.O. (2007). Urinary incontinence symptoms during and after pregnancy in continent and incontinent primiparas. *Int Urogynecol J Pelvic Floor Dysfunct,* Vol.18, (Apr 2007), pp. 147-151, ISSN 0937-3462

Thompson, J.F.; Roberts, C.L.; Currie, M. & Ellwood, D.A. (2002). Prevalence and persistence of health problems after childbirth: associations with parity and method of birth. *Birth,* Vol.29, No.2 (Jun 2002), pp. 83-94., ISSN 0730-7659

Torrisi, G.; Sampugnaro, E.G.; Pappalardo, E.M.; D'Urso, E.; Vecchio, M. & Mazza, A. (2007). Postpartum urinary stress incontinence: analysis of the associated risk factors and neurophysiological tests. *Minerva Ginecol,* Vol.59, No.5 (Oct 2007), pp. 491-498, ISSN 0026-4784

van Brummen, H.J.; Bruinse, H.W.; van der Bom, J.G.; Heintz, A.P. & van der Vaart, C.H. (2006). How do the prevalences of urogenital symptoms change during pregnancy? *Neurourol Urodyn,* Vol.25, No.2 (Aug 2006), pp. 135-139, ISSN 0733-2467

von Elm, E.; Altman, D.G.; Egger M.; Pocock S.J.; Gotzsche P.C. & Vandenbroucke J.P. (2007). The Strengthening the Reporting of Observational Studies in Epidemiology (STROBE) statement: guidelines for reporting observational studies. *Lancet* Vol.370, No.9596 (Des 2007), pp.1453-1457, ISSN 0140-6736.

Viktrup, L.; Lose, G.; ROlff, M. & Barfoed, K. (1992). The symptoms of stress incontinence caused by pregnancy or delivery in primiparas. *Obstet Gynecol,* Vol.79, No.6 (Jun 1992), pp. 945-949, ISSN 0029-7844

Viktrup, L.; Rortveit, G. & Lose, G. (2006). Risk of stress urinary incontinence twelve years after the first pregnancy and delivery. *Obstet Gynecol,* Vol.108, No.2 (Aug 2006), pp. 248-254, ISSN 0029-7844

Wesnes, S.L.; Hunskaar, S.; Bo, K. & Rortveit, G. (2009). The effect of urinary incontinence status during pregnancy and delivery mode on incontinence postpartum. A cohort study. *BJOG,* Vol.116, No.5 (Apr 2009), pp. 700-707, ISSN 1471-0528

Wesnes, S.L.; Rortveit, G.; Bo, K. & Hunskaar, S. (2007). Urinary incontinence during pregnancy. *Obstet Gynecol,* Vol.109, No.4 (Apr 2007), pp. 922-928, ISSN 0029-7844

Wijma, J.; Potters, A.E.; de Wolf, B.T.; Tinga, D.J. & Aarnoudse, J.G. (2003). Anatomical and functional changes in the lower urinary tract following spontaneous vaginal delivery. *BJOG,* Vol.110, No.7 (Jul 2003), pp. 658-663, ISSN 1470-0328

Wilson, P.D.; Herbison, R.M. & Herbison, G.P. (1996). Obstetric practice and the prevalence of urinary incontinence three months after delivery. *BJOG,* Vol.103, No.2 (Feb 1996), pp. 154-161, ISSN 0306-5456

Yang X, Zhang HX, Yu HY, Gao XL, Yang HX & Dong Y. (2010). The prevalence of fecal incontinence and urinary incontinence in primiparous postpartum Chinese women. *Eur J Obstet Gynecol Reprod Biol,* Vol.152, No.2 (June 2010), pp. 214-217, ISSN1872-7654

3

A Multi-Disciplinary Perspective on the Diagnosis and Treatment of Urinary Incontinence in Young Women

Mariola Bidzan[1], Jerzy Smutek[2,3], Krystyna Garstka-Namysł[4], Jan Namysł[5] and Leszek Bidzan[6]
[1]*Department of Clinical Psychology and Neuropsychology, Institute of Psychology, University of Gdansk*
[2]*Department of Obstetrics, Medical University of Gdansk*
[3]*Pro-Vita Private Medical Center for Urinary Incontinence, Gdansk*
[4]Department of Tourism and Recreation, *University of Physical Education, Poznan*
[5]*INNOMED - Poznan, Private Neurorehabilitation Centre*
[6]*Department of Developmental Psychiatry, Psychotic Disorders and Old Age Psychiatry, Medical University of Gdansk*
Poland

1. Introduction

Urinary incontinence (UI) has a multifactorial etiology, and as a rule lasts for many years (Abrams et al., 2002; Milart & Gulanowska-Gędek, 2002; Rechberger & Skorupski, 2005). It is most commonly seen in women (Foldspang & Mommsen, 1997; Rechberger, 2004; Rechberger & Skorupski, 2005; Garstka-Namysł, 2006, 2009). According to a recent epidemiological study (Minnasian, 2003), in a population of 230,000 people, the frequency of occurrence of UI was approximately 27.6% among women, as opposed to 10% among men. It is estimated that about 3% of men between the ages of 15 and 64 have UI-related problems, as compared to 7-10% of men over 64 (Evans, 2005). The prevalence of UI in women is likewise dependent on age: it affects nearly one-third of all women before menopause and over 45% after (Rogers et al., 2001a, 2001b). A detailed analysis of the occurrence of UI in various age brackets indicates that it affects 25% of women under 18, 18% under 29, and 37% between 35 and 54, whereas 39% of women with UI are over 55 years old (Bø, 2004). However, approximately 70-80% of women over 65 have UI (Milsom et al., 1993, 2001; Hannestad et al., 2000; Nygaard et al., 2003, 2004). This has been confirmed by several studies (cf. Diokno et al., 2004; Hunskaar et al., 2004; Furelly et al., 2003; Kirby et al., 2006; Rechberger & Tomaszewski, 2007).

On the basis of separate studies, sponsored by the National Association for Incontinence in the United Sates, it can be inferred that, among all diseases of social significance, UI is the most common. While 21% of American women suffer from arterial hypertension, 20% have depression, and 9% have diabetes, as many as 30% of women have UI (Resnick, 1998;

Broome, 2003). As mentioned earlier, it is estimated that the statistics are similar for European countries (Hunskaar et al., 2002). Since UI affects much more than 5% of the population, and has a significant impact on personal, family, and vocational functioning, it is considered a disease of social significance (Cioskowska-Paluch, 2000; Adamiak & Rechberger, 2005; Bidzan, 2008).

The spectrum of psychological problems associated with the symptoms of UI is particularly broad when the disease is at an advanced stage (Lagro-Janssen et al., 1992a, 1992b). Lalos et al. (2001) found that the life of persons with UI undergoes a diametrical change, which affects many aspects of life:

1. The manner and style of family life is changed, as is sexual activity (cf. Norton et al., 1988). As many as 25% of female patients experience some urine emission during sexual intercourse, while 35% have difficulties achieving orgasm (Veerecken, 1989). Moreover, UI can be a drain on the family budget, due to expenses entailed in treating and mitigating the symptoms (sanitary pads, diaper-panties, etc.).
2. Career plans are changed, vocational opportunities are limited, and sometimes it is impossible to work outside the home.
3. Social life (including quality of life, QOL) is impaired, with the loss of good social functioning and limitations on social contacts (cf. Brown et al., 1998a; Wein & Rovner, 1999; Anders, 2000; Thom, 2000; Tołłoczko, 2002; Smutek et al., 2004a; Bidzan et al., 2005a,b; Garstka-Namysł et al., 2007, 2008). It is estimated that ca. 35% of persons with UI are on disability pension, where one of the main reasons for an adjudication of disability is the significant degree of incontinence and the concomitant inability to maintain a job. This can cause a feeling of reduced self-worth, a loss of social position, a deterioration of mood, and social isolation, all of which serve to reduce subjective QOL (Norton et al., 1988).

For many patients UI continues to be shameful and stigmatizing; it may well be the "last taboo of the 21st century" (Roe & May, 1999; Thom, 2000; Bidzan, Smutek & Bidzan, 2005b). Treatment outcomes in UI, though systematically improving, are still unsatisfactory: there is too high a percentage of relapse, an insufficient understanding of the reasons for treatment failure, and non-compliance with recommended therapy. This has led to increasing interest in an multi-disciplinary approach to UI, in which the process of diagnosing and treating UI involves the joint efforts of urologists and uro-gynecologists with clinical psychologists, psychiatrists, neurologists and physiotherapists.

Psychological research to date has concentrated on the psychopathology of persons with UI, especially depression (Vereecken, 1989; Lew-Starowicz, 2002; Chiverton et al., 1996; Valvanne et al., 1996; Kinn & Zaar, 1998; Bodden-Heidrich et al., 1999; Zorn et al., 1999; Dugan et al., 2000; Watson et al., 2000; Zajda et al., 2000; Fultz & Herzog, 2001; Meade-D'Alisera et al., 2001; Broome, 2003; Nuotio et al., 2003; Nygaard et al., 2003; Bodden-Heidrich,2 004; Perry et al., 2006), anxiety, and mental discomfort (Chiara et al., 1998; Watson et al., 2000; Libalová et al., 2001; Bogner et al., 2002; Bogner & Gallo, 2002; Perry et al., 2006), as well as the impact of psychosocial factors on the course of UI, the coping methods used by patients, and treatment outcomes (Sand et al., 1999; Thom, 2000; Janssen et al., 2001; Shaw, 2001; Miller & Hoffman, 2006; Sand & Appell, 2006; Bidzan, 2008). In recent years many researchers have focused on the evaluation of Health Related Quality of Life (HRQOL) in persons with UI, including their psychosocial functioning, broadly understood

(Sutherst & Brown, 1980; Norton, 1982; Norton et al., 1988; Grimby et al., 1993; Grimby et al., 1997; Samuelsson et al., 1997; Wyman et al., 1997; Wyman, 1998; Chiarelli et al., 1999; Kelleher et al., 1997; Swithinbank & Abrams, 1999; Brown et al., 1999; Coyne et al., 2000; Kelleher, 2000; Coyne et al., 2003; Fultz & Herzog, 2001; Badia et al., 2004; Currie et al., 2006; Bidzan, 2008; Bidzan, 2011). It should be emphasized in this context that the evaluation of HRQOL has become in recent times the most important diagnostic and prognostic index for the functioning of patients, regardless of the disease (Majkowicz et al., 1997; Brown et al., 1999a; Swithinbank & Abrams, 1999; Woodman et al., 2001), and is recommended by the International Continence Society (Abrams et al., 2002; Williams, 2004).

The analyses performed to date have dealt with particular types and degrees of clinical intensity of UI, as well as particular symptoms (e.g. UI during intercourse) before and after the application of various treatment methods (Sutherst, 1979; Lamm et al., 1986; Hilton, 1988; Lagro-Janssen et al.,1992b; Samuelsson et al., 1997; DuBeau et al., 1998; Robinson et al., 1998; Temml et al., 2000; Carcamo & Lledo, 2001; Fultz & Herzog, 2001; Hägglund et al., 2001; Scarpero et al., 2003; Abrams, 2003; Bidzan et al., 2006a, 2006b; Skrzypulec et al., 2006; Bidzan, Smutek & Bidzan, 2010). Most of this research has pointed to a connection between the variable assessed by the psychologist and those assessed by the physician, although there have been differing conclusions as to the strength of these dependencies. New possibilities are emerging for psychotherapeutic intervention, and the opportunity now exists to improve the outcome of complex, holistic treatment. It should be noted, however, that research on these connections among younger women (in the 18-34 age bracket) is relatively scant (Debus-Thiede & Dimpfl, 1993; Dugan et al., 1998; Fultz & Herzog, 2001; Hägglund et al., 2001; Shaw et al., 2001; Papanicolau et al., 2005). Attention has been drawn to the fact that the consequences of UI in younger patients are more visible than in older persons (Debus-Thiede & Dimpfl, 1993; Dugan et al., 1998; Fultz & Herzog, 2001; Hägglund et al., 2001; Shaw et al., 2001; Papanicolau et al., 2005). This may be associated with the fact that difficulties in retaining urine are generally ascribed to aging, and are perceived as a typical complaint in the elderly (Dowd, 1991; Bush et al., 2001; Dugan et al., 2001; Davey 1993). A state that is perceived as being normal is less often treated, either by public opinion or by the persons involved, as exerting a negative impact on emotional and social functioning, than when the same state is perceived as a deviation from the norm. Moreover, both the lifestyle and the range of obligations (family duties, vocational responsibilities) change with age, a fact which may support greater adaptation to UI in older persons than in younger (Umlauf et al., 1996).

In this chapter, based on the results of earlier research, we would like to draw attention to the particular nature of the conditions surrounding UI in young women, and to advocate an multi-disciplinary approach (gynecology, urology, psychology, psychiatry, and physiotherapy) at every stage of the diagnosis and treatment of persons with UI. Based on our own experience with functional research on the lower urinary tract and the pelvic floor in a group of female patients reporting problems with urination, we shall present the most common discrepancies in the evaluation of the causes and the indications for treatment of UI.

All these discrepancies may occur even in patients with correctly performed standard diagnostic tests, because the latter are not always enough to reveal disturbances of functional origin. We discuss three diagnostic problems that in our opinion are most often encountered, and propose optimum solutions.

2. Low urethral pressure or abnormal urethra function

Our clinical observations suggest that as early as the preliminary patient history an awareness of the dependencies between the mental sphere and UI can enable the physician to avoid committing diagnostic errors and applying ineffective treatment methods. Particular striking were the discrepancies regarding young women (18-34 years old in our patients) treated with a diagnosis of high urethral pressure, with concomitant UI of greater or lesser intensity and disturbances of micturition. In our urodynamic clinic, we see a large number of patients previously treated surgically by urethral dilatation due to a diagnosis of high urethral pressure, and urodynamically normal detrusor profile. In many cases, however, the initial psychological interview, including a psychosexual biography (Bidzan, Smutek & Bidzan, 2010), suggested that the micturition disturbances might have existed since childhood. A questionnaire we have developed helped us to discover that these patients had frequently repressed from consciousness their memories of UI and bedwetting in childhood and youth, and in filling out the standard questionnaires had often denied that any such thing had occurred (or they had never been asked). They most often associated the onset of their complaints with childbirth or a bladder infection in childhood or adolescence. A detailed patient history (lack of neurological disorders), palpation of perineal muscles, an evaluation of muscle contraction in the pelvic floor and the state of conscious control of these muscles by surface electromyography, and a functional evaluation of the pelvic floor muscles using a transperineal ultrasonogram, along with data from the psychosexual biography, pointed to a diametrically different diagnosis even before urodynamic testing.

The majority of the symptoms reported by these patients (recurring urinary infections, episodic urinary retention, urinary incontinence, assisting urination by abdominal pressing, with a urodynamic image typical for a sub-vesical obstruction or disorders of sphincter-detrusor coordination) were caused by a state of permanent contraction (possible since childhood) of the pelvic floor muscles (Figures 1a,b). This mechanism, used sub-consciously for years to defend against UI and the feeling of the urge to urinate, makes it impossible for the pelvic floor muscles to relax normally, which is essential for unhampered urination. It should be emphasized that the inflow of urine to the upper urethra with low or dysfunctional pressure at moments of reduced urethral pressure can evoke the urinary reflex, which our patients (with urodynamically normal detrusor function) refer to as "sudden urges." The constant maintenance of increased muscle tone can cause not only difficulties with initiating voiding, but also overfilling, which gives a clinical picture of bladder outlet obstruction. The lack of normal relaxation of the pelvic floor muscles in virtually the entire group of patients with chronic low urethral pressure, and in those with abnormal changes in urethral closure pressure, definitely hampered sexual initiation, the maintenance of sexual activity satisfying for both partners, and the establishment of a lasting relationship, and for many patients caused constant discomfort in the urogenital region. These patients assessed their HRQOL much lower. During the first visit, after a patient history has been taken and the questionnaire developed by our team has been filled out, the patients are informed about the possible genesis of the problem, and they are taught to relax the pelvic floor muscles during palpation and a transperineal ultrasonogram in standing position, with visualization of muscle activity on the screen. Those patients who had trouble with mastering conscious muscle relaxation additionally benefited from EMG biofeedback exercises with a vaginal electrode. As a rule, during the uroflow testing towards the end of the first visit, the women voided their bladders without abdominal pressing, with normal flow and without retention, or, in the case of abnormal urethra function, with a wavy curve but without urinary retention. Urodynamic testing, including profilometry (performed 2-3 weeks after the first visit), with relaxed pelvic floor muscles, confirmed the suspicion of low urethral closure pressure (P clos max oscillated from 25 - 35 cm H_2O), or abnormal urethra function. We were able to discover in the same patients during the first visit, that the P clos max could reach 80 or 120 cm H_2O, if the patient were maintaining the pelvic floor muscles in constant tension.

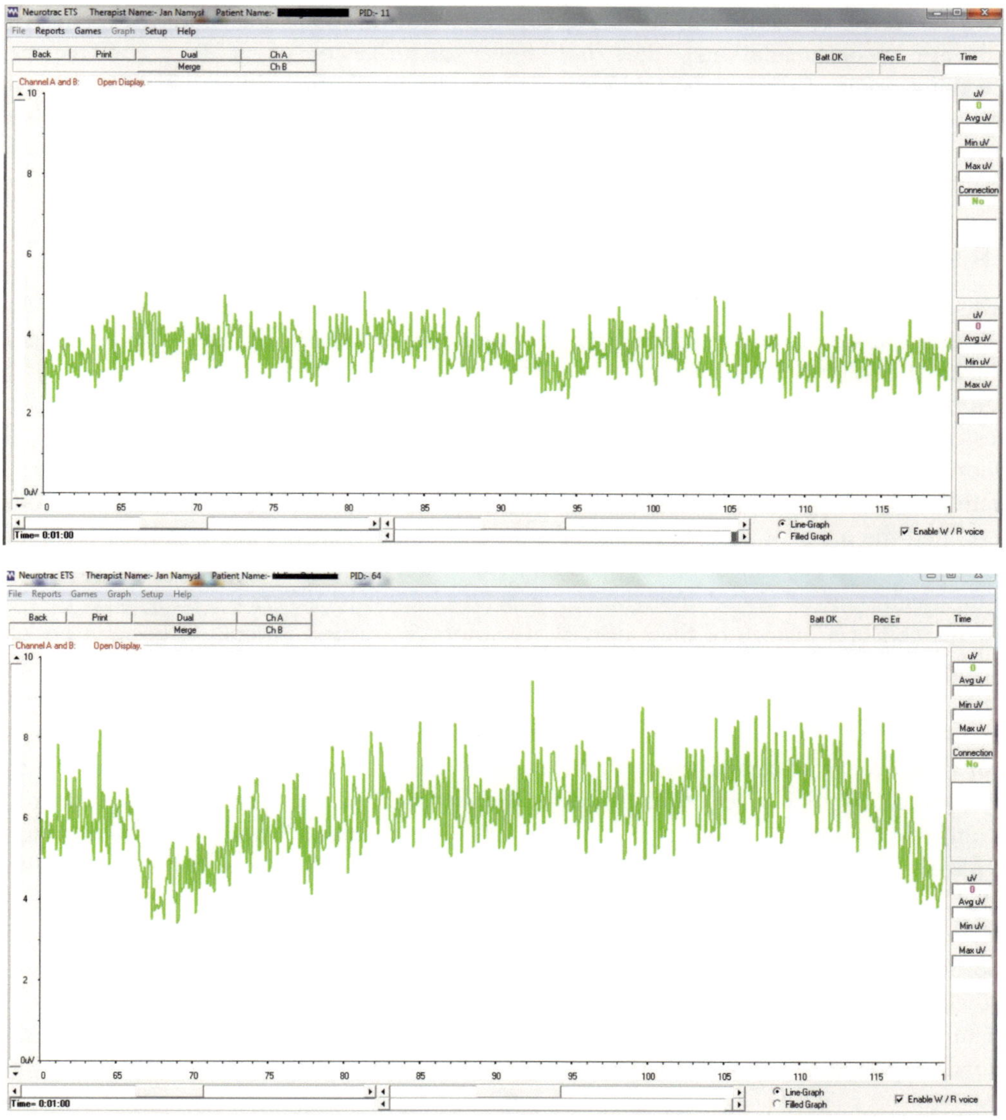

Fig. 1 a,b. EMG recordings of perineal muscle resting tone made in supine position with Veriprobe® vaginal probe and MyoPlus® EMG unit (Verity Medical Ltd) from different patients with increased muscle resting tone. Source: authors' own examinations.

This explains why in some previous investigations these women had been diagnosed with high urethral pressure. Most likely, when the previous urodynamic testing had been done without prior training in muscles relaxation with visualization of muscle function, these women had not relaxed the pelvic floor muscles even for a moment (first of all, they were unaware of the problem). The increased resting tone in the pelvic floor muscles, or slight muscle tone changes during the various phases of urodynamic testing, could lead to an incorrect diagnosis, despite the EMG record from the skin electrodes, which results from the limitations of this method of registration.

The great majority of patients in this group reported, that after the first visit (complying with our recommendations), they had fewer disturbances of voiding and recurrent infections. Some of them, who had periodic episodes of UI, decided on rehabilitation with electrical muscle stimulation (EMS) and EMG biofeedback therapy, or surgical treatment with sling procedures for better urethral support, supplemented by post-operative rehabilitation.

3. Reduced bladder sensation and increased bladder functional capacity

This same mechanism (many years of maintaining increased resting tone in the pelvic floor muscles) may also be developed by female patients whose bladders have increased functional capacity, with a weakened feeling of bladder fullness and urination reflex, and urethra with normal closing pressure. Just as in the group of patients with chronic low-pressure urethra or abnormal urethral pressure, these patients were unaware of the abnormal reactions involved in voiding, and had repressed any memories of involuntary micturition or bedwetting (due to overfilling) in childhood or adolescence. They most often associated the onset of symptoms with the most dramatic medical event in their childhood or adolescence (hospitalization for a urinary tract infection, or for difficulties in urinating), or the beginning of sexual intercourse, or with childbirth. When we suggested that the patients collect a history of their urinary disorders from their parents, it became possible during the next visit to confirm that episodes of UI, voiding problems, or urinary tract infections had occurred with varying intensity since childhood, and/or had occurred much more often than these women had reported during the first visit. Maintaining the pelvic floor muscles in a state of increased resting tone for many years had limited the number of episodes of UI due to overfilling, while the unconscious or sometimes recommended abdominal pressing had prevented undue urinary retention. It was only weakening or damage in the mechanisms of retaining urine, most often postnatal or iatrogenic, resulting from bladder emptying using the abdominal press, that over time had reduced the effectiveness of the mechanism used since childhood to cope with this form of voiding disorder. Static disturbances (whether postnatal or caused by other factors, such as changes in the posture of the pelvis, cf. Nguen 2000), regardless of the congenital weakening of the urinary reflex and the increased capacity of the bladder, can reveal congenital voiding disorders, previously masked by the defense mechanisms.

When there are no static disturbances, however, the unconscious use of abdominal pressing to support urination since childhood, due to constantly contracted muscles and a weakened urination reflex, has usually been rather effective in preventing urine retention and frequent infections. The strategy of behavior and ways of coping with bladder emptying, maintained over many years, give the patient a false sense of being in good health, and make it difficult to establish the cause-and-effect relationship of psychosomatic factors. Along with the appearance of static disturbances (e.g. due to childbirth or disturbances in the innervation of the pelvic floor muscles due to discopathy), the previous mechanism for voiding an overfilled bladder and reducing urine retention ceases to be effective, and difficulties with urination intensify. They are caused by the exacerbation of deformities (folding of the urethra), along with prolapse of the anterior vaginal wall when the effort is made to assist urination by abdominal pressing. In these patients, just as was the case in the group of patients with congenitally low or abnormal urethral pressure and with a normally sensitive and properly innervated bladder of the correct volume and an active urination reflex, there is an identical defense mechanism, i.e. permanently increased resting tone in the pelvic floor muscles. This mechanism is likewise the cause of psychosexual disturbances and a worse HRQOL. The lack of a diagnosis reached early enough using surface electromyography with vaginal electrode (or rectal electrode in children), produces a similar history of largely ineffective treatment. Unfortunately, some physicians still do not have the possibility to make an objective evaluation of the rest tone in the pelvic floor muscles with surface electromyography.

4. Underactive detrusor, bladder with increased cystometric capacity and underactive urination reflex

The patients with long standing underactive detrusor and a weakened urination reflex were subjected to the same diagnostic procedures as the first two groups, and were taught to relax the pelvic floor muscles. The effect of the proposed treatment, education, and exercises was particularly spectacular in this group, since after we had taught them to urinate with relaxation of the pelvic floor muscles and referred them for rehabilitation of the pelvis in cases where the disturbances were severe, further treatment was no longer necessary, and the symptoms of urinary dysfunction did not recur. The EMG recordings of perineal muscles rsting tone done with vaginal probe were much lower than in patients without rehabilitation (Figs. 2a,b).

Since the patients in this group had normal urethral closure pressure, there was no UI. If we found disturbances of statics and functional mechanisms producing a tendency to UI due to overfilling, e.g. kinking of the urethra, with reduction of hernia, we referred the patient for appropriate surgical treatment, supplemented by rehabilitation process.

5. Discussion

If we accept the criteria for the classification of dysfunctions of the lower urinary tract in the three groups of patients under discussion here, i.e. low urethral pressure/normal detrusor, abnormal urethral pressure/normal detrusor, and normal urethral pressure/underactive detrusor with increased capacity, the dysfunction was sufficiently mild and the defense mechanisms used sufficiently effective that the patients had not sought specialist medical care until additional factors had appeared, such as childbirth, reducing their ability to retain or pass urine. Ordinary medical care had been more oriented to symptomatic diagnosis and treatment. The complicated mechanisms underlying the appearance and development of UI and the broad background of psychosomatic conditions require adequate diagnostics and a thorough investigation of the etiopathology of pelvic floor muscle dysfunction, the absence of which retards properly targeted treatment and the choice of appropriate prevention methods.

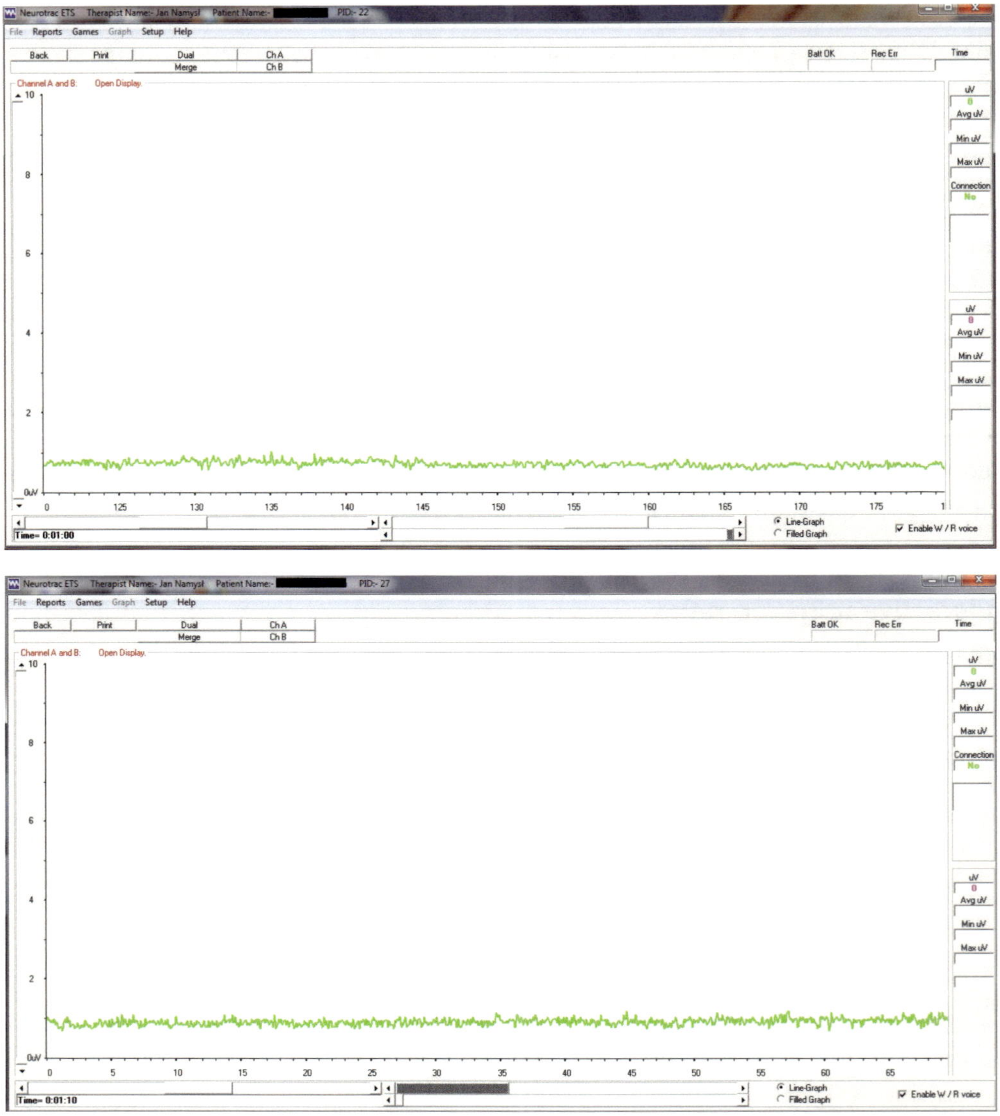

Fig. 2. a,bEMG recordings of perineal muscle resting tone made in supine position with Veriprobe ® vaginal probe and MyoPlus® EMG unit (Verity Medical Ltd) from different patients. A previously increased muscle resting tone tends to normalize after 8 weeks of rehabilitation using EMG biofeedback and functional electrostimulation. Source: authors' own examinations.

It is generally known that UI and urinary dysfunctions in childhood and adolescence are difficult medical problems in young women, though relatively rare, occurring less often than in adult women (Bø, 2004). The statistical data cover children and adolescents registered in medical facilities, with symptoms of the most severe urinary dysfunctions, primarily as a result of congenital defects of the spine and lower urinary tract. Milder (sub-clinical) and probably much more common disturbances remain undiagnosed, and thus they are mostly treated symptomatically. Years later, they are often diagnosed as the generally familiar risk factors in later phases of the life cycle: age, childbirth, overweight, genetic predispositions (Minassian et al., 2003; Nygaard et al., 2003; Rechberger & Skorupski, 2005). It would appear that the actual frequency of these dysfunctions in girls and young women may be much higher.

Among the essential factors producing the low rate of early diagnosis of dysfunctions in the lower urinary tract in girls are the lack of access to specialists who comprehend the complicated mechanisms for retaining and passing urine, the inadequacy of knowledge among pediatricians in respect to the diversity of urinary dysfunctions, and the lack of education for parents in respect to observing behaviors or abnormalities associated with bladder emptying in children. In our opinion, reliable scientific research on a representative sample would allow us to identify the needs and the principles for education and screening, in order to achieve earlier diagnosis and treatment of urinary dysfunctions in girls and young women. Like most authors, we believe that this results from the broad spectrum of personal variability and the functional norms generally accepted for the functional parameters, which do not entail specifying the normal resting tone of the pelvic floor muscles.

The constant maintenance of the pelvic floor muscles in increased resting tone is generally speaking one of the basic ways of coping with the problem of UI and severe static disorders. It is natural that, if only the muscles of the bladder and pelvis are not partially denervated or significantly weakened, a woman feels the degree of bladder fullness and the changes in intraabdominal pressure. Normal innervation of the lower urinary tract and normal muscle strength enable the autonomically controlled reactions of flexing the pelvis in response to a full bladder or increased intraabdominal pressure. In the case of the dysfunctions under discussion here, the conscious contraction of the pelvic floor muscles can facilitate the retention of urine in the collection phase and during exertion in all the basic types of UI seen in adult women (stress incontinence, urge urinary incontinence, and mixed). When this way of coping is maintained for many years (though often unconsciously, or consciously concealed by the patient), it is at least in part, along with neurogenic causes and disturbances of statics (postnatal, post-traumatic, spinal diseases, etc.) the cause of urinary dysfunctions, urine retention and recurrent infections. It can also lead to chronic constipation, difficulties with bowel movements, and fecal incontinence (Namysł & Garstka-Namysł, 2011). If squeezing the pelvic muscles has been the main reason for urinary dysfunction or discomfort in the urogenital region, once the patient has been made aware of the causes of her symptoms and taught to relax these muscles, spectacular treatment effects can be achieved: resolution of UI symptoms, and improved quality of sexual life, partner relations, and HRQOL in a very short time after the patient becomes aware of the reasons for the symptoms and rehabilitation has been implemented.

If functional testing of the pelvic floor muscles using surface electromyography confirms a neurogenic component, there are indications for implementing functional electrostimulation procedures with a neuroregenerative effect (Namysł & Garstka-Namysł, 2011). Expanding diagnostics with non-invasive surface electromyography, performed, depending on the subject's age, with rectal electrode in children, or (in women who have undergone sexual initiation) with a vaginal electrode, would facilitate early detection of increased muscle resting tone in the pelvic floor. Also, appropriately constructed psychological instruments at the preliminary interview stage (including a brief psychosexual biography, focused on the problems associated with UI), would help us change the treatment plan to obtain good outcomes in the large group of female patients previously diagnosed with, and unsuccessfully treated for, high urethral pressure. Thus the application in the diagnostic algorithm of the evaluation of the occurrence and intensity of the interaction (rather typical, as it seems at the present state of our knowledge) between the development of UI and urinary dysfunctions with mental functioning, facilitates the differentiation of risk groups among young female patients in the case of even a routine visit for recurrent lower urinary tract infections or sporadic episodes of UI (Bidzan, Smutek & Bidzan, 2010).

The awareness of these facts will help us avoid diagnostic errors, choose an appropriate therapy, and make use of multi-disciplinary interventions, including psychological help, or psychiatric help and rehabilitation in cases where it is needed.

6. Conclusions

These observations from our daily clinical practice point to the essential role of cooperation between urologists and a broad gamut of other specialists, especially uro-gynecologists, clinical psychologists, physiotherapists, and psychiatrists, in relation to patients in whom, despite several months of treatment, there are frequent relapses. They also make us aware of the need for physicians to expand their knowledge in the area of psychological factors associated with lower urinary tract symptoms and the holistic approach to treatment. And finally, they can also be a contribution to the ongoing discussion on the methodology of performing urodynamic tests (using profilometry), the need to apply surface electormyography of the pelvic floor muscles, acknowledged by numerous authors to be very useful (Garstka-Namysł, 2006, 2009; Garstka-Namysł et al., 2007, 2008), and the need to create multi-disciplinary teams and highly specialized centers for the diagnosis and therapy of urine retention disorders.

The lack of relaxation in the constantly contracted muscles of the pelvic floor can significantly impede a correct urodynamic diagnosis and cause a misdiagnosis regarding the activity of the urethra and the pelvic floor muscles.

Preparation of the patient for therapy by a multidisciplinary team, including a diagnostician, a psychologist, a psychiatrist and physiotherapist, specialized in the treatment of patients with urinary dysfunctions, can significantly increase the effectiveness of surgical treatment and limit relapses. A properly prepared questionnaire to evaluate quality of life, expanded with information about functional disorders in childhood or traumatic experiences in the urogenital area, can facilitate a correct diagnosis.

The visualization of the activity of the pelvic floor muscles in standing and prone position, using a transperineal ultrasonogram and surface electromyography, is of great help in the education and therapy of patients in order to improve urination.

Developing a plan of preventive and therapeutic activities, using education and rehabilitation, can prevent the development of full-symptom urinary incontinence and other negative symptoms of dysfunction in the muscles and nerves of the pelvic floor, leading to a deterioration of quality of life.

In our opinion, a multi-disciplinary approach to the therapy of urine retention dysfunctions and additional basic tests can contribute to a better understanding of the specific nature of different types of urinary incontinence in young women, reduce the number of diagnostic errors, hasten the implementation of correct treatment, reduce the recurrence of symptoms, provide a better understanding of the reasons for treatment failure, and increase the number of successfully treated women.

7. References

Abrams, P.; Cardozo, L.; Fall, M.; Griffiths, D.; Rosier, P.; Ulmsten, U.; van Kerrebroeck, P.; Victor, P. & Wein, A. (2002). ICS standardization of terminology of lower urinary tract function. *Neurourology and Urodynamics*, vol. 21, pp. 167-178

Adamiak, A. & Rechberger, T. (2005). Potencjalne możliwości zastosowania komórek macierzystych w uroginekologii. *Endokrynologia Polska*, vol. 6, pp. 994-997.

Anders, K. (2000). Coping strategies for women with urinary incontinence. *Best Practice & Research in Clinical Obstetrics & Gynaecology*, vol. 2, pp. 355-361

Badia, J.X.; Corcos, J.; Gotom, M.; Kelleher, C.; Lukacs, B. & Shaw, C. (2004). Symptom severity and QLQ scales for urinary incontinence. *Gastroenterology*, vol. 1, Suppl 1, pp. S114-123

Bidzan, M. (2011). Dynamika oceny jakości życia pacjentek z wysiłkowym nietrzymaniem moczu, In: *Rodzina i praca w warunkach kryzysu*, E. Bielawska-Batorowicz & L. Golińska, pp. 199-208, Wyd. UŁ, Łódź, Poland

Bidzan, M. (2008). *Jakość życia pacjentek z różnym stopniem nasilenia wysiłkowego nietrzymania moczu*, Oficyna Wyd. "Impuls", Kraków, Poland

Bidzan, M.; Smutek, J. & Bidzan, L. (2010). Psychosexual biography and the strategies used by women afflicted with stress urinary incontinence during intercourse: Two case studies. *Medical Sciences Monitor*, vol. 16, pp. CS6-10

Bidzan, M.; Dwurznik, J. & Smutek, J. (2005a). Jakość związku partnerskiego a poziom seksualnego funkcjonowania kobiet leczonych z powodu nietrzymania moczu w świetle wyników badania Skalą Jakości Związku DAS Spaniera oraz Kwestionariusza Zdrowia Kingsa, *Annales Universitas Mariae Curie –Skłodowska*, Vol. LX, Supl. XVI, 28, Sectio D, pp. 122 – 128

Bidzan, M.; Smutek, J. & Bidzan, L. (2005b). Nietrzymanie moczu - stygmatyzacją? Czy ostatnim tabu XXI wieku? *Annales Universitas Mariae Curie –Skłodowska*, Vol. LX, Supl. XVI., 29, Sectio D , pp. 129 -132

Bodden-Heidrich, R.; Beckmann, M.W.; Libera, B.; Rechenberger, I. & Bender, H.G. (1999). Psychosomatic aspects of urinary incontinence. *Archives of Gynecology and Obstetrics*, vol. 262, pp. 151-8

Bogner, H.R.; Gallo, J.J.; Swartz, K.L. & Ford, D.E. (2002). Anxiety disorders and disability secondary to urinary incontinence among adults over age 50. *International Journal of Psychiatry in Medicine*, vol. 2, pp. 141-154

Bogner, H.R. & Gallo, J.J. (2002). Urinary incontinence, condition-specific functional loss, and psychological distress. *Journal of the American Geriatrics Society*, vol. 7, pp. 1311

Bø, K. (2004). Urinary incontinence, pelvic floor dysfunction, exercise and sport. *Sports Medicine*, vol. 7, pp. 451-64

Broome, B.A.S. (2003). The impact of urinary incontinence on self-efficacy and quality of life. *Health and Quality of Life Outcomes*, vol. 1, pp. 35-40

Brown, J.S.; Subak, L.L.; Gras, J.; Brown, B.A.; Kuppermann, M. & Posner, S.F. (1998). Urge incontinence: the patient's perspective. *Journal of Women's Health*, vol. 7, pp. 1263-69

Brown, J.S.; Posner, S. & Stewart, A.L. (1999). Urge incontinence: new health-related quality of life measures. *Journal of the American Geriatric Society*, vol. 47, pp. 980-988

Bush, T.A.; Castellucci, D.T. & Phillips, C.A.D. (2001). Exploring women's beliefs regarding urinary incontinence. *Urologic Nursing*, vol. 3, pp. 211-218

Carcamo, C.R. & Lledo, R. (2001). Predictors of satisfaction with surgical treatment. *International Journal of Quality in Health Care*, vol. 3, pp. 267-69

Chiara, G.; Piccioni, V.; Perino, M.; Ohlmeier, U.; Fassino, S. & Leombruni, P. (1998). Psychological investigation in female patients suffering from urinary incontinence. *International Urogynecology Journal*, vol. 2, pp. 73-77

Chiarelli, P.; Brown, W. & McElduff, P. (1999). Leaking urine: prevalence and associated factors in Australian women. *Neurourology and Urodynamics*, vol. 18, pp. 567-577

Chiverton, P.; Wells, R.N.; Thelma, J.R.N.; Brink, C. & Mayer, R. (1996). Psychological factors associated with urinary incontinence. *Clinical Nurse Specialist*, vol. 5, pp. 229-233

Cioskowska-Paluch, G. (2000). Kłopoty z pęcherzem. *Wiadomości Zielarskie*, vol. 4, pp. 5-6

Coyne, L.; Schmier, J.; Hunt ,T.; Corey, R.,; Liberman, J. & Revicki, D. (2000). Developing a specific HRQL instrument for overactive bladder (abstract). *Value Health*, vol. 3, pp. 141

Coyne, K.S.; Zhou, Z.; Thompson, C. & Versi E. (2003). The impact on health-related quality of life of stress, urge and mixed urinary incontinence. *BJU International*, vol. 7, pp. 731-5

Currie, C. J.; McEwan, P.; Poole, C. D.; Odeyemi, I. A.; Datta, S. N. & Morgan C. L. (2006). The impact of the overactive bladder on the health-related utility and quality of life. *BJU International*, vol. 6, pp. 1267-72

Davey, G.C.L. (1993). A comparison of three cognitive appraisal strategies: the role of threat devaluation in problem-focused coping. *Personality and Individual Differences*, vol. 4, pp. 535-546

Debus–Thiede, G. & Dimpfl, T. (1993). Die psychische Situation der harninkontinenten Frau. *Zentralblatt für Gynäkologie*, vol. 7, pp. 332-335

Diokno, A.C.; Burgio, K.; Fultz, N.H.; Kinchen, K.S.; Obenchain, R. & Bump R.C. (2004). Medical and self-care practices reported by women with urinary incontinence. *American Journal of Managed Care*, vol. 10, pp. 69-78.

Dowd, T.T. (1991). Discovering older women's experience of urinary incontinence. *Research in Nursing and Health*, vol. 3, pp. 179-86

DuBeau, C.E.; Levy, B.; Mangione, C.M. & Resnick, N.M. (1998). The impact of urge urinary incontinence on quality of life: importance of patient's perspective and explanatory style. *Journal of the American Geriatrics Society*, vol. 6, pp. 683-92

Dugan, E.; Cohen, S.; Robinson, D.; Anderson, R.; Preisser, J.; Suggs, P.K.; Pearce, K.; Poehling, U. & McGann, P. (1998). The quality of life of older adults with urinary incontinence: determining generic and condition-specific predictors. *Quality of Life Research*, vol. 7, pp. 337-344

Dugan, E.; Cohen, S.J.; Bland, D.R.; Preisser, J.S.; Davis, C.C.; Suggs, P.K. & McGann, P. (2000), The association of depressive symptoms and urinary incontinence among older adults. *Journal of the American Geriatric Society*, vol. 48, pp. 413-416

Dugan, E.; Roberts, C.P.; Cohen, S.J.; Preisser, J.S.; Davis, C.C.; Bland, D.R. & Albertson, E. (2001). Why older community-dwelling adults do not discuss urinary incontinence with their primary care physicians. *Journal of the American Geriatrics Society*, vol. 4, pp. 462-465

Evans, D. (2005). Lifestyle solutions for men with continence problems. *Nursing Times*, vol. 2, pp. 61-64

Foldspang, A. & Mommsen S. (1997). The International Continence Society (ICS) incontinence definition: is the social and hygienic aspect appropriate for etiologic research? *Journal of Clinical Epidemiology*, vol. 9, pp. 1055-1060

Fultz, N.H. & Herzog, A.R. (2001). Self-reported social and emotional impact of urinary incontinence. *Journal of the American Geriatric Society*, vol. 7, pp. 892-899

Furelly, E.; Fianu-Jonasson A.; Larsson G. & van Kerrebroeck, P. (2003). Zuidex® treatment of SUI – impact on quality of life (King's Health Questionnaire). *Proceedings Abstract Book*, International Continence Society 33rd Annual Meeting, Florence, 5-9 October 2003, pp. 249-251

Garstka-Namysł, K. (2006). Surface electromyography (sEMG) and SEMG-biofeedback utility in therapy of muscle activity disorders s. *Polish Journal of Sports Medicine*, vol. 22, pp. 52-59

Garstka-Namysł, K.; Bręborowicz, G.H. ; Pilaczyńska-Szcześniak, Ł.. ; Huber J.; Sajdak, S.; Pisarska, M.; Witczak, K.; Sroka, Ł. & Witkowska, A. (2006). Functional stimulation of perineal muscles in women with urinary incontinence after gynecological surgery and its effect on quality of life changes. *Fizjoterapia Polska*, vol. 2, pp. 124-132

Garstka-Namysł, K.; Huber J.; Pisarska, M.; Bręborowicz, G.H. & Pilaczyńska-Szcześniak, Ł.. (2008). Change in the assessment of sexual intercourse of women after gynecological operations caused by disorders of micturition under the influence of electrostimulation of pelvis floor muscles and oververtebral electrostimulation. *New Medicine*, vol. 12, pp. 8-12

Garstka-Namysł, K. 2009. The role and use of surface electromyography (sEMG) for objective diagnostics of perineal muscles and as a method of conservative therapy of stress urinary incontinence (SUI). *Studies in Physical Culture and Tourism*, vol. 16, no. 3, pp. 233-239

Grimby, A.; Milsom, J.; Molander, U.; Wiklund, I. & Ekelund P. (1993). The influence of urinary incontinence on the quality of life of elderly women. *Age and Ageing*, vol. 2, pp. 82-89

Grimby, A. & Svanborg A. (1997). Morbidity and health related quality of life among ambulant elderly citizens. *Aging*, vol. 5, pp. 356-364

Hägglund, D.; Walker-Engström, M.L.; Larsson, G. & Leppert, J. (2001). Quality of life and seeking help in women with urinary incontinence. *Acta Obstetricia et Gynecologica Scandinavica*, vol. 11, pp. 1051-1055

Hannestad, Y.S.; Rortveit, G.; Sandvic, H. & Hunskaar, S. (2000). A community-based epidemiological survey of female urinary incontinence: the Norwegian EPINCONT study. Epidemiology of incontinence in the County of Nord - Trondelag. *Journal of Clinical Epidemiology*, vol. 53, pp. 1150-57

Hilton, P. (1988). Urinary incontinence during sexual intercourse: a common, but rarely volunteered symptom. *British Journal of Obstetrics and Gynaecology*, vol. 95, pp. 377-81

Hunskaar, S.; Burgio, K.; Diokno, A.C.; Herzog, A.R.; Hjälmĺs, K. & Lapitan M.C. (2002). Epidemiology and natural history of urinary incontinence (UI), In: *Incontinence. 2nd International Consultation on Incontinence*, 2nd edition, Abrams, P.; Cardozo, L.; Khoury, S. & Wein, A., pp. 65-201, Health Publication Ltd., Plymouth

Hunskaar, S.; Lose, G.; Sykes, D. & Voss S. (2004). The prevalence of urinary incontinence in women in four European countries. *BJU International*, vol. 4, pp. 324-30

Janssen, C.C.; Lagro-Janssen, A.L. & Felling, A.J. (2001). The effects of physiotherapy for female urinary incontinence: individual compared with group treatment. *British Journal of Urology International*, vol. 3, pp. 201-206

Kelleher, C.J.; Cardozo, L.D.; Khullar, V. & Salvatore S. (1997). A new questionnaire to assess the quality of life of urinary incontinent women. *British Journal of Obstetrics and Gynaecology*, vol. 104, pp. 1374-79

Kelleher, C.J. (2000). Quality of life and urinary incontinence. *Bailliere's Best Practice and Research. Clinical Obstetrics and Gynaecology*, vol. 2, pp. 363-379

Kinn, A.C. & Zaar, A. (1998). Quality of life and urinary incontinence pad use in women. *International Urogynecology Journal and Pelvic Floor Dysfunction*, vol. 2, pp. 83-87

Kirby, M.; Artibani, W.; Cardozo, L.; Chapple, C.; Diaz, D.C.; De Ridder, D.; Espuna-Pons, M.; Haab, F.; Kelleher, C.; Milsom, I.; Van Kerrebroeck, P.; Vierhout, M. & Wagg A. (2006). Overactive bladder: the importance of new guidance. *International Journal of Clinical Practice*, vol. 10, pp. 1263-1271

Lagro-Janssen, T.; Smits, A. & Van-Weel, C. (1992a). Urinary incontinence in women and the effects on their lives. *Scandinavian Journal of Primary Health Care*, vol. 3, pp. 211-216

Lagro-Janssen, T.; Debruyne, F.M. & Van-Weel, C. (1992b). Psychological aspects of female urinary incontinence in general practice. *British Journal of Urology*, vol. 5, pp.499-502

Lalos, O.; Berglund, A.L. & Lalos, A. (2001). Impact of urinary and climacteric symptoms on social and sexual life after surgical treatment of stress urinary incontinence in women: a long-term outcome. *Journal of Advanced Nursing*, vol. 3, pp. 316- 327

Lamm, D.; Fischer, W. & Maspfuhl B. (1986). Sexuality and urinary incontinence. *Zentralblatt für Gynäkologie*, vol. 108, pp. 1425-1430

Lew-Starowicz, Z. (2002). Zdrowie seksualne Polaków 2002. *Medycyna po Dyplomie*, vol. 11, pp. 16-21

Libalova, Z.; Feyereisl, J.; Martan, A.; Cepický, P.; Halaška, M.; Krosta, L.; Váchová, D.; Balcarová, J. & Pecená, M. (2001). Psychologie incontinence moce I. Srovnani zen Psychologie urgentni Psychologie stesovou inkontinenci pred zahájenim terapie. *Ceska Ginekologia*, vol. 3, pp. 171- 4M

Majkowicz, M.; de Walden-Gałuszko, K. & Trojanowski, L. (1997). Rola oceny funkcjonowania społecznego, psychicznego i strefy duchowej w globalnej ocenie jakości życia (w świetle badań kwesionariuszem QLQ-C30 i PIL propozycje modyfikacji kwestionariusza. *Psychoonkologia*, vol. 1, pp. 78-85

Meade-D'Alisera, P.; Merriweather, T.; Wentland, M.; Fantl, M. & Ghafar M. (2001). Depressive symptoms in women with urinary incontinence: a prospective study. *Urologic Nursing*, vol. 21, pp. 397–400

Milart, P. & Gulanowska-Gędek, B. (2002). Nietrzymanie moczu u kobiet w okresie pomenopauzalnym. *Nowa Medycyna - Hormonalna Terapia Zastępcza* (wydanie specjalne), vol. 9, pp. 31-36

Miller, J. & Hoffman E. (2006). The causes and consequences of overactive bladder. *Journal of Women's Health*, vol. 3, pp. 251-260

Milsom, I.; Ekelund, P.; Mokander, U.; Arvidsson, L. & Areshoug, B. (1993). The influence of age, parity, oral contraception, hysterectomy and menopause on urinary incontinence in women. *Journal of Urology*, vol. 149, pp. 1459-1462

Milsom, I.; Abrams, P.; Cardozo, L.; Roberts, R.G., Thüroff, J. & Wein, A.J.(2001). How widespread are the symptoms of an overactive bladder and how are they managed: a population based prevalence study. *BJU International*, vol. 87, pp. 760-766

Minassian, V.A., Drutz, H.P. & Al-Badr, A. (2003). Urinary incontinence as a worldwide problem. *International Journal of Gynecology & Obstetrics*, vol. 82, pp. 327-338

Namysł, J. & Garstka-Namysł, K. (2011). Rehabilitacja pacjentów z nietrzymaniem stolca, In: *Leczenie chorób proktologicznych w okresie ciąży i porodu*, Kołodziejczak, M., Wyd. Borgis, Warsaw (in press)

Norton, C. (1982). The effects of urinary incontinence in women. *International Rehabilitation in Medicine*, vol. 4, pp. 9-14

Norton, P.A.; MacDonald, L.D.; Sedgwick, P.M. & Stanton, S.L. (1988). Distress and delay associated with urinary incontinence, frequency and urgency in women. *British Medical Journal*, vol. 297, pp. 1187-1189

Nuotio, M.; Jylhä, M.; Luukkaala, T. & Tammela, T.L.J. (2003). Urinary incontinence in a Finnish population aged 70 and over. *Skandinavian Journal of Primary Health Care*, vol. 21, pp. 182- 187

Nygaard, I.; Turvey, C.; Burns, T.L.; Crischilles, E. & Wallace, R. (2003). Urinary incontinence and depression in middle–aged United States women. *Obstetrics and Gynecology*, vol. 101, pp. 149-156

Nygaard, I.E. & Heit, M. (2004). Stress urinary incontinence. *Obstetrics and Gynecology*, vol. 104, pp. 607-620

Papanicolaou, S.; Hunskaar, S.; Lose, G. & Sykes, D. (2005). Assessment of bothersomeness and impact on quality of life of urinary incontinence in women in France, Germany, Spain and the UK. *British Journal of Urology International*, vol. 96, pp. 831-838

Perry, S., McGrother, C.W. & Turner K. (2006). An investigation of the relationship between anxiety and depression and urge incontinence in women: development of a psychological model. *British Journal of Health Psychology*, vol. 3, pp. 463-482

Rechberger, T. (2004). Wysilkowe nietrzymanie moczu u kobiet. Jak leczyć skutecznie? *Kwartalnik NTM*, vol. 1, pp. 4-5

Rechberger, T. & Skorupski, P. (2005). Nietrzymanie moczu - problem medyczny, socjalny i społeczny, In: Nietrzymanie moczu u kobiet. Diagnostyka i leczenie, T. Rechberger & J. Jakowicki, pp. 29-38, Wyd. BiFOLIUM, Lublin, Poland

Rechberger, T. & Tomaszewski, J. (2007). Epidemiologia, znaczenie kliniczne i leczenie pęcherza nadreaktywnego: solifenacyna - nowa opcja terapeutyczna. *Ginekologia po Dyplomie*, vol. 1, pp. 50-57

Robinson, D.; Pearce; K.F.; Preisser, J.S.; Dugan, E.; Suggs, P.K. & Cohen S.J. (1998). Relationship between patient reports of urinary incontinence symptoms and quality of life measures. *Obstetrics and Gynecology*, vol. 2, pp. 224-228

Roe, B. & May C. (1999). Incontinence and sexuality: findings from a qualitative perspective. *Journal of Advanced Nursing*, vol. 3, pp. 573-579

Rogers, G.R.; Kammerer-Doak, D.; Villarreal, A.; Coates, K. & Qualls, C. (2001a). A new instrument to measure sexual function in women with incontinence and/or pelvic organ prolapse. *American Journal of Obstetrics and Gynecology*, vol.. 4, pp. 552-8

Rogers, G.R.; Villarreal, A.; Kammerer-Doak, D. & Qualls C. (2001b). Sexual function in women with and without urinary incontinence and/or pelvic organ prolapse. *International Urogynecology Journal*, vol. 12, 361-365

Samuelsson, E.; Victor, A. & Tibblin, G.A. (1997). A population study of urinary incontinence and nocturia among women aged 20-59 years. *Acta Obstetricia et Gynecologica Scandinavica*, vol. 76, pp. 74-80

Sand, P.K.; Staskin, D.; Miller, J.; Diokno, A.; Sant, G.R.; Davila, G.W.; Knapp, P.; Rappaport, S. & Tutrone R. (1999). Effects of a urinary control insert on quality of life in incontinent women. *International Urogynecology Journal and Pelvic Floor Dysfunction*, vol. 2, pp. 100-105

Sand, P.K. & Appell, R.(2006). Disruptive effects of overactive bladder and urge urinary incontinence in younger women. *American Journal of Medicine*, vol. 119, Suppl. 1, pp. 16-23

Shaw, C. (2001). A review of the psychosocial predictors of help-seeking behaviour and impact on quality of life in people with urinary incontinence. *Journal of Clinical Nursing*, vol. 1, pp. 15-24

Shaw, C.; Tansey, R.; Jackson, C.; Hyde, C. & Allan, R. (2001). Barriers to help seeking in people with urinary symptoms. *Family Practice*, vol. 1, pp. 48-52

Smutek, J.; Grzybowska, M.; Bidzan, M. & Płoszyński, A. (2004). Nietrzymanie moczu u kobiet. Strategie radzenia sobie z problemem gubienia moczu w czasie współżycia,

Annales Universitas Mariae Curie -Skłodowska, Vol.LIX, Supl. XIV, Sectio D, pp. 180-186

Steciwko, A. (2002). *Wybrane zagadnienia z praktyki lekarza rodzinnego.* Tom 4: *Nietrzymanie moczu – problem interdyscyplinarny, choroby gruczołu krokowego,* Wyd. Continuo, Wrocław, Poland

Sutherst, J.R. (1979). Sexual dysfunction and urinary incontinence. *British Journal of Obstetrics and Gynaecology,* vol. 86, pp. 378-8

Sutherst, J. & Brown M. (1980). Sexual dysfunction associated with urinary incontinence. *Urology International,* vol. 35, pp. 414-416

Swithinbank, L.V. & Abrams, P. (1999). The impact of urinary incontinence on the quality of life of women. *World Journal of Urology,* vol. 17, pp. 225-229

Temml, C.; Haidinger, G. & Schmidbauer J. (2000). Urinary incontinence in both sexes: prevalence rates and impact on quality of life and sexual life. *Neurourology and Urodynamics,* vol. 19, pp. 259-271

Thom, D.H. (2000). Overactive bladder: epidemiology and impact on quality of life. *Patient Care,* Winter Suppl., pp. 6-14

Tołłoczko, T. (2002). Nietrzymanie moczu - problem społeczny i kliniczny. *Terapia,* vol. 4, pp. 4-6

Umlauf, M.G.; Goode, P.S. & Burgio K.L. (1996). Psychosocial issues in geriatric urology: problems in treatment and treatment seeking. *Urologic Clinics of North America,* vol. 23, pp. 127-136

Valvanne, J.; Juva, K., Erkinjuntti, T. & Tilvis, R. (1996). Major depression in the elderly: a population study in Helsinki. *International Psychogeriatrics,* vol. 3, pp. 437-43

Vereecken, R.L. (1989). Psychological and sexual aspects in different types of bladder dysfunction. *Psychotherapy and Psychosomatics,* vol. 3, pp. 28-134

Watson, A.J.; Currie, L.; Curran, S. & Jarvis G.J. (2000). A perspective study examining the association between the symptoms of anxiety and depression and severity of urinary incontinence. *European Journal of Obstetrics & Gynecology & Reproductive Biology,* vol. 88, pp. 7–9

Wein, A.J. & Rovner, E.S. (1999). The overactive bladder: an overview for primary care health providers. *International Journal of Fertility,* vol. 44, pp. 56-66

Williams K. (2004). Stress urinary incontinence: treatment and support. *Nursing Standards,* vol. 31, pp. 45-52

Woodman, P.J.; Misko, C.A. & Fischer J.R. (2001). The use of short-form quality of life questionnaires to measure the impact of imipramine on women with urge incontinence. *International Urogynecology Journal,* vol. 12, pp. 312-331

Wyman, F.J.; Fantl, J.A.; McClish, D.K.; Harkins, S.W.; Uebersax, J.S. & Ory M.G. (1997). Quality of life following bladder training in older women with urinary incontinence. *International Urogynecology Journal,* vol. 8, pp. 223-229

Wyman, F.J. (1998). Quality of life of older adults with urinary incontinence. *Journal of the American Geriatrics Society,* vol. 6, pp. 778-779

Zajda, J.; Połujański, J. & Zbrzeźniak M. (2000). Leczenie nietrzymania moczu u kobiet - problem społeczny, ekonomiczny i leczniczy. *Nowa Medycyna,* vol. 5, pp. 76-81

Zorn, B.H.; Montgomery, H.; Pieper, K.; Gray, M. & Steers, W.D. (1999). Urinary incontinence and depression. *Journal of Urology*, vol. 162, pp. 82-84

4

Effects of Pelvic Floor Muscle Training with Biofeedback in Women with Stress Urinary Incontinence

Nazete dos Santos Araujo[1,*], Érica Feio Carneiro Nunes[1], Ediléa Monteiro de Oliveira[1], Cibele Câmara Rodrigues[2] and Lila Teixeira de Araújo Janahú[3]

[1]*Amazonia University,*
[2]*Federal University of Pará,*
[3]*College of Amazonia,*
Brazil

1. Introduction

This chapter addresses the effects of training of the pelvic floor muscles using an electromyographic biofeedback equipment as a tool for treatment in women with stress urinary incontinence.

The Stress Urinary Incontinence (SUI) is defined by the International Continence Society (ICS) as involuntary loss of urine during physical effort with sneezing and coughing, and it is considered a consequence of the weakness of the pelvic floor[1,2]. It is the most common type of urinary incontinence and its prevalence can vary from 12% to 56% depending on the population studied and the diagnostic criterion adopted[3,4]. In Brazil the prevalence of complaints of stress urinary incontinence is around 35% [2].

Approximately 1/3 of women of the research presented mixed complaints, i.e., urinary loss during stress associated with irritative symptoms, such as increased urinary frequency, urinary urgency, nocturia, urgency incontinence and/or enuresis[3].

Nowadays there are several risk factors for the onset of sui, and we can realize that the literature often relates it to obesity, menopause, smoking, parity, types of delivery and exercise. The white ethnicity is also related to risk factors; In an American study, when the authors compared white to black people, it appears an higher incidence for the first group (white one), varying from 23 to 32% and a lower incidence to the second group, with na average from 16 to 18% [5, 6,7].

It is known that SUI compromises the quality of life (QOL) of women of different ages[5,6]. However, many women with UI believe that sporadic involuntary urinary loss is a normal part of the aging process and, also because they find it embarrassing, they do not refer to its impact on their daily activities or report these symptoms to their doctors[8].

*Corresponding Author

In the literature, there are some questionnaires to assess quality of life of women with SUI, but the King's Health (KHQ) is the most commonly used in Brazil, which is validated in Portuguese and evaluates the presence of UI symptoms AND ITS relative impact, leading to more consistent results[9].

Many factors are involved in the SUI physiopathology, especially the rotational descent of the urethra, a functionally shorturethra, pudendal nerve lesions, fascia laceration, pelvic floor muscle (PFM) ruptures, intrinsic urethral mechanism deficiency and bladder neck hypermobility[10].

PFM functional detoriation, or weakness is an important factor causing SUI[11]. Physical therapy is considered a first line option for the rehabilitation of the pelvic floor muscles. Regarding to the conservative treatment, Kinesiotherapy is considered as level 1 evidence of its beneficial effects in SUI women (ICI 2009), but when we talk about operative interventions, Slings are the level 1 evidence. The most commonly used treatment modalities are pelvic floor muscle training (PFMT) to strengthen the PFM, vaginal electrostimulation, biofeedback (BF), vaginal cones and behavioral therapy, including information, education, awareness and advice[12].

Electromyographic biofeedback (EMG BF) can be used to measure, assess and treat PFM dysfunctions and is one of the potential treatment modalities used for the rehabilitation of pelvic floor muscles[10], once in its clinical use allows the patient to obtain informations about the physiological process of contraction, which used to be unknown in most of the cases. it facilitates the motor control of the pelvic floor muscles, favoring the re- education through a visual or hearing feedback generated by electromyography 13.

2. Methodological description

This was a randomized clinical trial research delevoped in the city of Belém, state of Pará, Brazil. the aim of this research was to study the effects of PFMT with EMG BF on bladder neck mobility, motor activity of PFM with EMG, PFM strength, levator ani muscle thickness and the quality of life of women with SUI, involving 50 women, 25 in each group, complaining of SUI was carried out. The relevant baseline characteristics are shown in Table 1.

The inclusion criteria were women aged from 30 and 55 years, with negative urine test and urodynamic diagnosis of SUI due to bladder neck hypermobility, pressure of stress-induced urine loss (PSIUL) higher than 90 cm of H_2O. Patients with SUI due to intrinsic insufficiency with PSIUL of less than 60 cm, those who have undergone previous SUI surgery and those who presented vaginal prolapse of any degree in the physical examination were excluded. All the patients were referred by urologists or gynecologists, who requested and executed the urinary sediment and quantitative urine culture, urodynamic study and ultrasound test. The sample was randomized using sealed envelopes to choose the patients who would receive EMG BF and the ones who would be part of the control group. The control group was offered the same treatment given to Gbio after the end of the study. The Gbio underwent thirty-minute training sessions twice a week for eight weeks [14].

The ultrasound was conducted by the Toschiba-Nomio equipment (Tokyo, 2004) to measure urethral mobility (in centimeters) and the thickness of the levator ani muscle (in centimeters). Urethral mobility was measured by the transvaginal technique using a convex endocavitary probe with a frequency of 6.5 MHz and the thickness of the levator ani muscle was measured by the transabdominal technique using a 3.5 MHz transducer. This test was conducted while the bladder contained a maximum of 50 ml of urine[15] and by the same specialist in diagnostic imaging.

After referral, the patients were assessed by the same specialized physical therapist before and after the study. PFM strength was done by digital vaginal palpation using the Ortiz[16] scale to assess PF muscle strength. PFM EMG motor activity was measured with PHENIX equipment (Vivaltis, Paris, France), model USB-4 through a 5-cm long and 5.5-cm wide vaginal probe, dampened with KY Johnson gel. The probe was introduced 3 cm inside of the vagina's introitus. The PFM electric signal was registered in microvolts (μv) by two 1-cm rings located in the probe, captured and viewed by patients on the computer screen.

The electrical signal of the PFM was registered in microvolts (μv), with the use of an individual intravaginal probe with the patient lying in supine position, flexed legs and feet supported by a stretcher after instruction the patient was asked to perform 3 maximal PFM contractions. The highest registration of the contraction was selected as starting point for the treatment that was registered by and transmitted to the computer through a visual signal. The King´s Health Questionnaire (KHQ) was also applied.

The King´s Health Questionnaire (KHQ) assesses both the presence of urinary incontinence and its relative impact. It consists of 30 questions distributed across nine domains: general health, impact on life, role limitations, physical limitations, social limitations, personal relationships, emotions, sleep/energy and severity (coping) measures[17]. There is also a scale of symptoms: increased urinary frequency, nocturia, urgency, bladder overactivity, SUI, nocturnal enuresis, incontinence during sexual intercourse, urinary infections and bladder pain. Each domain receives a individual score; therefore, there is not an overall score. Scores vary from zero to 100 and the higher the score, the worse the quality of life associated with that domain[17].

Before they started treatment, Gbio patients received information on the function of pelvic floor muscles and were informed of the importance of continuing their exercises and functional training, so, adaptation into daily life activities. In addition to the EMG BF-assisted exercises, patients were advised to do the same exercises at home to strengthen the PFM through slow and rapid contractions, being told to do three series of 10 contractions in the supine, sitting and orthostatic positions three times a day with a duration of 5-10 seconds, the contraction per subject was verified through an initial assessment of each individual[18]. They were also encouraged to undergo functional PFM training, i.e. to contract this muscle group during stress activities and increased intra-abdominal pressure.

The same EMG BF that was used to test the electromyographic activity of the PFM was also used to train the Gbio. The EMG BF was connected to a computer, equipped with specific software. Two pre-established programs with alternate contraction and relaxation periods were used: a twenty-minute program (85 rapid contractions and 34 slow contractions including) and a ten-minute program (including 54 rapid contractions and 24 slow contractions) [19]. The women watched the contractions on the computer screen receiving visual feedback. Recent literature reviews show there is no a consensus regarding what kind of training program would be the most effective [20,21]. This study's protocol was based on the review of Hay-Smith et. al, in which the maximum number of daily contractions requested from patients was estimated at between 36 and 200 [21,22].

Descriptive statistics, with mean and standard deviation, were used to analyze the data. The normality of the sample was evaluated by the Shapiro-Wilk test and the homogeneity variance by the Levene test. The inter-group data were analyzed using Student's t test for independent samples, when there was heterocedasticity we applied the Mann-Whtiney U test. Categorical variables were tested by the chi-square test. The significance level alpha = 0.05 were considered to reject the null hypothesis. The data were put into an Excel database and analyzed with SPSS, version 14.0[23].

3. Results

Relevant baseline and KHQ characteristics before the treatment, presented in Table 1, showed that there were no present statistically significant differences between both groups.

	Gc	Gbio	Value-p
General characteristics			
Age (years)	445.5 ±5.6	45.8 ±5.2	0.3957
Number of children	2 ±1	2 ±1	0.8757
Time of incontinence (years)	3.9 ±3.8	3.5 ±2.1	0.0776
EMG-test (μV)	9.36 ±5.66	7.76 ±5.06	0.2977
Muscular strength (me, min, max)	3 (1 - 4)	3 (1 - 4)	0.1519
Thickness (mm)	11.55 ±1.77	11.01 ±1.97	0.3139
Urethal mobility (mm)	16.97 ±4.40	16.10 ±7.04	0.3467
Kings Health Questionnaire			
General health	25 (0 - 75)	25 (25 - 75)	0.1282
Impact on life	50 (0 - 100)	33.3 (0 - 66.6)	0.3781
Role limitations	33.3 (0 - 100)	0 (0 - 77)	0.3987
Physical limitations	0 (0 - 100)	33.3 (0 - 100)	0.2959
Social limitations	16.6 (0 - 83.3)	26.6 (0 - 80)	0.4231
Personal relationships	33. 3 (0 - 100)	0 (0 - 66.6)	0.6208
Emotions	16.6 (0 - 66.6)	0 (0 - 66.6)	0.6766
Sleep and energy	0 (0 - 100)	22.2 (0 - 100)	0.6139
Severity (coping)	16.6 (0 - 100)	26.6 (0 - 100)	0.4492

Student's t test and Mann-Whitney's test
me: mean; min: minimum value; max: maximum value; EMG: Electromyographic.

Table 1. Relevant baseline characteristics and KHQ domains - data obtained before intervention, Gc (n=25) and Gbio (n=25).

Based on statistically significant differences in all the characteristics assessed (Table 2), comparison of anatomic and functional characteristics between the groups after intervention showed that treatment was associated with changes in the configuration of anatomic and functional structures of the PF.

	Gc	Gbio	Value-p
Anatomo-functional characteristics			
EMG-test (μV)	9.40 ±5.99	15.28 ±8.52	0.0068*
Muscular strength (me, min, max)	3 (1 - 4)	4 (2 - 4)	0.0009**
Thickness (mm)	11.66 ±1.65	13.27 ±2.12	0.0044*
Urethal mobility (mm)	17.67 ±4.53	9.26 ±3.01	<0.0001*
Kings Health Questionnaire			
General health	25 (0 - 75)	25 (0 - 50)	0.3933
Impact on life	50 (0 - 100)	33.3 (0 - 66.6)	0.0305**
Role limitations	33.3 (0 - 66.6)	0.0 (0 - 33.3)	0.0099**
Physical limitations	33.3 (0 - 100)	0.0 (0 - 33.3)	0.0010**
Social limitations	0.0 (0 - 77)	0.0 (0 - 66.6)	0.3084
Personal relationships	0.0 (0 - 100)	0.0 (0 - 50)	0.0426**
Emotions	33.3 (0 - 100)	11.1 (0 - 44.4)	0.2444
Sleep and energy	16.6 (0 - 83.3)	(16.6 (0 -66.6)	0.8311
Severity (coping)	26.7 (0 - 80)	6.6 (0 - 73)	0.0021**

* Student's t test

** Mann-Whitney

me: mean; min: minimum value; max: maximum value; EMG: Electromyographic.

Table 2. Gc (n=25) and Gbio (n=25) after the treatment.

4. To show the bladder neck mobility

Figures below show transvaginal ultrasound from bladder neck during rest and effort phases, before and after treatment with EMG BF. Figures 1 and 2 : ultrasound before treatment. Figures 3 and 4: ultrasuond post- treatment.

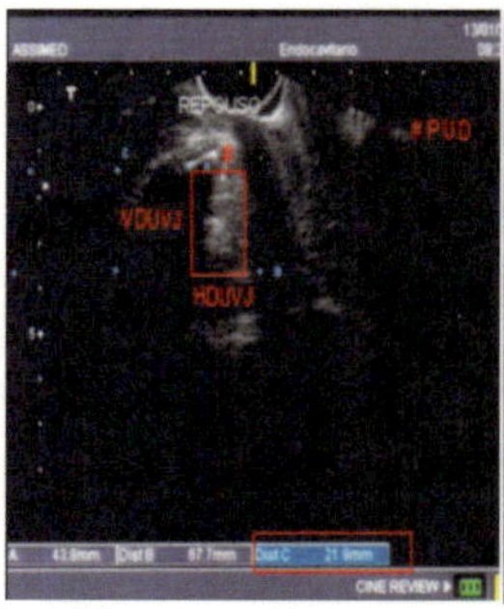

Fig. 1. Rest

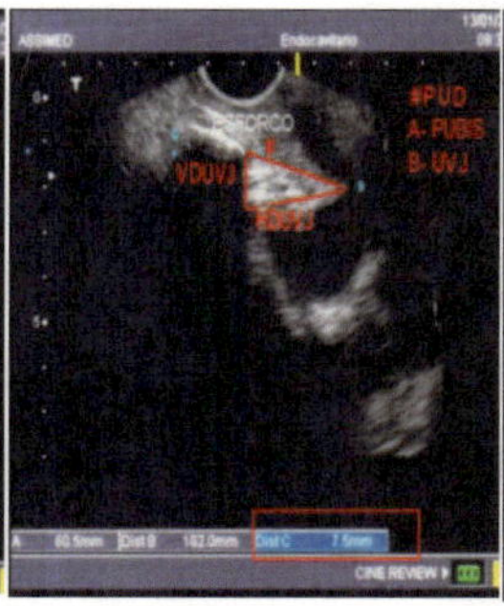

Fig. 2. Effort

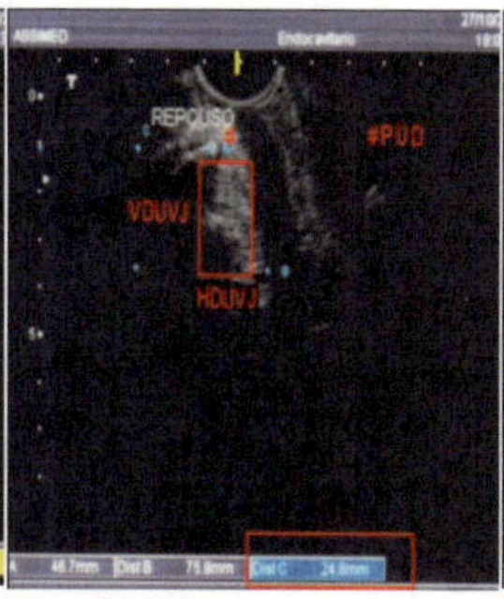

Fig. 3. Rest

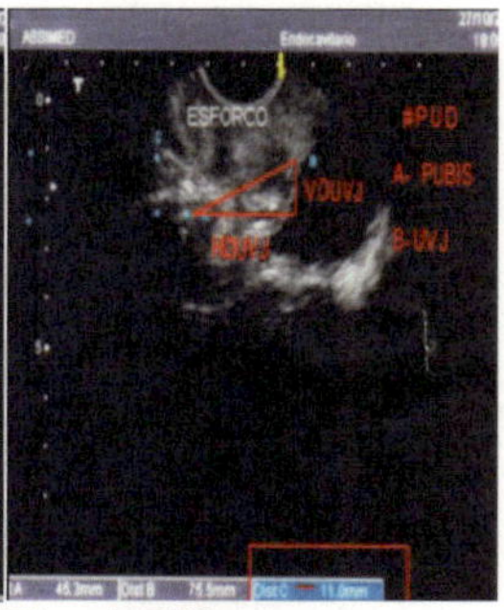

Fig. 4. Effort

HDUVJ: Horizontal Distance from Urethrovesical Junction; PUD: Pubo-Urethral Distance; UVJ: Urethrovesical Junction; VDUVJ: Vertical Distance from Urethrovesical Junction.

The EMG test presented a statistically significant difference (p= 0.0068) between the groups; Gbio (15.28 ±8.52 μV) presented higher levels of PF motor activity than Gc (9.40 ±5.99 μV).

The assessment of pelvic floor muscular strength showed a statistically significant difference (p = 0.0009): Gbio (mean = 4) was higher than Gc (mean = 3).

In Gbio the levator ani muscle thickness (13.27 ±2.12 mm) was statistically significant bigger compared to Gc (11.66 ±1.65 mm) (p= 0.0044).

Bladder neck mobility was statistically significant less in the Gbio group (9.26 ±3.01 mm) than in Gc (17.67 ±4.53 mm) (p = 0.0044*).

The intergroup KHQ analysis showed significant differences in 5 domains. In the impact on life domain (p = 0.0305), Gbio (mean = 33.3%) presented lower levels compared to Gc (mean = 50%); in the role limitations domain, there was a significant improvement (p = 0.0099) in Gbio (mean = 0.0%), but not in Gc (mean = 33.3%); in the physical limitations domain, the result was statistically significant (p = 0.0010), since Gbio (mean = 0.0%) showed fewer limitations than Gc (mean 33.33%); in the personal relationships domain (p = 0.0426), the mean for both groups was the same (0.0%), but no Gbio individual had scores higher than 50%; and in the severity (coping) measures, there was also a significant difference (p = 0.0021), with a mean of 6.6% in Gbio, versus a mean of 26.7% in Gc.

On the other hand, general health, social limitations, emotions and sleep/energy did not show a statistically significant difference between groups after treatment.

Comparison between groups of KHQ urinary scale symptoms (Table 3) shows that urinary frequency, nocturia and SUI were statistically significantly different after intervention

Symptoms	Gc Intensity				Gbio Intensity				Value-p
	slight (%)	Moderate (%)	Severe (%)	NRA (%)	Slight (%)	Moderate (%)	Severe (%)	NRA (%)	
Frequency	56	36	0	8	32	24	8	36	0.0337*
Nocturia	52	32	0	16	40	8	8	44	0.0261*
Urgency	36	40	0	24	36	12	4	48	0.0796
Urge incontinence	60	12	0	28	40	12	0	48	0.3141
Stress urinary incontinence	28	56	16	0	52	4	0	44	<0.0001*
Nocturnal enuresis	8	4	0	88	4	0	0	96	0.4916
Sexual intercourse incontinence	20	12	0	68	12	0	0	88	0.1261
Frequent infections	12	0	0	88	16	0	0	84	0.9999
Bladder pain	4	0	0	96	8	4	0	88	0.4916

*Chi-square
NRA: omitted response

Table 3. Urinary symptoms in Gc (n=25) and Gbio (n=25) after intervention.

Regarding urinary frequency (p = 0.0337*), Gbio presented lower percentages in the "low" (32%) and "moderate" (24%) categories, versus 56% "low" and 36% "moderate" for Gc. However, the "severe" category presented an inversion, with Gbio (8%) exceeding Gc (0%).

Nocturia was statistically significantly different (p = 0.0261) between the groups, Gbio presented lower percentages in the "low" (40%) and "moderate" (8%) categories, versus 52% "low" and 32% "moderate" for Gc. However, the "severe" category presented an inversion, with Gbio (8%) exceeding Gc (0%).

When we analyze SUI results, we observe a statistically significant improvement (p<0.0001) in the "low" (52%) and "moderate" (4%) and "severe" (0%) intensities in Gbio, versus "low" (28%), "moderate" (56%) and "severe" (16%) intensities for Gc.

The other symptoms did not present any statistically significant difference between the groups.

5. Discussion

The results of this study indicate that the training of pelvic floor muscles through EMG BF can lead to changes in the anatomic and functional structures of PF, since there were statistically significant differences in all the assessed characteristics of the incontinent women treated.

When compared to healthy women, decrease of surface electromyographic activity in women with SUI, urgency incontinence and mixed incontinence has been found, which suggests a deterioration of the neuromuscular function in these women[24]. In this study, we observed that the quantification of muscular activity carried out through the EMG test showed statistically significant increase (p = 0.0068) after treatment in Gbio, which suggests that BF can restore PF neuromuscular function.

In this study, compared to Gc, PFM strength presented a statistically significant change (p = 0.0009) after BF treatment. However, we did not objectively quantify the SUI reduction. In a study of 52 women, aged from 24 to 64 (mean 45.4 years) suffering from SUI, a positive correlation between the increase in PFM maximum strength and the reduction in urine loss during stress was demonstrated [25], and in another study by Rett at al[26], who included a sample of 26 women with SUI a significant improvement in pelvic floor muscular strength, from 0 (zero) or 1 (one) to 2 (two) or 3 (three) was seen. Yet, the profile of the patients in both studies was different.

Regarding the thickness of the levator ani muscle, Bernstein[27] demonstrated through transabdominal ultrasonography a significant reduction in the thickness of the levator ani muscle in women over 60 compared to that of younger women. According to this author, the levator ani muscle was significantly thicker in healthier women than in those with urinary incontinence and this problem can be eliminated through physical therapy, as corroborated by this study, which showed a statistically significant increase in the thickness of the levator ani muscle in Gbio (p = 0.0044), but not in Gc, which did not have any statistically relevant improvement.

The investigation of the effectiveness of ultrasound in assessing bladder neck descent in the SUI diagnosis still presents contradictory results and unclear responses. Urethral hypermobility can occur in patients without UI and the reason to extent urethral hypermobility has been related to (the severity) of UI remains unclear [28,29]. However, regardless the cause of SUI, nowadays, there is some consensus also to measure urethral hypermobility[30]. Recently, ultrasound seems to play an important role in the study of the urethral vesical junction(UVJ) and the proximal urethra (PU), also because it is a simple, low-cost, innocent and easily repeatable technique[30,31,32].

In this study, there was a statistically relevant reduction in urethral mobility ($p<0.0001$) in Gbio after the treatment compared to Gc. These results contradict that of a study with transvaginal electrostimulation in a group of 23 women suffering from SUI who did not show a significant difference in bladder neck mobility before and after treatment ($p= 0.30$)[33]. However, our data are in line with the studies of Balmforth et al[34], which comprised 97 women (49.5±10.6 years) and demonstrated a positive and significant association of the improved position of the bladder neck and the anatomical and functional improvement of the pelvic floor, accompanied by an improvement in the quality of life as measured by the KHQ.

Regarding the impact on the quality of life of the SUI patients in this study, in the intergroup comparison considering the KHQ domains there was a positive response in the following ones: incontinence impact on life ($p = 0.0305$), activity of daily life limitations ($p = 0.0099$), physical limitations ($p = 0.0010$), personal relationships ($p = 0.0426$) and severity (coping) measures ($p = 0.0021$) in Gbio. Similar results were obtained by other studies[9,30]. It is worth to notice that the impact of these symptoms on the life of each patient is closely related to the individual perception these women have of the severity, type and amount of loss, in addition to each individual's cultural context[35].

This study showed that the most prevalent symptoms were SUI, urinary frequency and nocturia, and that, after treatment, the Gbio presented a reduction or elimination of these symptoms compared to the Gc, in line with the findings of the Rett study[26], in which a sample of 26 women of reproductive age with SUI showed a significant response to the use of EMG BF, with a decrease of urinary symptoms, especially urinary frequency, nocturia, urinary urgency and urine loss during stress.

We concluded that the EMG BF for the PFM can lead to changes in anatomo-functional changes in the PF assessed in this study, with a positive influence on the quality of life of these women, although we cannot prove there was a reduction in SUI since we did not use a quantitative instrument to measure the decrease of urinary loss. Considering the results, this study was of huge importance regarding the use of ultrasound as an objective instrument on the evaluation of the efficacy of EMG BF on the reduction of urethral mobility, which is one of the important factors that is directly related to SUI.

6. References

[1] Abrams P, Cardozo L, Fall M, Griffiths D, Rosier P, Ulmsten U. et al (2003) The standardization of terminology of lower urinary tract function: report from the standardization of terminology sub-committee of the International Continence Society. Urology 61:3-49.

[2] Korelo RIG, Kosiba CR, Grecco L, Matos RA. Influência do fortalecimento abdominal na função perineal,associado ou não à orientação de contração do assoalho pélvico, em nulíparasFisioter Mov. 2011 jan/mar;24(1):75-85.

[3] Hannestad YS, Rortveit G, Sandvik H, Hunskaar A (2000) A community-based epidemiological survey of female urinary incontinence: the Norwegian epicont study. J Clin Epidemiol 53:1150-7.
[4] Toledo DD'A; Dedicação AC; Saldanha MES; Haddad M; Driusso P. Physical therapy treatment in incontinent women provided by a Public Health Service. Fisioter. mov. (Impr.) vol.24 no.2 Curitiba Apr./June 2011
[5] Coyne KS, Zhou Z, Thompson C, Versi E (2003) The impact on healthrelated quality life of stress, urge and mixed urinary incontinence.BJU Int 92(7):731-5.
[6] Papanicolaou S, Hunskaar S, Lose G, Sykes D (2005) Assessment of bothersomeness and impact on quality of life of urinary incontinencein women in France, Germany, Spain and UK. BJU Int 96(6):831-8.
[7] Antunes,MB, Manso VMC, Andrade NVS. e Análise dos sinais e sintomas da incontinência urinária de esforço em mulheres de 25 a 50 anos praticantes de atividades físicas em academias. Ensaios e Ciência, Vol. 15, No 1 (2011)
[8] Pages I-H, Jahr S, Schaufele MK, Conradi E (2001) Comparative analysis of biofeedback and physical therapy for treatment of urinary stress incontinence in women. Am J Phys Med Rehabil 80:494–502.
[9] Sousa JG; Ferreira VR; Oliveira RJ; Cláudia Elaine CestariAvaliação da força muscular do assoalho pélvico em idosas com incontinência urináriaFisioter. mov. (Impr.) vol.24 no.1 Curitiba Jan./Mar. 2011
[10] Ortiz OC (2004) Stress urinary in gynecological practice. Int J Gynecol Obstet 86:6-16.
[11] James AA-M, Denise H, J OL D (2001) The functional anatomy of the female pelvic floor and stress continence control system. Scans J urol Nephrol Suppl (207):1-125
[12] Culligan JP, Heiter M (2000) Urinary incontinence in women: evelaution and management. Am Fam Physician 62:2433-4
[13] Seleme, M (2002) As técnicas reeducativas em uroginecologia. Rev Fisio&terapia 33:33-34.
[14] Cammu H, Van NM (1995) Pelvic floor muscle exercise: 5 years later. Urology 45:113-8.
[15] Dietz HP, Wilson PD (1999) The influence of baldder volume on the position and mobility of the urethro-vesical juntion. Int Urogynecol J Pelvic Floor Dysfunct 10:3-6.
[16] Ortiz OC (2004) Stress urinary in gynecological practice. Int J Gynecol Obstet 86:6-16.
[17] Tamanini JTN, D'ancona CAL, Botega NJ, Netto NR (2003) Validação do "King's Health Questionnaire" para o português em mulheres com incontinência urinária. Rev Saúde Pública 37(2):203-211.
[18] Glavind KNORH, Walter, S (1996) Biofeedback and physiotherapy versus physiotherapy alone in treatment of genuine stress urinary incontinence. Int Urogynecology J Pelvic Floor Dysfunct 7(6):339-43.
[19] Hay-Smith EJC, Bo K, Berghmans ICM, Hendriks HJM, Debie RA, Van Waalwijk van Doorn, ESC (2001) Pelvic floor muscle training for urinary incontinence in women. Cochrane Database Syst Rev Review.
[20] Berghmans B, Bo K, Bernards N, Nol B, Marga G-M, Nettie B at al (2003) Clinical practice guidelines for the physical therapy of patients with urinary incontinence. Rev Urodinãmica & uroginecologia 6(1):1-28.
[21] Hay-Smith, EJC, Ryan K, Dean S (2003) The silent, private exercise: experiences of pelvic floor muscle training in sample of women with stress urinary incontinence. Physiotherapy 93:53-61.

[22] Bo K, Talseth T, Holme I (1999) Single blind, randomized controlled trial of pelvic florr exercise, electrical stimulation, vaginal cones and no treatment in management of genuine stress incontinence in women. BJM 318:487-93.
[23] Rosner B (1986) Fundamentals of Biostatistics. 2nd Ed. Massachusetts: PWS Publishers 442-80.
[24] Gunnarsson M, Mattiasson A (1999) Female stress, urge and mixed urinary incontinence are associated with a chronic and preogessive pelvic floor/vaginal neuromuscular disorder: an investigation of 317 health and incontinent women using vaginal surface electromyography. Neurourol Urodyn 18:613-21.
[25] Bo K (2003) Pelvic floor muscle strength and response to pelvic training for stress urinary incontinence. Neurourol Urodyn 22(7):654-8.
[26] Rett MT, Simoes JA, Herrmann V. et al (2007) Management of stress urinary incontinence with surface electromyography-assisted biofeedback in women of reproductive age. Physical Therapy 87(2):136-142.
[27] Bernstein IT (1997) the pelvic floor muscles: muscle thickness in healthy and urinary incontinent women measured by a perineal ultrasonography with reference to the effect of pelvic floor training estrogen receptor studies. Neurourol Urodyn 16:237-75.
[28] Otcenasek M, Halaska M, Krcmar M, Maresova D, Halaska MG (2002) New approach to the urogynecological ultrasound examination. Eur J Obstet Gynecol Reprod Biol 103(1):72-74.
[29] Rovner ES, Wein AJ (2003) Evaluation of lower urinary tract symptoms in females. Curr Opin Urol 13(4):273-8.
[30] Weil EH, van Waalwijk van Doom Es, Heesakkers Jp, Meguid T, Janknegt RA (1993) Transvaginal ultra-sonography: a study with healthy volunteers and women with genuine stress incontinence. Eur Urol 24:226-30.
[31] Brandt FT, Albuquerque CDC, Lorenzato FRB, Lopes DSG, Cunha ASC, Costa RF. A importância da ultra-sonografia transvulvar na avaliação de parâmetros anatômicos relevantes no tratamento de mulheres com incontinência urinária de esforço. Radiol Bras 2007;40(6):371–376
[32] Sartori JP; Martins JAM; Castro RA; Sartori MGF; Girão MJBC, Sling de aponeurose e com faixa sintética sem tensão para o tratamento cirúrgico da incontinência urinária de esforço feminina. Rev. Bras. Ginecol. Obstet. vol.30 no.3 Rio de Janeiro Mar. 2008
[33] Herrmann V, Potrick BA, Palma PCR, Zanettini CL, Marques A, Júnior NRN (2003) Eletroestimulação transvaginal do assoalho pélvico no tratamento da incontinência urinária de esforço: avaliações clínica e ultra-sonográfica. Rev Assoc Med Bras 49(4): 401-5.
[34] Balmforth JR, Montle J, Bidmead J, Cardozo L (2006) A prospective observational trial of pelvic floor muscle training for female stress urinary incontinence. BJU Int 98(4): 811-7.
[35] Rett MT, Simões JA, Herrmann V, Gurgel MSC, Moraes SS (2007) Women's life quality after physical therapy treatment for stress urinary incontinence. Rev. Bras. Ginecol Obstet 29(3):134-40.99

5

Incontinence: Physical Activity as a Supporting Preventive Approach

Aletha Caetano
Faculdade de EducaçãoFísica- Universidade Estadual de Campinas - UNICAMP
Brazil

1. Introduction

Aerobic exercises, as well as those for muscle strength and flexibility, might play a positive role in preventing and treating heart diseases, hypertension, osteoporosis, obesity and diabetes, to name a few, especially when practiced on a regular basis, under supervision and properly adapted to each individual (Carrol & Dudfield, 2004). Furthermore, the benefits brought by physical activity reach as far as the emotional aspects of the individual and help prevent the negative effects of stress, reduce tensions, enhance mood, lower the symptoms of stress and anxiety (Gorayeb & Turibio, 1999), and, eventually, improve health and boost the quality of life. According to the American Heart Association, the lack of physical activity can lead to a higher mortality and morbidity rate (America Heart Association, [AHA], 2007) Disengagement in physical activities is quite often associated to sedentary habits which might lead up to degenerative-chronic diseases, offering great risk to the population as a whole (Who, 1995). There are evidences that the incidence of these pathologies, plus other health conditions, including diabetes mellitus, osteoporosis, some cancers, obesity, the maintenance of body mass index (BMI) and hypertension, can be reduced by encouraging a more active life style, based on a constant and regular physical practice.

Urinary incontinence is a disease which interferes with the practice of physical activities, mostly among women; since physical workouts may trigger involuntary episodes and urinary leaking, incontinent women are likely to be caught on an embarrassing and uncomfortable spot while exercising (Brown & Miller, 2001; Caetano et al., 2009a). This is a huge limitation for the practice of physical exercises by women (especially those with moderate to severe incontinence), and dangerous for female health (Nygaard et al., 2005; Stach-Lempinem et al., 2004). Significant morbidity and mortality prevalence has been reported among women with urinary incontinence (Mullins & Subak, 2005). Putting it this way, quitting physical activities and sports practice might lead up to a sedentary life style, a major risk for and cause of several diseases.

Given that, this chapter aims to: (1) review publications on important available data about urinary incontinence as related to sports and physical activities.; (2) based on a systematic program of physical activities, introduce strategies which enable the Physical Education instructor and other professionals to take supplementary action in order to help prevent urinary incontinence in women and lower its prevalence rate.

2. Urinary incontinence

Urinary Incontinence was first seen as a disease by the International Classification of Diseases (ICD/WHO) in 1998; up until then, it was treated as a symptom. The International Continence Society currently defines urinary incontinence as "a complaint of any unintended urinary leaking" (Abrams et al., 2003). It is estimated that 200 million people across the world show some sort of urinary incontinence. Its incidence is twice as higher in women, due to anatomic reasons, hormonal changes and as an after-effect of pregnancies and baby deliveries which can relocate and weaken the pelvic muscles. (Simeonova et al., 1999). According to Ortiz (2004), one out of 4 women has already had an episode of urinary leaking. When considering the kind of population under study (features such as age, professional activity, incidence of chronic diseases, menopause), the kind of diagnosis applied, and the definition used during the investigations, urinary incontinence prevalence may range from 10% to 55% in 15 to 64 year-old females (Hunskaar et al., 2004). About 38% of elderly females urinary leaking intense enough to be classified as a "urinary incontinence problem" within this group (Nygaard et al., 2007a). Just the same, the greatest incidence of urinary incontinence typically occurs in the years prior to or after the menopause, reaching its highest peak in 45 to 49 year-old women. Despite this high prevalence, less than 50% of these female patients look for medical treatment. Reasons for this might be as complex as shame and/or embarrassment and the belief that urinary incontinence, simply comes along with the ageing process (Mullins & Subak, 2005).

Not only does urinary incontinence imply medical consequences, but high expenses and negative emotional effects as well. It has been shown that this condition demands a cost which might range from 16 to 26 billion dollars a year, including days off at work and the use of sanitary napkins and diapers (Hu et al., 2004). Emotional damages can be even more devastating, as most incontinent women hardly ever share this problem and usually prefer to deal with it on their own, "silently". About 80% of women with severe urinary incontinence show symptoms of depression, high anxiety and low self-esteem, including loneliness and sadness. Moreover, the embarrassment and shame that come along are responsible for their quitting social activities and sports as well as for their lack of sexual interest (Fultz et al.; 2003; Norton et al.; 1988), which might exacerbate negative emotions and feelings.

Among the different types of urinary incontinence, the most commonly identified are stress urinary incontinence, urge-incontinence and mixed incontinence. The first is most frequently seen in 25 to 49 year-old females. Mixed urinary incontinence is more common in middle-aged women (40 to 60 years old) while urge-incontinence is mostly identified in elderly women (Minassian et al., 2003). Stress urinary incontinence appears to be more frequent in physically active female, those who practice sports and/or exercise regularly.

2.1 Stress urinary incontinence

Guyton & Hall (1997), characterize two main phases in urination: bladder filling or storage is the first, when there is an increase in the bladder wall pressure above limits; the voiding (urine flow) reflex occurs in the second phase, when the bladder is emptied and there should be a conscious signal of urinary urge. It is an autonomous reflex, integrated in the spinal cord which can be inhibited or facilitated by cortex centers or by the brainstem. In order to maintain urinary continence, the bladder must be complacent capable of storing hundreds of milliliters in volume, the urethra must be preserved and in a normal position, innervations must be intact, which is crucial for the sphincters integrity. A properly long urethra is also important, as it allows urethral mucosal coaptation which mechanically prevents the flowing of urine or the voiding. (Wei et al., 1999).

However, the female urinary continence mechanism is also supported by a healthy perineum structure, such as muscle and fascias (tissues) which provide structural framework for the internal organs as well as the closure of the pelvic opening. (Ashton-Miller & DeLancey, 2001). The perineum comprises all soft tissues that circle the pelvis and keep viscera in the upright position. In a simplistic analogy, the pelvic floor is compared to *the foundations of a house, the diaphragm would be the ceiling and the abdominal muscles would make the front and side walls, while the spinal muscles and cord would make the back walls" (Grosse & Sengler, 2002). The pelvic floor muscles encompass three different layers (or plans), known as deep, middle and superficial. All layers, but the superficial, have voluntarily active muscle parts which can help keep continence when proper and supervised training takes place.

The deep layer consists of the main pelvic diaphragm, comprised by two muscles: the levator ani and the ischiococcygeus. The outward section of the levator ani is called elevator, its sphincter-like (consists of two hammock-like muscles - the pubococcygeus and the iliococcygeus) and has the support of the ischiococcygeus muscles; the inward section is formed by the pubovaginal and puborectal muscles. For the physical trainer, the levator ani is crucially important, as the pelvic floor muscle strength and quality can be improved by exercising this muscle.

The layer in the middle has three muscles: two deep transverse and the external urethral sphincter. The latter has the shape of a ring, circles the mid-third of the urethra and plays a fundamental role in the maintenance of continence. It's made of non-fatigable slow fibers which form the intra-urethral section plus a group of stretched muscles formed by slow fibers, fast and strong but highly fatigable fibers, called peri-urethral section. Despite being formed by striated fibers, the external sphincter is always in a state of contraction, helping to keep the pressure in a balanced level; in addition, it helps eliminate involuntary urinary flow as urinary needs can be controlled by strong and quick contractions.

Stress urinary incontinence is classified as the involuntary urine leaking as a result of physical exercises, physical efforts, sneezing and/or coughing (Abrams et al., 2002). It occurs when the urethral sphincter cannot withstand the urinary flow resulting from physical activities that increase intra-abdominal pressure; whenever a weakness or flaw occurs in the pelvic floor, there is an incorrect pressure transmission for the physical efforts, thus damaging the urinary continence mechanism and leading up to an unintended urinary leaking. This kind of incontinence is probably due to anatomic reasons; hypoestrogenism; after-effects of baby deliveries and pregnancies which might relocate and weaken the pelvic floor muscles. Other causes of stress urinary incontinence in women are: obesity; chronic diseases; gynecological surgeries; bowel obstruction; caffeine ingestion; smoking; hereditary reasons; medicinal drug ingestion (for example, alpha-adrenergic) and physical exercises.

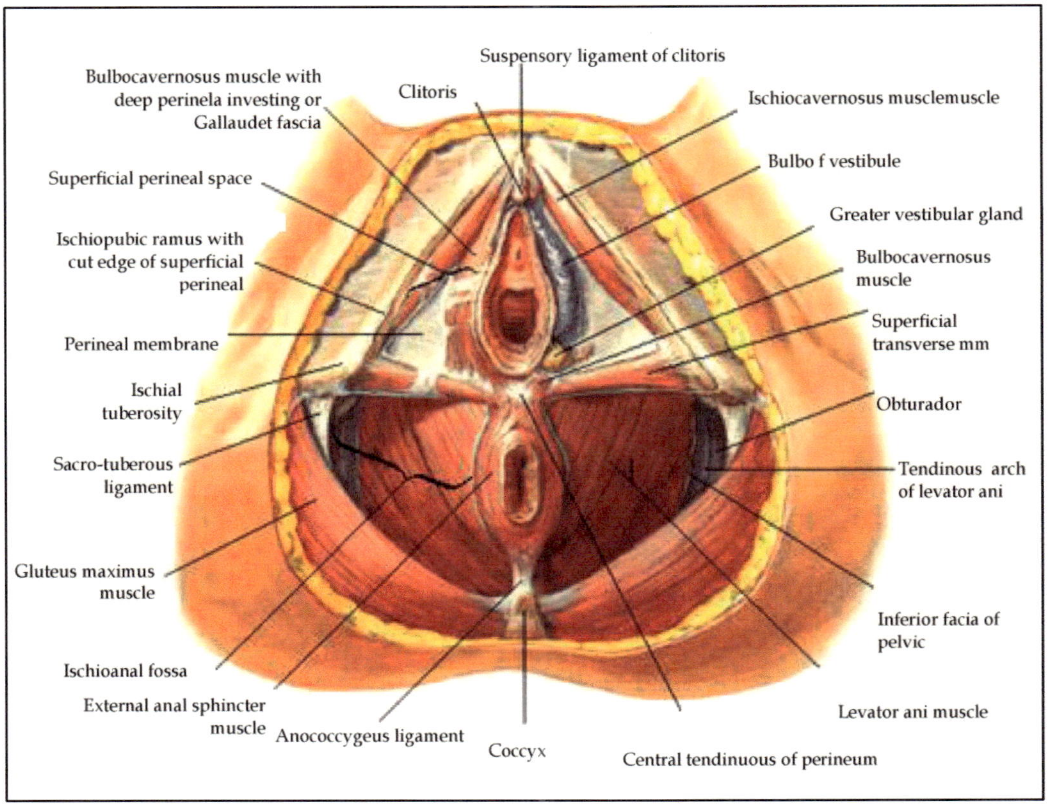

Fig. 1. Pelvic Floor Muscle -Source- Atlas of Human Anatomy(Frank H.Netter, 2010).

As mentioned earlier, stress urinary incontinence has lately been more frequently identified in physically active women. Though not conclusive, studies on this issue have reported that great effort and high impact exercises can enhance the chances for the development and worsening of stress urinary incontinence.

3. Relationship between urinary incontinence and sports and physical exercise

3.1 Physical exercises as a risk factor for stress urinary incontinence

Authors do believe that high impact exercise can represent a risk factor to the development of stress urinary incontinence (Bump & Norton, 1998; Nygaard et al., 1994; Bo, 1992), however, studies and researches on the relationship between stress urinary incontinence and physical activities and sports are still quite rare and little is known about the impact of several exercises and sports on the pelvic floor. Previous studies showed two different hypothesis for the way high impact exercises affect the pelvic floor. One of them states that physical exercise may strengthen the pelvic floor muscles and, thus, help prevent stress urinary incontinence as it bolsters the muscles in charge of the continence. The second one, on the other hand, argues that physical exercises may overburden, strain and weaken the pelvic floor muscles and consider strenuous and high impact exercises (Bo, 2004b) as a risk factor for urinary incontinence. It is worth reminding that both hypothesis are related to young nulliparous elite athletes. Just the same, amenorrhea resulting from intense workout, eating disorders and/or both can foster urinary incontinence in athletes.

Some studies have associated urinary incontinence in nulliparous athletes with impact strength assimilation resulting from some activities. Long jumps allow the feet to touch the ground and may generate a maximum reaction force 16 times higher than body weight (Hay, 1993). This impact, a consequence of high impact exercises, may affect the continence mechanism by modifying the amount of strength transmitted to the pelvic floor. The shock transmission force, which occurs between the feet and the ground and is transferred to the pelvic floor, may foster incontinence in young nulliparous females, who do high impact exercises (Nygaard et al., 1996; Nygaard, 1997). Recently, O'Dell et al. (2007), analyzed the abdominal pressure during the use of hydraulic exercise machine; weight-lifting; floor exercises and jogging and comparing those exercise with abdominal pressure resulting from coughing in several individuals, the authors found out that, though different among subjects, the pressure on the pelvic floor during physical activities was lower than during coughing. Ree et al., (2007), verified that young nulliparous females with urinary incontinence symptoms showed fatigue in the PFM after performing strenuous physical activities for 90 minutes. According to the authors, studies about the impact of long term strenuous physical exercises on the pelvic floor among elite athletes should be carried out, once there has been a significant prevalence of stress urinary incontinence in this group (Bo, 2004a).

3.2 Urinary incontinence prevalence in women

3.2.1 Athletes

Studies on the relationship between urinary incontinence, sports and physical activities and the prevalence of this condition in elite athletes date back from the 90s. Since then, they have gradually called the attention of professionals from different areas of expertise. As aforementioned, longitudinal systematic studies are still necessary, in order to identify the pelvic floor reactions while long term sports and physical activities are being performed, considering different intensities and frequencies. All the same, up until now, researches have indicated that urinary incontinence complaints are quite common among elite athletes. The examined studies showed 6% to 80% urinary incontinence prevalence among 12 to 22 year-old athletes, depending on which sport was practiced. Gymnastics, running and trampoline were the ones with the most urinary leaking complaints. (Bo, 2004b; Bump & Norton 1998; Eliasson et al., 2002; Jiang et al., 2004; Nygaard, et al., 1994; Nygaard et al., 1996;).

Nygaard et al., (1994), studied 156 athletes with an average age of 19,9 years; 28% said they had experienced urinary leaking while practicing a sport. The most frequently mentioned was gymnastics (67%), followed by basketball (66%), tennis (50%), hockey (42%), trekking (29%), swimming (10%), volleyball (9%), softball (6%) and, lastly, golf (0%). Jumping, high impact landings (or hitting the ground with high impact) and running were the physical activities with the highest incidence of urinary leaking. The jumping exercises with legs open, were a major complaint for 30% of the athletes, followed by tight-leg jumps (28%). In the same research, around 40% of the athletes reported urinary leaking while practicing sports in high school and 17% in junior high school. Another study showed that the athletes also complained about urinary leaking not only during sports practice but also while performing every-day activities. The author identified that over half of 291 athletes, with an average age of 22.8 years, reported urinary leaking in both situations (Thyssen at al., 2002). It is interesting to mention that most of the athletes participating on this research, who complained about urinary leaking only while practicing sports, admitted it, happened only during practice and not during competitions. The authors believe this is probably due to "a ritual" of emptying the bladder and of drinking less liquid before competitions.

Urinary incontinence prevalence was also compared between a group of 660 athletes, belonging to a junior and senior national team (of 38 different sports) and a control group of 765 non-athlete females (Bo & Borgen, 2001). Their age ranged from 15 to 39 years. The majority was nulliparous, only 4% had had children. As for the non-athletes, one third had already given birth. Hence, data about childbirth must be taken into consideration and were more significant in the control group. There was no meaningful difference in the urinary incontinence prevalence in athletes and non-athletes: 41% and 39%, respectively. 27% of the athletes complained about urinary leaking while coughing, sneezing and laughing; 29% reported incontinence during physical activities and 15% during sudden moves or standing up.

The highest prevalence of urinary incontinence complaints during exercises was detected among trampoline professionals; 80% out of 35 nulliparous athletes, average age 15 (12-22 years old), complained about incontinence while jumping on the trampoline (Elliason et al., 2002). Athletes who complained about incontinence reported that urinary leaking was first noticed after two and a half years of practice. In this study, urinary incontinence was associated to the years of practice, age and duration and frequency of training. Incontinent athletes were older and had more frequent and longer trainings than athletes who had no symptoms of incontinence. During tests, incontinent athletes had more difficulty with voluntary voiding control by contracting the pelvic floor muscles than the other group with no incontinence symptoms. These athletes are likely to have been exposed to constant effort and impact; on the long run, due to the lack of training, the muscles responsible for continence lost their strength, leading up to urinary incontinence. In a more recent study, the same author (Eliasson et al., 2008) identified a high urinary incontinence prevalence in trampoline athletes (18-44 years old) during a competition. The author divided the athletes in two groups, according to the exercise intensity; 85 women performed high impact jumps and 220 performed low impact jumps. Among those who complained about urinary incontinence while practicing the sport, 76% still complain about the same symptoms; of these, 57% belong to the high impact jump group and 48% to the low impact jump group. The author also detected prospective reasons for urinary incontinence development in this group; similarly to his prior study (Elliasson et al., 2002), the author reported that the frequency and intensity of the exercises, age of first menstrual period, bowel obstruction and inability of voiding control were important factors for urinary incontinence. Hence, the practice of this sport (trampoline) without simultaneous and proper training for the strengthening of pelvic floor muscles may represent a risk factor for urinary incontinence onset, during and after the aforesaid practice.

A retrospective study including 104 athletes who were in the Olympics, in the 60s up until 1976, detected that 35% reported urinary leaking during high impact activities, such as gymnastics and trekking. Swimming was considered a low impact sport, responsible for only 4.5% of the complaints. (Nygaard, 1997). All the same, the author concluded that high impact activities do not lead up to a significant urinary incontinence in the adulthood of the women belonging to the studied group. Actually, in a more recent retrospective study, authors investigated urinary incontinence complaint in 331 retired athletes as compared to a 640 female control group. Currently, 36.5% of the athletes complained about stress urinary incontinence and 36.9% of the control group had the same complaint. There was no meaningful difference between the two groups. Yet, after a more thorough and specific analysis on the athletes, the results indicated that urinary incontinence, when identified during the sports practice, can be a strong signal of future urinary problems in adulthood (Bo & Borgen, 2001).

Another issue, not less important and that must be taken into consideration in the complex relation of urinary incontinence prevalence among professional athletes is the much less studied eating disorder. This condition was detected in 20% of the athletes and only in 9% of the control group. As for stress urinary incontinence, it was reported by 49% of the athletes and by 38.8% of the control group. Urinary incontinence in women with eating disorders is likely to be associated with self-induced vomiting (a particular feature of such a disorder), which applies significant and repetitive pressure over the pelvic floor and, eventually, damages it. High impact sports practice without proper supervision might promote urinary incontinence in athletes with eating disorders (Bo & Borgen, 2001; Hextal et al.,1999). New researches should be carried out in order to identify the relationships between both urinary incontinent and eating disorder symptoms, considering different sports and physical activities

3.2.2 Non-athletes

Similarly to the aforesaid about professional athletes, not until 2008 were studies and researches on urinary incontinence and sports and physical activities among non-athletes conducted. These few researches studied 18 to 65 year-old women, non-professional athletes, who mostly complained about incontinence while running and doing high impact sports; still, urinary leaking was also observed during everyday activities. Bo et al. (1989) observed a major difference between participants who practiced physical activities and those who didn't. Two different groups were compared: students whose major was physical education and others majoring in nutrition. (A=22.9; 19-59). Aspects such as age, childbirth and different physical exercises were considered. About 26% of the physical education students reported urinary leaking as compared to 19% of the nutrition students. According to the authors, this was not significant. However, when physical education students worked out more than three times a week, urinary incontinence prevalence increased up to 31%, a major difference when compared to the 10% presented by sedentary nutrition students. Nygaard et al., (1990) studied 326 women, 20-65 years old, (A=38,5) who exercised regularly; 47% had already noticed some kind of urinary leaking throughout life. In this study, no important connection was established between urinary incontinence and profession, educational background, weight, height or menopause. About 33% of the women reported incontinence while exercising. These women usually exercised three times a week during 30 to 60 minutes. Incontinence was most frequent while running; 38% of the women complained about urinary leaking while doing high impact aerobic exercises.

Another study including 3,364 women, 18 to 60 years old, detected that 1 out of 7 were incontinent while performing any kind of physical activity. (36). High urinary incontinence prevalence is also identified in women who belong to the US Army and US Air Force (Davis, 1999; Fischer & Berg, 1999). 31% out of the 563 female soldiers under observation complained about urinary leaking during physical and field drilling. Around 40% of them also complained about it during recreational activities. Aerobic exercises ranked highest in complaints (42%), followed by running (35%), weight-lifting (18%), jogging (21%), biking (8%), swimming (5 %) and lastly, golf (3%).

Salvatore et al., (2009) recently studied 679 female soldiers aiming to check urinary incontinence prevalence during recreational activities. The authors reported that stress urinary incontinence was detected in 14.9% of the subjects; out of this total, 31.7% complained about incontinence during sports practice and 10.4% considered their incontinence severe enough to limit or discourage their activities. The sport with the most complaints, (16.6%) was basketball, followed by running (15%). Body Mass Index and childbirth were connected to urinary linking. Also, data about studies on physical exercises and sports instructors were found. The first study with Physical Education teachers was done by (Santos, et al., 2009). We studied nulliparous students, 19 to 26 years old. 20.7% of them had already had urinary leaking before while practicing their sport and ranked it as a 2.3 leaking (in a scale of 0 to 10), being no problem at all and 10 being a severe problem). In this study, we came to the conclusion that, though urinary incontinence was quite frequent, the group didn't consider it a problem. More recently, 685 Pilates and Yoga instructors, with an average age of 32.7 years (18 to 68 years old) were studied; the authors identified a 26,4% prevalence of incontinence complaints. Among incontinent women, 15.3% reported urinary leaking during physical activities and 10.9% while sneezing or coughing. Hence, pelvic floor training is recommended not only for athletes and women who leisurely practice sports or physical activities, but also for instructors, coaches, trainers and teachers (Bo et al., 2011; Santos, et al., 2009.)

3.3 Urinary incontinence impact on physical activity

Unexpected and involuntary episodes of urinary leaking which may happen during physical activities may put incontinent women on an embarrassing and uncomfortable spot. According to studies, nearly 20% females give up (Nygaard et al., 1990) or limit their favorite sports and physical activities due to urinary incontinence. (Salvatore et al., 2009). A longitudinal study on female health (Australian Longitudinal Study on Women's Health-(ALSWH) reported that 27% females who practiced physical exercises showed urinary incontinence symptoms(> 40%were middle aged women and 16% were young or elderly); a percentage which supports previously discussed studies. Most incontinent women said they gave up sports practice due to their incontinence. According to the authors, the highest incidence of disengagement was among ≥ to 48 year-old women. Some authors consider that this might be even higher among women in the post menopause (Eliasson et al., 2002; Salvatore et al., 2009). Furthermore, the greater the concerns towards incontinence during exercise performances, the higher the frequency of urinary leaking episodes (Fultz et al., 2003) leading to an increase in giving up physical activities. More specifically, severe urinary incontinence symptoms strongly hamper the practice of physical activities, (Brown & Miller,

2001; Nygaard et al., 2005), increasing sedentary habits and exposing the population to health conditions associated with sedentary life styles.

On the other hand, encouraging physical activities can have a positive effect on incontinent women's attitude towards exercising. However successful urinary incontinence treatment was, women who had always exercised, continued doing so. Likewise, those who had never exercised before did not change their habits. According to information gathered from women who participated in the research, the more active ones looked for medical treatment because they wanted to lower and prevent urinary incontinence and, thus, keep up with their exercises (Stach-Lempinen et al., 2004).This attitude might be associated to a high motivation in doing physical activities. According to Bo et al., (1989), more motivated women tend to take urinary leaking for granted, while the less motivated ones make a big deal out of it. Professional athletes seem to be more motivated for sports and physical activities and perform more stressing exercises than those who practice sports leisurely. The first continue practicing, despite incontinence and other problems (Nygaard et al., 2005). Researches have found that women who did not quit physical activities because of urinary incontinence, worked out a way to prevent urinary leaking while exercising. Their usual strategies were: the use of sanitary napkins and diapers, emptying the bladder before practice and competitions, liquid ingestion restrictions, and choosing a different exercise to perform. This last strategy means that exercises which might facilitate urinary leaking (jumping, running) are avoided, and these women start to practice low impact sports, such as walking, biking and swimming (Nygaard et al., 1990; Thyssen et al., 2002). Besides these strategies, women studied by Salvatore et al., (2009) chose exercises to strengthen the pelvic floor muscles as a way to prevent incontinence during physical activities. These "adaptation" strategies, however, did not seem to be effective enough to prevent that they quit exercising. Several times, sanitary napkins cannot avoid urinary leaking and, after the first incontinence, women tend to give up physical practice (Tata, 1998).

In a prospective study of 314 women with pelvic organ prolapse and stress urinary incontinence, the authors investigated if women who had undergone sacrocolpopexy surgery a year before, changed physical activities. One year after the surgery, 36% of the women increased the intensity of the exercises, 18% lowered and 47% kept the same intensity. The authors reported that most women who considered that the pelvic floor organ prolapse could prevent or restrict exercising changed their view after the surgery.

However, it is worth saying that a few participants kept on limiting their physical activities, despite de surgery, due to fear of prolapse recurring and to their doctor's advice (Nygaard et al., 2007b; Nygaard et al., 2008).Bottom line, when women themselves limit the frequency and intensity of physical exercises, they drift apart from the benefits of a systematic practice for their overall health.

4. Benefits of physical exercises for urinary incontinence

4.1 Pelvic floor muscle training

The most widely known exercises which prevent and treat urinary incontinence were created by Dr. Arnold Kegel in the fifities. This American gynecologist was the first to scientifically use exercises to strengthen the pelvic floor muscles in order to improve urinary incontinence mechanisms. These exercises improve the perineum muscle contraction, giving it more power (strong and fast), increase urethral compression against the pubic symphysis, increase intra-urethral pressure when intra-abdominal pressure is increased, help pelvic muscle hypertrophy and increase the volume of such muscles. Hence, structural support of this body area becomes more effective and prevents the urethra from descending when intra-abdominal pressure increases and, consequently, decreasing urinary leaking. Kegel (1948), observed that, apart from decreasing urinary incontinence, his exercises had positive effects on female sexual desire. His exercises are, therefore, based on the strengthening of the pelvic floor muscles (Palma & Ricetto, 1999). The pelvic floor muscles should support the viscera in the upright position and maintain urinary continence as well. So, they should be kept strong and in perfect condition. Still, in order to effectively perform these exercises, Levi-D'Ancona (2001) states that incontinent women should learn to contract and relax these muscles, once they are not usually used, and that many women have difficulties with their voluntary contraction (Moen et al., 2007).

Since Kegel first published the development of these exercises, they have been widely used and quoted in medical academic literature; however, as of then, it is also possible to find not only different techniques and systematization (that is, frequency, intensity, repetitions and associations) but also different instructions given to patients in scientific literature. According to theory on the development of exercises to treat stress urinary incontinence, the aim is to boost pelvic floor muscle (PFM) strength, coordination, speed and resistance in order to keep structures in an adequate position whenever there is an effort which causes intra-abdominal pressure increase and, thus, keeping a proper urethral closure strength. (Ashton-Miller et al., 2001).

In literature, it's possible to find different protocols to strengthen the pelvic floor through exercises. Most studies follow protocols with instructions based on quick and slow contractions, in 3 steps, ranging from 8 to 12 repetitions; isometric contractions with maximum contraction held for 6 to 8 seconds, 2 to 4 times a week. According to different authors, PFM strength increased after a period which varied from 4 weeks to 6 months. Another procedure used to strengthen the PFM is training only with isometric contractions with maximum contraction for a period of 6 weeks to 6 months. The study also advised women to perform the exercises at home; according to others, women had better attend weekly or monthly group training; some advise a doctor's appointment once in 6 months and others see no need for group training or appointment with a doctor. Most protocols or training methods were reported as positive for the improvement or cure of incontinence symptoms presented by some of the subjects of their studies. "Skill training" is also a procedure which may help strengthen and train the PFM; it implies the learning of motor skills which favor a more effective contraction time of the PFM before an activity that increases abdominal pressure followed by a possible urinary leaking (whenever there are injured and/or weakened muscles). Bo et al., have named this a motor learning approach. Though "skill training" has been quoted as useful for PFM training, few information on the specificity of these exercises have been made available. Other studies (Arvonen et al., 2000; Balmforth et al., 2004; Dumoulin et al., 2004; Hay-Smith et al., 2002; Parkkinen et al., 2004;) Turkan, 2005), even match up PFM strengthening exercises with "skill training", getting positive results, but as the reports don't follow a standard protocol, comparisons become invalid. The role of the abdominal muscles has also been discussed, as far as PFM training and strengthening are concerned (Cammu & Nylen, 1998; Johnson, 2001; Pieber et al., 1995). However, studies available in literature do not reach an agreement, and as evidence is not strong enough, abdominal muscle training is not included in the treatment of urinary incontinence (Bo et al., 2009).

The benefits of PFM training and strengthening could be seen when they were performed with no other technique (reference); or when combined with techniques such as biofeedback; electrical stimulation; with vaginal weight or cones; with the combination of two techniques, such as biofeedback + electrical stimulation; and also with the combination of three techniques: biofeedback + electrical stimulation + with vaginal weights and cones. More detailed data on the researches aforementioned can be found in publications by Neumann et al. (2006). Notwithstanding, no study linking PFM training and strengthening to a systematic exercise program outside the therapeutic context was identified during this review.

4.2 Pelvic floor exercises during sports practice

Only a few researches in which training for the pelvic floor muscle strengthening has simultaneously occurred during sports practice were pointed out. As aforesaid, there is little knowledge about how pelvic muscles work during sports and physical activity practice. According to some authors, most physical activities do not involve pelvic muscle voluntary contraction during the performance of exercises which increase intra-abdominal pressure. Thus, women who exercise do not have stronger pelvic muscles than the ones who do not; actually, the more active women have reported greater incontinence while doing strong-effort and high-impact exercises than those who do not exercise regularly (Bo, 2004b). Athletes should be taught to contract those muscles previously or simultaneously to impact exercises and sports practice. Instructions on this matter are needed because previous studies indicated that one third of females either contract their pelvic muscles incorrectly or have difficulty with doing so. In three different studies, around 30% of female subjects reported inability to interrupt urinary flow (Bevenute et al., 1987; Bo et al., 1988; Kegel, 1952). This "inability" is associated with urinary leaking. After women were "taught" to contract their PFM while coughing, the authors noticed a significant incontinence reduction; still, no mention to whether women had the same training during sports practice was made (Brown & Miller, 2001). According to another study, 17 out of 23 women reported a decrease in urinary leaking during jumping and running, after exercising the PFM. All the same, just like the aforementioned study, it was impossible to identify if the PFM exercises were done during and simultaneously to sports practice (Bo, 2004a). More recently, researchers reported a reduction and even a suspension of incontinence complaints in 3 nulliparous athletes (29-33 years old). They had had training for strengthening PFM with specific exercises along with biofeedback; electrical stimulation and vaginal cones. Yet, though athletes were advised to work on the contractions at home every day, this instruction was not described simultaneously to their physical activity and sports practice (Rivalta et al., 2010).

4.3 Systematic proposal of physical activities for women in general, including pelvic floor exercises

Due to the lack of researches in Physical Education or of a multidisciplinary project which discussed a PFM strengthening exercise program and considering that physical exercises are likely to become a risk factor for urinary incontinence symptoms, we decided to create a physical activity program with PFM exercises (Fig.2). It was first developed in 2003, and improved and applied to a female group afterwards, as part of a research. Its results showed a reduction of incontinence complaints and an improvement of participants' body image (Caetano et al., 2009b). This research project included specific exercises for PFM, plus proprioception exercises (to get a better perception of the pelvis), breathing exercises, recreational activities (such as games and plays), stretching exercises, warm-up exercises (aerobic activities), upper and lower limb, abdominal and gluteus strengthening exercises and relaxation exercises.

This research aimed mainly at creating strategies for the Physical Education professional to develop PFM strengthening exercises during physical exercise and sports practice with students who might or might not have complaints about urinary incontinence, in order to prevent or reduce its symptoms. The Physical Education professionals usually work at venues such as clubs, rehabilitation centers, gyms, schools, indoor or outdoor courts and companies; they also work as sports and fitness coaches for female professional athletes; this means their work involves a wide-ranging population group, which requires PFM exercises suitable to different ages as well as physical activities and exercises focusing on each individual's needs.

One of this systematization first concerns was to characterize the inclusion of PFM exercises in physical exercise and sports practice as a non-therapeutic action under the assumption that the engaged muscles also contain voluntary fibers, contracted according to the individual's will, the same way as upper and lower limbs, pectoral, abdominal, gluteus and calf muscles. The PFM contractions, however, can only be "felt", not observed. Thus, as these muscles are somehow "unknown", most women find it difficult to perform and sense the contractions. Given this, the first step to be taken by women, both, athletes and non-athletes, prior to PFM training, should include proprioception exercises so as to achieve a conscious "recognition" of those muscles and a complete cohesion of this area ("asleep" up until then) with the whole body, favoring the PFM training.

Pelvic Floor Muscles contractions can be obtained by specific procedures, in which these are the only exercised muscles; PFM can also be contracted simultaneously to other exercises which mainly focus on other muscles' strengthening. Simultaneity is handy, especially when there are strong-effort and high-impact exercises, whether competitively or leisurely. PFM simultaneous exercising is possible during body-building activities using specific equipment, free weight-lifting exercises, gym classes, mini-trampoline practice, steps, hydro-gymnastics; and aerobic exercises.

As aforesaid, though some procedures were created in order to help professionals to work with PFM contraction exercises, quite a few researches follow standardized guidelines. Both our proposal and our research follow the instructions published by the Association of Women's Health Obstetrics and Neonatal Nurses (Agency for Health Care Policy and Research, [AWHONN]). According to this protocol, PFM strengthening exercises should include 40 to 50 contractions per session, with a sequence of 8 to 12 slow and quick contractions, where contractions are slow and isometric, 5 seconds long at the beginning and lasting for 10 seconds later on. Long term and daily training can, however, allow more contractions per class or training session, which was detected during our research, in which

1- hour classes were routinely given twice a week for a four-month period (Caetano et al, 2009b)

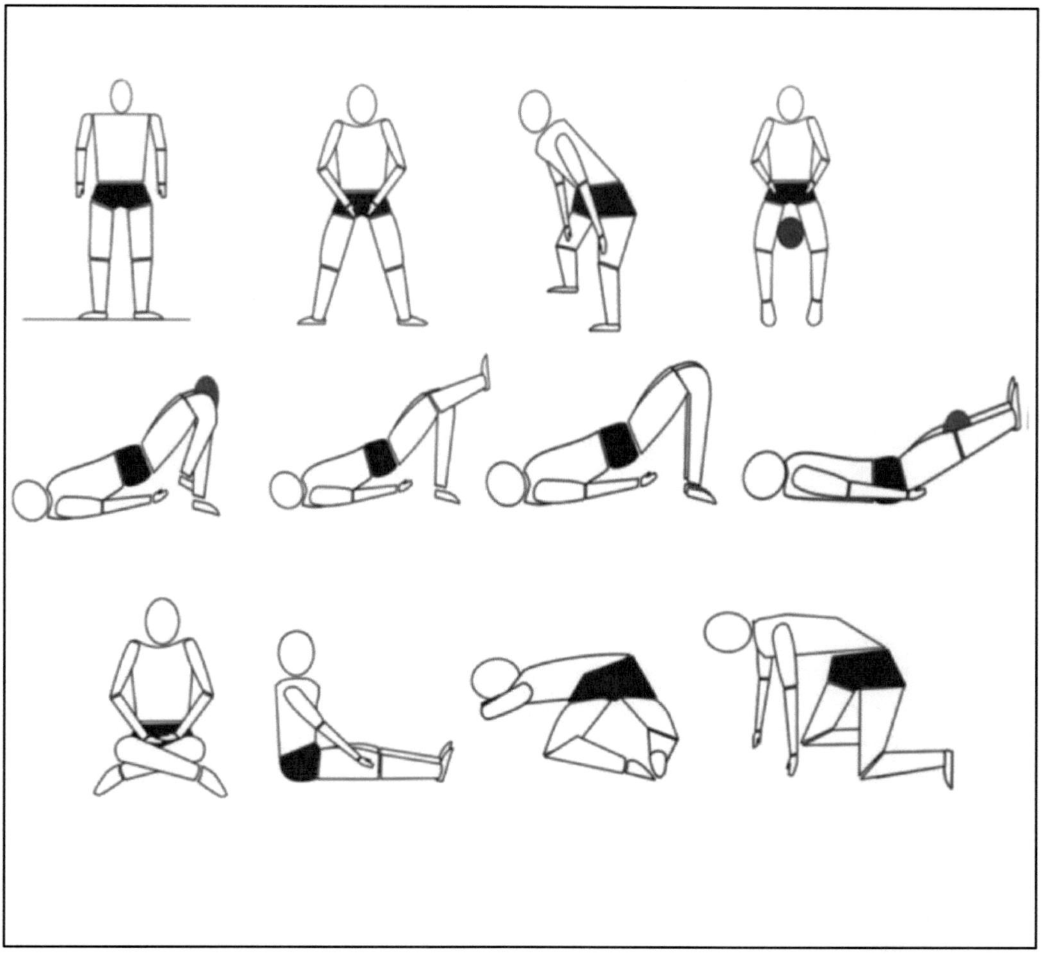

Fig. 2. Pelvic Floor Muscle Exercises (By Artur Paulo Caetano & Nicholas Silva Caetano). Source: Caetano, A.S. et al.,(2004). Physical Activity Proposal for Stress Urinary Incontinent Women. Lecturas Educacion Fisica y Deportes [online journal] Available: URL: http://www.efdeportes.com/efd76/mulheres.

5. Conclusions

After reviewing the data about the main relationships between urinary incontinence and physical activity and sports practice referred to in this chapter, we identified a high prevalence of urinary incontinence symptoms in women who exercise, significantly higher in young athletes; we also noticed that strong-effort and high-impact exercises are a major cause of incontinence complaints. Though literature is still inconclusive on this matter, these exercises seem to represent a risk factor for the development of urinary incontinence or are likely to aggravate pre-existing symptoms. Just the same, little is known about the pelvic floor reactions during several physical activities and also during long term physical practice. Researches aiming to identify pelvic floor reactions to different mid and long term physical exercises should be carried out in the future.

Through our project and a proposal of physical activities (Aletha et al., 2009b) which included PFM training and strengthening exercises, we were able to point out that, besides the results showing a reduction of incontinence complaints and an improvement in the participants' body image, it is also possible to create strategies to be used by Physical Education professionals who train incontinent women. A systematic and integrated physical activity program as described in the previous item allow incontinent women to get a better health and quality of life perception, specially towards their own body image and towards a decrease in incontinence complaints, with a reduction of the amount and frequency of urinary leaking.

Unfamiliarity with the connection between urinary incontinence and physical activity creates a gap in the education of Physical Education professionals and, hence, in their teaching practice. Leaving PFM exercises out of global exercising programs does not seem reasonable, as those muscles are part of every woman's functional activity and deserve attention. Coaches and physical trainers should encourage female athletes and non-athletes to contract the pelvic muscles while exercising because women are quite unlikely to think about it without guidance. Every woman, athlete or not, must stimulate these muscles so as to identify and contract them during gym classes and aerobic exercises, in order to prevent or reduce urinary incontinence and improve bladder control. The coach should always ask his/her athletes about incontinence symptoms resulting from strong-effort and high-impact exercises so as to contribute with strategies which help solve or minimize the problem. Moreover, the coach should help his/her student or athlete become aware of urinary incontinence and of its connection with high impact exercises and sports and make them realize how important it is to strengthen the muscles responsible for female urinary continence. Hence, once they have a coach or instructor who is prepared to discuss these issues, students and athletes will find it safe to share their incontinence first symptoms or existing problems with them. These actions can change physical activity and sports practice into a supporting and even preventing intervention in the treatment of urinary incontinence, helping to reduce prevalence rates and to prevent incontinent women to quit physical activities, making sure they enjoy the benefits of such practice. Controlled studies carried out on future researches are needed, in order to investigate how physical activities, specific PFM exercises included, can bring benefits people with urinary incontinence in the mid and long run.

6. Acknowledgments

Faculdade de Educação Física- Universidade Estadual de Campinas- UNICAMP.
Maria Helena Baena de Moraes Lopes.
Maria da Consolação G.C.F. Tavares.
Artur Paulo Caetano.
Nicholas Silva Caetano.
Andrea Castillo.

7. References

Abrams, P.; Cardoso, L.; Fall, M.; Rosier. P.; Ulmsten, U.; Van Kerrebroeck, P.; Victor, A. & Wein, A. (2003). M. The standardization of terminology of lower urinary tract function: report from the standardization sub-committee of The International Continence Society. *Urology*, Vol.61, No.1 (January), pp. 37-49, ISSN: 0090-4295.

Agency for Health Care Policy and Research (AHCPR), (1996). *Overview urinary incontinence in adults clinical practice guideline update*, Retrieved Jun., 7, 2011. Available from: http://www.ahcpr.gov/clinic/uiovervw.htm.

America Heart Association (AHA). (2007).In: *Facts and statistics*. Retrieved Jun 7, 2011, Available from http://www.americanheart.org/presenter. jhtml?identifier=2321.

Ashton-Miller, J.; Howard, D. & DeLancey, J.O. (2001) The functional anatomy of the female pelvic floor and stress incontinence control system. *Scandinavian Journal of Urology Nephrology Supplementum* Vol 207, (March), pp.1-7, ISSN: 0300-8886.

Arvonen, T.; Fianu-Jonasson, A. & Tyni-Lenne, R. (2000). Effectiveness of two conservative modes of physical therapy in women with urinary stress incontinence. *Neurourology and Urodynamic,*Vol.19, No.5, (September), pp. 591-599, ISSN: 0733-2467.

Balmforth, J.; Bidmead, J.; Cardozo, L.; Hextall, A. Kelvin, B. & Mantle J. (2004). Raising the tone: a prospective observational study evaluating the effect of pelvic floor muscle training on bladder neck mobility and associated improvement in stress urinary incontinence. *Neurourology and Urodynamic*, Vol., 23, No.5-6, (August) pp.553-554, ISSN: 0733-2467.

Bevenuti, F.; Caputo, G.M. & Bardinelli S. (1987). Reeducative treatment of female genuine stress incontinence. *American Journal Physical Medicine*, Vol.66, No.4, (August) pp.155-168, ISSN: 0002-9491.

Bo.; K.; Larsen, S. & Oseid, S.(1988). Knowledge about and ability to correct pelvic floor muscle exercises in women with urinary stress incontinence. *Neurourology and Urodynamic*, Vol.7, No.2, (November) pp.261-272, ISSN: 0733-2467.

Bo, K.; Hagen, R.; Kvastein, B. & Larsen, F. (1989). Female stress urinary incontinence and participation in different sport and social activities. *Scandinavian Journal of Sports & Science*, Vol.11, No.1, pp.117-121, ISSN: 1600- 0838.

Bo, K. (1992). Stress urinary incontinence, physical activity and pelvic floor muscle strength training. *Scandinavian Journal of Medicine & Science in Sports,* Vol.2, No.4, (December), pp.197-206, ISSN: 1600-0838.

Bo, K. & Borgen, J.S. (2001). Prevalence of stress and urge urinary incontinence in elite athletes and controls. *Medicine and Science in Sports and Exercise*, Vol.33, No.11, (November), pp.1797-802, ISSN: 0195-9131.

Bo, K. (2004a).Pelvic floor muscle training is effective in treatment of female stress urinary incontinence, but how does it work? *International Urogynecology Journal and Pelvic Floor Dysfunction*, Vol.15, No.2, pp.76-84, ISSN: 0937-3462

Bo, K. (2004b). Urinary incontinence, pelvic floor dysfunction, exercise and sport. *Sports Medicine*, Vol.34, No.7, pp.451–464, ISSN: 0112-1642.

Bo,K.; Morkved, S.; Frawley, H. & Margaret, S. (2009). Evidence for Benefit of Transversus Abdominis Training Alone or in Combination With Pelvic Floor Muscle Training to

Treat Female Urinary Incontinence: A Systematic Review. *Neurourology and Urodynamics*, Vol.28, (February), pp.368–373, ISSN: 0733-2467.

Bo.,K.; Bratland-Sanda, S. & Borgen, J.S. (2011). Urinary Incontinence Among Group Fitness Instructors Including Yoga and Pilates Teachers *Neurourology and Urodynamics*, Vol. 30, No.3, (March), pp.370–373, ISSN: 0733-2467.

Brown, W. & Miller, Y. (2001). Too wet to exercise? Leaking urine as a barrier to physical activity in women. *Journal of Science and Medicine in Sport*, Vol.4, No.4, (December, pp. 373-378, ISSN: 1440-2440.

Bump, R. & Norton, P. (1998). Epidemiology and natural history of pelvic floor dysfunction. *Obstetrics and Gynecology Clinics of North American*,Vol.25, No.4, (December), pp.723-746, ISSN: 0889-8545.

Caetano, A.S.; Tavares, M.C.G.C.F.; Lopes, M.H.B.M. (2009a). Urinary incontinence and physical activity practice. *Revista Brasileira de Medicina do Esporte*, Vol.13, No.4, (Jul), ISSN: 1517-8692.

Caetano, A.S.; Tavares, M.C.G.C.F.; Lopes, M.H.B.M & Poloni, R.L. (2009b).Influence of Physical Activity in the Quality of Life and Self Image of Incontinent Women. *Revista Brasileira d Medicina do Esporte*, Vol. 15; No.2, (March), ISSN: 1517-8692.

Cammu, H.; & Van Nylen, M. (1998). Pelvic floor exercises versus vaginal weight cones in genuine stress incontinence. *European Journal of Obstetrics and Gynecol*ogy and *Reprodution Biolology*, Vol.77, No.1, (March), pp.89-93, ISSN: 0301-2115.

Carrol, S.; Dudfield M. (2004). What is the relationship between exercise and metabolic abnormalities? A review of the metabolic syndrome. *Sports Medicine, Vol.*34, No.6, pp. 371- 418, ISSN: 0112-1642.

Davis, G. (1999). Urinary incontinence among female soldiers. *Military Medicine*, Vol.164, No.3, (March), pp.182-187, ISSN: 0026-407.

Dumoulin, C.; Lemieux, M.C.; Bourbonnais, D.; Gravel, D.; Bravo, G. & Morin, M. (2004). Physiotherapy for persistent postnatal stress urinary incontinence: A randomized controlled trial. *Obstetrics and Gynecol*ogy, Vol.104, No.3, (September), pp.504-510, ISSN: 0029-7844.

Eliasson, K.; Larsson, T. & Mattsson, E. (2002). Prevalence of stress incontinence in elite trampolinists. *Scandinavian Journal of Medicine & Science in Sports*, Vol.12, No.2, (April), pp.106-110, ISSN: 1600-0838.

Eliasson, K.; Edner, A. & Mattsson, E. (2008). Urinary incontinence in very young and mostly nulliparous women with a history of regular organised high-impact trampoline training: occurrence and risk factors. *International Urogynecology Journal and Pelvic Floor Disfunction*, Vol.19, (January), pp.687–69, ISSN: 0937-3462.

Fischer, J,R. & Berg, P.H. (1999). Urinary incontinence in United States Air Force female aircrew. *Obstetrics and Gynecology*, Vol.94, No.4, (October), pp.532-536, ISSN: 0029-7844.

Fultz, N.; Burgio, K., Diokno, A.C.; Kinchen, K.; Obenchain, R. & Bump, R. (2003). Burden of stress urinary incontinence for community-dwelling women. *American Journal of Obstetrics Gynecology*, Vol.189, No.5, (November), pp.1275-1282, ISSN: 0029-7844.

Gorayeb, N.; Turibio L.B.N. (1999). *O exercício: preparação fisiológica, avaliação médica, aspectos especiais e preventivos*, Atheneu, ISBN: 857379139, São Paulo, Brazil.

Grosse, P.D. & Sengler, J. (2001). *Reeducação Perineal.* Manole ISBN: 85-204-1162-2,São Paulo, Brazil.

Guyton, A. C. & HALL, J.E. (1997) *Fisiologia Humana e Mecanismos das Doenças* Guanabara Koogan ISBN: 85-201-0201-8, Rio de Janeiro, Brazil.

Harris, R.L.; Cundiff, G.W, & Coates, K.W. (1998). Urinary incontinence and pelvic prolapse in nulliparous women. *Obstetrics and Gynecology,* Vol.92, No.6, (December), pp.951-954, ISSN: 0029-7844.

Hay, J.G. (1993). Citius, altius, longius (faster, higher, longer): the biomechanics of jumping for distance. *Journal of Biomechanics,* Vol.26, No1, pp.7-21, ISSN: 0021-9290.

Hay-Smith, E.J.C.; Herbison, G.P. & Wilson, P.D. (2002). Pelvic floor muscle training for women with symptoms of stress urinary incontinence: A randomised trial comparing strengthening and motor relearning approaches. *Neurourology and Urodynamic,* Vol.21, No.4, (Jul) pp.371-372, ISSN: 0733-2467.

Hextall, A.; Majid, S. & Cardoso, L. (1999) A prospective controlled study of urinary symptoms in women with several anorexia nervosa. *Neurourology and Urodynamic,* Vol.18, No.4, (August), pp.398-409, ISSN: 0733-2467.

Hu., T.W.; Wagner, T.H.; Bentkover, J.D.; Leblanc, K.; Zou, S.Z. & Hubt, T. (2004). Costs of urinary incontinence and overactive bladder in the United States: a comparative study. *Urology,* Vol.63, No.3, (March), pp.461-465, ISSN: 0090-4295.

Hunskaar, S.; Lose, G. & Sykes D. (2004) The prevalence of urinary incontinence in four European countries. *British Journal of Urology International,* Vol.93, No.3, (September), pp. 324-330, ISSN: 0007-1331.

Jiang, K.; Novi, J.M.; Darnell, S. & Arya, L.A. (2004). Exercise and urinary incontinence in women. *Obstetrics and Gynecology Survey,* Vol.59, No.10, (October), pp.717-721, ISSN: 0029-7828.

Johnson, V.Y. (2001). Effects of submaximal exercise protocol to recondition the pelvic floor musculature. *Nursing Research,*Vol.50, No.1, (January), pp.33-41, ISSN: 0029-6562.

Kegel, A.H. (1952). Stress incontinence and genital relaxation. *Ciba Clinical Symposia,* Vol.4, No.2, (February), pp.35-52 ISSN: 0362-5060.

Kegel, A.H (1948). Progressive resistance exercise in the functional restoration of the perineal muscles. *American Journal of Obstetrics and Gynecology,* Vol. 56, No.2, (August), pp.238–248, ISSN: 0002-9378.

Levi D'ancona, C.A. (2001). Diagnostico da Incontinência Urinária na Mulher, In: *Aplicações Clinicas da Urodinâmica.* C.A. Levi D'ancona & N. JR., Rodrigues Netto, (Ed.), Atheneu, ISBN: 8573793538, São Paulo, Brazil.

Minassian, V.A.; Drutz, H.P.& Al-Badr, A. (2003). Urinary incontinence as a worldwide problem. *International Journal of Gynecology and Obstetrics,* Vol.82, No.3, (September), pp. 327-338, ISSN: 0020-7292.

Moen, M.; Noone, M.; Vassallo, B.; Lopata, R.; Nash, M.; Sum, B. & Schy, S. (2007) Knowledge and performance of pelvic muscle exercises in women. *Female Pelvic Medicine & Reconstructive Surgery,* Vol.13, No. (March) pp.113–117, ISSN: 2151-8378.

Mullins, C.D.; Subak, L.L. (2005). New perspectives on overactive bladder: quality of life impact, medication persistency, and treatment costs. *American Journal Management Care, Vol.* 11, No.4, (July), pp.101-102, ISSN: 1088-0224.

Neumann, P.B.; Grimmer, K.A. & Deenadayalan, Y. (2006). Pelvic floor muscle training and adjunctive therapies for the treatment of stress urinary incontinence in women: a systematic Review. *BMC Women's Health,* Vol.6, No.11, (June), pp.1-28, ISSN: 1472-6874.

Norton, P.A.; Macdonald, L.D.; Sedgwinck, P.M. & Stanton, S.L. (1988) Distress and delay associated with urinary incontinence, frequency and urgency in women. *British Medical Journal,* Vol.297, (November), pp. 1187-1189, ISSN: 0959-8146.

Nygaard, I.E.; Delancey, J.O.& Arnsdorf L. (1990) Exercise and incontinence. *Obstetrics and Gynecology,* Vol.75, No.5, (May), pp.848-51, ISSN: 0029-7844.

Nygaard. I.E.; Thompsson, F.L. & Svengalis S.L. (1994) Urinary incontinence in elite nulliparous athletes. *Obstetrics Gynecology,* Vol.84, No,2, (August), pp.183-187, ISSN: 0029-7844.

Nygaard, I.E.; Glowacki. C. & Saltzman, C.L. (1996) Relationship between foot flexibility and urinary incontinence in nulliparous varsity athletes. *Obstetrics and Gynecology,* Vol. 87, No.6, (June), pp. 1049-1051, ISSN: 0029-7844.

Nygaard,I.E. (1997) Does prolonged high-impact activity contribute to later urinary incontinence? A retrospective cohort study of female Olympians. *Obstetrics and Gynecology,* Vol.90, no.5, (November), pp.718–722, ISSN: 0029-7844.

Nygaard, I.E.; Girts, T.; Fultz, N.H.; Kinchen, K.; Pohl, G. & Sternfeld, B. (2005). Is urinary incontinence a barrier to exercise in women? *Obstetrics and Gynecology,* Vol.106, No.2, (August), pp. 307-314, ISSN: 0029-7844.

Nygaard I.; Thom, D.H. & Calhoun, E.A. (2007a). Urinary Incontinence in women. In: *Urologie Diseases in America, MS.* Litwin & C.S. Saigal (ed.). US Department of Health and Human Services, Public Health Service, National institutes of Health, National Institute of Diabetes and Digestive and Kidney Diseases. Government Printing Office, 2007; NIH Publication No. 07-5512; 159-191, Washington, DC; US.

Nygaard, I.; Handa, V.; Brubaker, L.; Borello-France, D.; Wei, J.; Wells, E. & Weber, A.M. (2007b). Physical activity in women planning sacrocolpopexy. *International Urogynecology Journal and Pelvic Floor Dysfunction,* Vol.18, (May), pp. 33–37, ISSN: 0937-3462.

Nygaard, I.; Handa, V.L.; Brubaker, L.; Borello-France, D.; Wei, J.; Wells, E. & Goode, P. (2008). Changes in physical activity after abdominal sacrocolpopexy for advanced pelvic organ prolapsed for the Pelvic Floor Disorders. *American Journal of Obstetrics & Gynecology,* Vol.198, (May), pp.570.e1-570-575, ISSN: 0002-9378.

O'Dell, K.; Morse, A.N.; Crawford, S.L. & Howard, A. (2007). Vaginal pressure during lifting, floor exercises, jogging, and use of hydraulic exercise machines. *International Urogynecology Journal and Pelvic Floor Dysfunction,* Vol.18, No.12, pp. 1481–1489, ISSN: 0937-3462.

Ortiz, O.C. (2004). Stress urinary incontinence in gynecological practice. *International Journal of Gynecology and Obstetrics.* Vol.86, No.1 (August), pp.6-16, ISSN: 0020-7292

Palma, P.C.R. & Reccetto, C. L. Z. (1999). Incontinência Urinária de Esforço na Mulher, In: *Urologia Prática,* N.R.JR. Netto, (Ed.), Atheneu, ISBN: 9788572417174. São Paulo, Brazil.

Parkkinen, A.; Karjalainen, E.; Vartiainen, M. & Penttinen, J. (2004). Physiotherapy for female stress urinary incontinence: Individual therapy at the outpatient clinic versus home-based pelvic floor training: A 5 year follow up study. *Neurourology Urodynamic,* Vol. 23, No.7, (September), pp.643-648, ISSN: 0733-2467.

Pieber, D.; Zivkovic, F.; Tamussino, K.; Ralph, G.; Lippitt, G. & Fauland, B. (1995). Pelvic floor exercises alone or with vaginal cones for the treatment of mild to moderated stress urinary incontinence in premenopausal women. *International Urogynecology Journal Pelvic Floor Dysfunction,* Vol.6, No.1, pp.14-17, ISSN: 0937-3462.

Ree, M.L.; Nyggard, I. & Bo, K. (2007). Muscular fatigue in the pelvic floor muscles after strenuous physical activity. *Acta Obstetricia et Gynecologica Scandinavica,* Vol.86, No.7, (December), pp.870 876, ISNN: 0001-6349.

Rivalta, M.; Sighinolfia, M.C.; Salvatore, M.; De Stefano, S.; Francesca, Torcasio, F. & Giampaolo,B. (2010). Urinary Incontinence and Sport: First and Preliminary Experience With a Combined Pelvic Floor Rehabilitation Program in Three Female Athletes. *Health Care for Women International,* Vol.31, (April), pp.435–443, ISSN: 0739-9332.

Salvatore, S.; Serati, M.; Laterza; R.; Uccella, S.; Torella, M. & Bolis, P.F. (2009). The impact of urinary stress incontinence in young and middle-age women practicing recreational sports activity: an epidemiological study. *British Journal of Sports Medicine,* Vol. 43, (September), pp.1115–1118, ISSN: 0306-3674.

Santos, E.S.; Caetano, A.S.; Tavares, M.C.G.C.F. & Lopes, M.H.B.M. (2009). Urinary incontinence among physical education students. *Revista da Escola de Enfermagem USP,* Vol. 43; No. 2, (november), pp. 307-312, ISSN: 0080-6234.

Simeonova, Z.; Milson, I. & Kullendorf A.M. (1999). The prevalence of urinary incontinence and its influence on the quality of life in women from urban Swedish population. *Acta Obstetricia et Gynecologica Scandinavica,* Vol.78, No. 6, (June), pp. 546-51, ISSN: 0001-6349.

Stach-Lempinen, B.; Nygard, C.H.; Laippala, R.M.; Metsanoja, R. & Kujansuu, E. (2004). Is physical activity influenced by urinary incontinence? *Obstetrics and Gynecology,* Vol.111, No.5, (April), pp.475-480, ISSN: 0020-7292.

Tata, G.E. (1998). Incontinência, In: *Fisioterapia na Terceira Idade,* B. Pickles; A. Compton; R. Cott; J. Simpson & A. Vandervoort, Santos, ISBN: 572882189, São Paulo, Brazil.

Turkan, A.; Inci,Y. & Fazli D. (2005). The short term effects of physical therapy in different intensities of urodynamic stress incontinence. *Gynecology Obstetric Investigation,* Vol. 59, No.1, pp.43-48, ISSN: 0378-7346.

Thyssen, H.H.; Clevin, L. & Olosen S. (2002). Urinary incontinence in elite female athletes and dancers. *International Urogynecologic Journal and Pelvic Floor Dysfunction,* Vol.;13, No.1, pp.15-17, ISSN: 0937-3462.

Wei, J.; Raz, S. & Young, G.P.H. (1999). Fisiopatologia da Incontinência Urinária de Esforço. In: *Urologia Feminina,I.* Rubinstein (ed.), BYK, ISBN, São Paulo, Brazil.

WHO/FIMS (1995). Committee on Physical Activity for Health: Exercise for health. *Bullettin of the World Health Organization: The International Journal of Public Health,* Vol. 73, pp. 135-136, ISSN: 0042-9686.

6

Elderly Women and Urinary Incontinence in Long-Term Care

Catherine MacDonald
Saint Francis Xavier University
Canada

1. Introduction

The prevalence of urinary incontinence (UI), although difficult to define due to underreporting, is estimated to affect over 13 million Americans, and greater than 50% of residents residing in long-term care (LTC) facilities (Bennet, 2008; Earthy & Nativ, 2009; Parker, 2007). It has been estimated that the cost of UI in Canadian LTC facilities is approximately $3000.00 to $10,000.00 per year for each resident experiencing UI (Earthy & Nativ, 2009). The Canadian Continence Foundation (2005) reported that one in four middle-aged and older women are affected by UI. By the year 2050, the number of women likely to experience UI will increase by 46% (Romanzi, 2010). The increasing prevalence of UI in long term-care facilities from 55% to 65% over the past 10 years is alarming, and requires careful consideration by healthcare providers and policy-makers (MacDonald & Butler, 2007; Sahyoun, et al., 2001).

UI is a multidimensional healthcare issue that should be viewed from various perspectives and contexts, as a condition requiring operational, clinical, strategic, and interdisciplinary focus (Klusch, 2003). However, the current state of the knowledge maintains that much of the existing literature continues to explore UI from the contexts of the medicalization of UI, the physical and economic burdens of UI, the marginalization of elderly women experiencing UI in long- term care, and healthcare providers' attitudes, approaches, and strategies to managing UI in LTC. There were few references found that discussed how elderly women managed their UI, and the effects of UI on the quality of life (QoL) from the women's lived experiences. To date the psychosocial effects of urinary incontinence for elderly women has received minimal attention in the current research literature. Physiological complications and the implications for symptom management of UI are the predominant research issues being addressed. The following chapter presents an account of the current state of knowledge with each of the aforementioned topics discussed in relation to elderly women in LTC. The chapter will begin by defining UI, and end with a necessary discussion of healthcare practices, education, and research related to elderly women and UI in LTC.

2. Background

UI is a prevalent health issue adversely affecting the quality of life, well-being and psychosocial aspects of elderly women's lives residing in LTC (Bradway et al., 2010;

Howard & Steggall, 2010; Palmer, 2008). UI has been documented as a primary reason for institutionalization and admission to LTC facilities, and documented to negatively impact social, sexual, and physical activities of elderly women (Lifford et al., 2008; Stewart, 2010; Wilson, 2003). Yet, UI has been acknowledged as an inconvenience, rather than being a health issue requiring adequate healthcare resources (Hu, 1990; MacDonald & Butler, 2007; Norton & Brubaker, 2006). Given that, UI is not life threatening to women, often results in UI care not being viewed as a priority, therefore, it is repeatedly under-reported, under-treated, and often mismanaged (McDermott, 2010 Norton & Brubaker, 2006). UI has been labelled a "silent epidemic" and a worldwide health issue that commonly affects women (Beji et al., 2010).

Although UI has devastating physical and psychological effects on individuals, family, friends, and caregivers (McDermott, 2010; Wilson, 2003), society continues to stigmatize and associate UI with as inevitable component of ageing that is considered normal, and effortlessly managed (Bennet, 2008; Bradway et al., 2010). As suggested in the literature, this stigma has the potential to isolate women and render them silent about their experiencing of UI, hence, women accept UI as being a normal part of life (Borrie et al., 2002, Howard & Steggall, 2010; MacDonald & Butler, 2007; Robinson, 2000). This in turn, potentially may prevent women from accessing supportive healthcare services and seeking appropriate measures to assist in the prevention or management of UI (Bennet, 2008; Parker, 2007; Hagglund & Ahlstrom, 2007). The stigma of UI is further compounded by some healthcare professional trivializing UI in comparison to other healthcare issues and "by incorrectly describing it as a non-hierarchical index of functional status" (Wilson, 2003, p.752). While frequently cited as the primary reason for admission of elderly women to LTC, the impacts of UI are continually misunderstood, downplayed, under-reported, under-treated, silenced and not well defined (Borrie et al., 2002; Norton & Brubaker, 2006; Zeznock et al., 2009).

3. UI defined

The term UI can be defined in multiple and diverse ways by different groups and individuals (Palmer, 1996). The International Continence Society (ICS) has defined UI as a condition of involuntary urine loss that is objectively demonstrable and is a social or hygienic problem (Thakar & Stanton, 2000). This definition implies that UI can have a detrimental effect on the lives of those experiencing the condition (Hunskaar & Vinsnes, 1991). The ICS is an international society for medical professionals, concerned with furthering education, scientific research, clinical practice and removing the stigma of incontinence (ICS, 2011). The ICS has developed definitions and terminology for researchers pertaining to UI types, assessment, and diagnosis in an attempt to standardize UI discourse. The ICS has a global health focus committed to improve the QoL for individuals affected by urinary, bowel, and pelvic floor disorders through education, research, and advocacy.

Another group to consider when defining UI is administrators and managers in LTC facilities. According to Palmer (1996), administrators in LTC may define UI with respect to controlling the economic expenditures that is required to manage the issue. Budgeting monies for UI products, linens, and staffing to manage toileting, soiling, and skin breakdown is of primary concern to LTC administrators and managers (MacDonald & Butler, 2007). In my previous experience as a Director, Resident Care and site manager in an urban, LTC setting in Eastern Nova Scotia, Canada, discussions of UI frequently occurred in relation to the economic burden of managing the problem. Procedures and strategies were designed to maintain costs of products used for UI, with little consideration given to comfort or appropriateness of interventions from the resident's perspective or the overall impact on QoL.

Some healthcare providers and caregivers in LTC may define UI in terms of the demanding workload and the timely investments dedicated to physical management of changing incontinent products, voiding schedules, and soiled linens and clothing changes (Brink, 1990, Palmer, 1996). Furthermore, UI maybe viewed by some healthcare professionals as low on the priority list of healthcare needs, and not a prudent expenditure of precious time and energy (Bayliss & Salter, 2004). In an attempt to reduce or eliminate UI, it has been documented that some healthcare providers and caregivers in LTC spend productive time implementing fluid management strategies and double incontinent products worn in an attempt to deal with the issue of UI (Brink, 1990). Physicians on the other hand, may define UI in regards to assessment, diagnosis, medical and/or surgical technologies and management, and pharmacological treatments (Day et al, 2010). This definition incorporates the philosophy of controlling and/or curing UI for those individuals experiencing the condition and tends to medicalize UI. Conversely, elderly women experiencing UI in LTC may subjectively define UI with respect to psychological, social, economic or physical implications and contexts (DuBeau et al., 2006; Getliffe et al., 2007; Hagglund & Ahlstrom, 2007; Howard & Steggall, 2010; Lifford et al, 2008; MacDonald & Butler, 2007; McDermott, 2010; Norton & Brubaker, 2006; Palmer, 1996; Parker, 2007; Wilson, 2003; Zeznock et al, 2010). The loss of bodily control, decrease in activities of daily living, social isolation, skin infections and dermatitis, falls, cost of incontinent products, and embarrassment maybe considered important in a UI definition to elderly women (MacDonald & Butler, 2007; McDermott, 2010; Nix & Haugen, 2010; Palmer, 2008; Parker, 2007; Stewart, 2010; Wilson, 2003). Also, it has been well documented in the literature that elderly women experience feelings of being less attractive and different from others resulting in shame, depression, and loss of self-confidence and inferiority, which must be considered when defining UI from the individuals perspective (Gallagher, 1998; Goldstein et al., 1992; Grimgy et al., 1993; Lifford et al, 2008; Palmer, 2008; Hunskaar & Vinsnes, 1991).

The diversity in definitions, terminology, and perspectives pertaining to UI can lead to confusion and ambiguity about the health issue, which in turn impacts upon UI care. The lack of common, cohesive and holistic definitions and terminology relating to UI makes it difficult for healthcare professionals, caregivers, researchers, educators and those experiencing UI to communicate and conceptualize issues, solutions, and interventions (Palmer, 1996; Zeznock et al, 2010). Moreover, clear, common, and cohesive UI definitions and terminology could provide individuals with an opportunity to give voice and meaning to their experiences of living with UI, and subsequently influence their care (Hagglund & Ahlstrom, 2007). Thus, myths and ideas of UI being a normal part of ageing could be dispelled, while increasing the possibility of making UI an important healthcare issue that requires timely attention and resources.

The author suggests that definitions and terminology about UI may be expanded to encompass the social determinants of health and the broader impact of cultural, political, and economic contexts that influence individuals' experiences with UI. There is also a need to combine the cost factors related to the management of UI in long- term care, with the fiscal and human burden (cost) to women experiencing UI, to determine appropriate practices. What it means to experience UI and the impact on QoL, given the associated management strategies imposed on elderly women within LTC, is a critical concern for the delivery of holistic and individual continence care. Knowledge about the impact of UI on an individual's sense of self, and how that translates to the delivery of continence care has received minimal attention in the research literature. The need for healthcare providers to become more knowledgeable about the issues that effect the delivery of care related to UI requires an in depth analysis beyond budget consideration, to acknowledge the overall burden to elderly women experiencing UI in LTC. Thus, it is suggested by the author that UI may be viewed from a broader perspective encompassing the social, physical, economic, cultural, and political contexts rather than focusing primarily on a narrow perspective that can further lead to the medicalization of UI.

4. Medicalization of UI

UI has been associated with several disease processes and is reported to be one of the major causes of admission to long- term care facilities (Beji et al., 2010; Bradway et al., 2010; Coward et al., 1995; Du Moulinet al., 2009; Edwards, 2001; MacDonald & Butler, 2007; Norton & Brubaker, 2006; Thom et al, 1997). Yet, there is minimal research regarding the psychosocial impact of UI on elderly women. UI creates a multidimensional healthcare problem, which has become medicalized as evidenced by the predominance of diagnostic and treatment regimes. Further, UI is often associated with co-morbidity and invasive procedures such as urodynamic studies, catheterizations and pelvic examinations, particularly in the elderly (Norton & Brubaker, 2006; Resnick, 1992). However, for over twenty years, literature has suggested that incontinence in the elderly is curable with medical and/or surgical interventions (Resnick). The elderly population may be a more vulnerable group relative to the fear of impending surgery or invasive diagnostic treatments that require hospitalization (Mitteness, 1990), which consequently poses a threat to maintaining independence. Being independent and able to control UI is of vital importance to elderly women's perception of themselves (Birgersson et. al, 1993). The following are some examples of research demonstrating the medicalization of UI.

Thom et al. (1997) in a review of 5,986 medical records of men and women aged 65 years and older examined the associations between medically diagnosed UI and factors such as; risk of several disease conditions, hospitalizations, nursing home admissions and mortality. Results indicated that the risk of hospitalization was 30% higher for women. There was also an increased risk of UI with a diagnosis of Parkinson's disease, dementia, stroke, depression and congestive heart failure for both women and men. In addition, the likelihood of nursing home admission secondary to UI was twice as high for women while the risk of mortality was a not significant. These results demonstrate a medical approach to institutionalized care when managing UI, which is more likely to impact women.

Hunskaar and Vinsnes (1991) used the Sickness Impact Profile (SIP) questionnaire to assess the QoL of women with UI according to age, symptom group, volume of urinary leakage, and duration of incontinence. Thirty-six women between 40-60 years and forty women aged 70 years or more were randomly selected from a medical clinic. Women were categorized into two subgroups, either urge to void or stress incontinence, as defined by the SIP.

Findings revealed that UI in women adversely affects QoL. Major differences were found when age and symptoms were analyzed such that women who had the urge to void identified symptoms associated with greater impairment than the symptoms defined by women who had stress incontinence. However, age had a greater influence on the impact of stress incontinence. Elderly women reported little effect of stress incontinence in terms of impairment while younger women believed stress incontinence had a significant effect on the overall QoL.

Norton & Brubaker (2006) discussed UI in terms if being under-reported and under-treated. The authors cited that in women "urine storage and emptying is a complex coordination between the bladder and urethra, and disturbances in the system due to child birth, aging or other medical conditions can lead to urinary incontinence" (p.5). Further, that stress and urge UI, the two main types of UI in women, can be evaluated and clinically assessed by most primary physicians. They go on to discuss the pathophysiology, epidemiology, symptoms, signs, urodynamic diagnosis and treatment options for different types of UI in women. However, the authors do mention in the assessment and management of UI in primary care, the importance of acknowledging stigma or effect on QoL of the woman, and to initiate non-surgical options depending on the type of UI and overall goals for treatment.

Lifford, et al. (2008) used a prospective study design to examine the epidemiology of UI in older women. The authors cited that "establishing the epidemiological of UI can aid in identification of populations at risk, and help to target medical screening, prevention, and treatment" (p.1191). The study setting was a Nurses' Health Study that was established in 1976 when 121,700 female registered nurses in 11 United States responded to a survey pertaining to their medical history and lifestyles. Between 2000 and 2002 women were requested to complete two questions to evaluate their frequency of UI experienced and extent of urine leakage. Then, the rates of UI incidents and progression or remission of UI were calculated, and estimated relative risks of UI and associated risk factors completed by logistic regression. Results indicated women with no urine leakage at baseline reported 9.2% experiencing leakage at least once a month after 2 years. The women experiencing leakage at least weekly had an incidence of 3.6% with stress UI being the greatest incidence followed by mixed and urge UI. Stress UI in the women was found to decrease with age, while urge and mixed UI increased with age. With regards to the prevalence UI in the year 2000, findings indicated that 32.1% of the women experiencing leakage once a month progressed to experiencing leakage at least once a week over follow-up. Furthermore, 8.9% of women with frequency leakage in 2000 indicated an improvement to monthly leakage or less, while 25 had experienced complete remission. Conclusions from the study revealed that the UI incidence is high in older women, with the progression from occasional to frequent leakage being very common, while urge UI increases with age and has limited effective treatment modalities. Therefore, it was proposed that more research on UI prevention in older women needs to be conducted.

5. The burdens of UI on QoL of elderly women

UI imposes devastating psychosocial, physical and economical burdens for elderly women (DuBeau et al., 2006; Getliffe, et al., 2007; Hagglund & Ahlstrom, 2007; Howard & Steggall, 2010; Lifford et al, 2008; MacDonald & Butler, 2007; McDermott, 2010; Norton & Brubaker, 2006; Palmer, 1996; Parker, 2007; Wilson, 2003; Zeznock et al, 2010). Elderly women's emotional health can be negatively affected by experiencing UI (Gallagher, 1998; Howard & Steggall, 2010; McDermott, 2010). The following are some studies that will demonstrate the burdens of UI on the QoL of elderly women. Gallagher (1998) used a descriptive correlation research design to explore the relationship between urogenital distress and the psychosocial impact of UI in elderly women living in apartment complexes in Toledo, Ohio. The sample was comprised of 17 women over the age of 60 who experienced UI at least once a week. Findings indicated that there was a strong relationship between urogenital distress and the psychosocial impact of UI in elderly women. The author further reported that UI negatively impacted physical, social and emotional aspects of health. These findings are consistent with other studies that have identified factors that support a negative effect of UI. Another example, a quantitative study by Norton (1982) focused on the degree and extent of restrictions imposed by UI, using a sample of 55 women aged 22-78 who attended a urodynamic clinic. Results from the study demonstrated that incontinence did have far-reaching psychosocial effects and contributed to women feeling anxious, embarrassed and unwilling to participate in a wide range of activities. To what extent age impacted on these restrictions and the psychosocial effects of UI was unclear given the wide variance in ages in this sample.

Whyman et al. (1987) measured the psychosocial impact of UI on 69 women living in the community, aged 55 and older using the Incontinence Impact Questionnaire (IIQ).The IIQ consisted of 26 items which asked women to rate the extent to which urine leakage affected their activities of daily living, social interactions and perceptions of self. Findings revealed that incontinence affects primarily women's perceptions of self. Daily activities most affected occurred when the availability of restrooms was unknown, and when women were unfamiliar with surroundings or engaged in physical recreation.

To acquire an understanding of older women's experience of UI in the community, Dowd (1991) interviewed seven women aged 58-79. Findings suggested that older women's experiences with UI posed a threat to their self-esteem. In addition, these older women employed a number of self-care strategies to control and normalize their UI into daily routines, thus maintaining their self-esteem and dignity. Although this study did address the psychosocial impact of UI in older women, the author neglects to identify or discuss the actual types of self-care strategies the women used to maintain self-esteem.

Sandvik et al. (1993) in a study of 187 women aged 19-91, investigated the psychosocial consequences of UI using a 38 item questionnaire mapping demographic data, medial history and toileting habits. Findings cited that 80% of the women interviewed considered UI to be more than a minor problem. The effect of age on these findings was not reported, which is a major limitation in interpreting the findings. These researchers defined three major concepts relating to the psychosocial impact of UI, mental distress, practical inconveniences, and social restrictions. Mental distress caused by UI included, fear of smelling, fear of discovery, feelings of despair, feeling dirty, feeling of inferiority, lack of self confidence, fear of being alone, loss of joy, and shame. Practical inconveniences caused by UI included smell, disturbed sleep, skin irritation, extra laundry, and added expenses. For women living in long- term care the "practical inconveniences" of smell and skin irritations are potential psychological burdens when attending socials, visiting with friends and families, or eating in the dining room. The social restrictions caused by UI included; lifting, laughing, travelling, dancing, shopping, wearing desired clothes, and entertaining guests.

Rolls (1997) explored the night time sleeping patterns of 18 residents living in a nursing home and the factors that impacted on sleep. Findings indicated that factors such as; environmental noise, lights, staff conversation, performance of routine incontinence care, and repositioning of residents who were immobile were major contributors to sleep disruption. Consequently, individualized incontinence care routines were considered as critical to promote sleep. In addition, Rolls (1997) asserted that residents experience more agitation during the day if awaken by night staff to perform incontinence care and repositioning. Thus, a lack of sleep due to the changing of incontinence products at night is a burden affecting the QoL of individuals living in LTC.

DuBeau et al. (2006) conducted a retrospective quantitative study using a Minimum Data Set (MDS) database involving 5 states (Kanas, Maine, Mississippi, New York and South Dakota) in the USA from 1994-1996. The purpose of the study was to determine whether nursing home residents with UI experienced worse QoL than continent residents, whether the relationship between QoL differs across cognitive and functional impairment, and to determine whether a change in continence status is associated with a change in QoL. The participants were aged 65 years and older. QoL was measured according to the MDS derived social engagement scale. Findings reported that UI was significantly associated with worse QoL in residents experiencing moderate cognitive and functional impairment, and new or worsening UI experienced over a 6 month period was associated with worse QoL. The authors suggested that this research evidence supports strong rationale for targeting interventions and strategies for those residents experiencing UI, while presenting an incentive to improving continence care.

Howard & Steggall (2010) in a descriptive literature review explored the relationship between UI, QoL and barriers to help-seeking behaviour in women. The authors indicated that factors such as severity of UI, type of UI, age, and actual QoL scores seemed to contribute to how UI impacts women's QoL. Reliable evidence concluded that increased severity of UI is as a predictor of impact on QoL (Huang et al., 2006; Yu et al., 2003). Yet, with increasing age the prevalence and severity of UI increases, but in younger women the impact of UI on QoL was found to be more significant than in their older counterparts (Monz et al., 2007). The major cue for seeking help for UI appears to have been the QoL score itself. This is supported by Yu et al. (2003) in their findings that indicated that QoL and women's perceptions of whether they viewed UI as a disease or not, were factors that affected women's help-seeking behaviour.

5.1 Physical and economic burdens of UI

Not only do elderly women experience psychosocial impacts of UI, but the importance of physical and economic burdens that UI can impose should not be overlooked. UI predisposes elderly women to physical side effects such as rashes, dermatitis, skin infections, decubitus ulcers, and urinary tract infections (Du Moulin et al., 2009; Getliffe et al., 2007; Goldstein et al, 1992; Nix & Haugen, 2010; Schnelle, 1991). There is also an increased risk of falls associated with UI in the elderly, due to wet and slippery floors from dribbling and impaired mobility due to wearing bulky or poor fitting incontinence products (Hu, 1990; Loughrey, 1999; Parker, 2007). This was evidenced in my own nursing practice in LTC. Incidents of residents falling occurred while toileting by slipping on their own incontinent products or urine. For some, the outcome was traumatic requiring treatment and/or hospitalization for lacerations and fractures. This proved to be an enormous physical burden for the elderly and the healthcare system, despite being preventable with proper supervision and appropriate symptom management of UI.

UI imposes tremendous economic burdens on individuals and their families. UI is one of the primary reasons for breakdown in care giving relationships for the elderly, and often results in nursing home placement (Du Moulin et al., 2009; Coward et al., 1995; Hu, 1990). Given our aging population and longer life expectancy of women, it is the aging woman who will be at the greatest risk for requiring additional care for UI, and the potential increased for associated nursing home placement to long- term care facilities (Sharpe, 1995; Stewart, 2010; Wilson, 2003).

Over a twenty years ago Hu, (1990) asserted that there are costs associated with routine incontinence care included; labour, supplies, and laundry in LTC facilities. The burden of managing UI in long- term care been estimated to be more than 3 billion dollars annually in the USA (Wilson, 2003). In Canada, the average cost for supplies and nursing care for a senior with UI residing in LTC is between $3,000-$10,000 per year (Earthy & Nativ, 2009). Budget conscious administrators provide residents with the most cost-effective incontinence products, supplies, and staffing. Therefore, elderly women in long- term care facilities incur a personal cost for buying preferred incontinence products, and personal hygiene items to hide embarrassing odour associated with UI (Getliffe et al., 2007; Stewart, 2010). In turn, these disposalable incontinence and personal hygiene products are considered a burden for the environment, and may not be permitted for use in health related facilities and long -term care agencies (MacDonald & Butler, 2007). Moreover, scent-free policies instituted in many LTC facilities compounds the issue of elderly women attempting to hide embarrassing odours associated with being incontinent.

UI has pyschosocial, physical, and economic burdens which impact on elderly women in today's society as evidenced in the literature (Beji et al, 2010; Borrie et al, 2002; Coward et al., 1995; Dowd, 1991; Earthy & Nativ, 2009; Goldstein, 1992; Gallagher, 1998; Hu, 1990; Lifford et al, 2008; MacDonald & Butler, 2007; McDermott, 2010; Norton, 1982; Parker, 2007; Resnick, 1997; Sandvik et al., 1993; Schnelle, 1991; Simons, 1985; Wilson, 2003;). Research is required that explores how elderly women's perceive the impact of this event on their overall QoL and sense of well-being. For healthcare providers working in long- term care to be instrumental in reducing the economic, physical, and psychosocial burden of UI they need to consider the perception of the residents and plan incontinence care in a way that promotes QoL and assists in decreasing the marginalization of elderly women experiencing UI.

5.2 The marginalization of elderly women

Western society focuses on youthfulness as evidenced in media images of anti-ageing cosmetics, wrinkle-smoothing creams and hair dyes (Bernard, 1998). Historically, elderly women have rarely been portrayed as attractive females, and were commonly viewed as asexual or incapable of sexual expression (Steinke, 1988). Sexual behaviour was believed to be inappropriate, hence taboo for older adults (Smedley, 1991). Consequently, gender and age have continued to marginalize elderly women in our society. Ageism creates a negative attitude towards the elderly, while reinforcing social oppression (Bernard, 1998). Blair and White (1998) suggested that compelling evidence exists concerning stereotyping related to gender bias and ageism, which contributes to a lack of health maintenance services for older women. The present healthcare system reinforces this attitude by the lack of interest and resources for speciality practices in geriatrics (Wilson, 2003). Some healthcare providers diminish the significance of UI (Wilson, 2003) and some healthcare providers are seen as being unhelpful (Bradway, 2004), which in turn impacts upon women's seeking help for UI. UI is often found to be ignored by some healthcare providers due to their lack of education or expertise to address the healthcare issue, which are limiting factors negatively impacting service development and delivery (Getliffe & Dolman, 2007; Zeznock et al., 2009). Ignoring UI and negative demeaning attitudes towards the elderly, and the withholding treatments based on biased judgements and prognoses for the elderly are pervasive among some healthcare professionals and policy decision-makers (Mardon et al., 2006; Sharpe, 1995). The use of "baby talk" to elderly women by nursing staff in long- term care facilities reaffirms the negative perceptions of the elderly person's functional ability, perpetuating "women to women ageism" (Bernard, 1998; Sharpe, 1995). Bernard (1998) found that some healthcare providers, including nurses, possess more ageism attitudes than the population at large, a situation which dramatically impacts on the marginalization of elderly women. For elderly women, healthcare providers' stereotypical beliefs about aging increase the probability that their concerns will be devalued (Sharpe, 1995; Wilson, 2003). For that reason, elderly women may hesitate to discuss their UI with physicians, nurses, and other healthcare providers who possess ageist and sexist attitudes. Further, UI is considered to be a social taboo and stigmatizing, which is often another reason for women to not seek healthcare or delay in seeking healthcare services for their UI (Hagglund et al, 2003; Howard & Steggall, 2010). Walters et al. (2001) cited that withdrawal, resignation and low expectations were found to be dominant reasons for women not seeking assistance for their UI. Further, Horrocks et al. (2004) in a grounded theory study of twenty participants over 65 years old added that reasons for not seeking help for UI were independent management of UI, reactions to incontinence and attitudes to ageing and health. When individuals did seek help for incontinence the themes media influences and contact with primary care emerged.

Tauton et al. (2005) found that the attitudes of some healthcare providers' negatively impacted incontinence care, as they viewed UI as being time consuming and sometimes frustrating. Subsequently, patients were passively managed instead of being actively treated for UI. This is consistent with MacDonald & Butler (2007) who noted that the attitudes of staff providing care directly to women with UI in long-term care affected their UI experience, particularly when the staff were busy. This is supported by one woman in the study mentioning that her experience with UI in LTC was influenced directly by how busy the staff were when she rang to be toileted. Walters et al. (2001) acknowledged that even when some elderly do consult with healthcare providers there are high rates of unmet needs experienced. It was also found that healthcare providers often do not inquire about UI, even when individuals are at high risk (Du Moulin et al., 2009).

Zeznock et al. (2009) in a qualitative descriptive study of 17 women living with UI in Alaska found that although most women did seek out healthcare providers' their encounters with healthcare providers were varied with both negative and positive experiences. Many of the women in the study viewed encounters with healthcare providers as being a significant factor in their experiences of living with UI, particularly if those encounters were negative. Negative encounters with healthcare providers precluded women from seeking future healthcare pertaining to their incontinence. Likewise, Hagglund and Ahlstrom (2007) in a phenomenological hermeneutic approach interviewed 14 women with UI in Sweden. One of the findings pointed out that some women had experienced a less satisfying encounter when they sought help for their UI. In some instances, women felt that they were treated nonchalantly by healthcare providers, and were not being taken seriously. Also, some women felt that they were wounded by the manner in which they were treated by some healthcare providers, but they did have a respectful experience when they accessed another healthcare provider.

Yet, some healthcare providers have found have to positively influence those experiencing UI (Borrie et al., 2002; MacDonald & Butler, 2007). One example is Borrie et al (2002) , who reported the use of specialized nurses (nurse continence advisors) with education and training in managing UI to positively impacted UI care, and reduced the incidence of UI, and use of incontinence pads in Ontario, Canada. The nurse continence advisors used behavioural interventions and lifestyle counselling, which proved to be a cost- effective management strategy consistent with recommendations and guidelines of the Canadian Continence Association. Given the shifting of demographics of our population, the extent to which healthcare providers' attitudes and behaviours exists in the delivery of care to the elderly, and specifically to women, requires close scrutiny and careful examination by healthcare providers and the public.

5.3 Managing UI in LTC

Distinct odours and piles of clean diapers are considered the hallmarks of nursing homes (Tulloch, 1989). The paucity of research and literature relating to UI in long- term care makes it difficult to change these images as the hallmarks of long -term care. There is obviously a need for more exploratory work to describe living and management of UI in long -term care. Managing the burden of UI in LTC is a major concern to administrators and healthcare providers. The increased availability of incontinence products augments the "cultural knowledge" that UI is a normal process for which pads and briefs are the best solution (Mitteness, 1990). The use of disposable absorbent products such as adult diapers or briefs, underpads and panty liners are major strategies for managing wetness for elderly women with UI in long- term care (Brink, 1990; Palmer, 2008; Wagg et al, 2004; Watson et al., 2003). The purpose of these disposable incontinence products are to "soak up" urine or contain incontinence for the dignity and comfort of the resident, protect clothing, furniture, floors and bedding, while simultaneously controlling odour (Brink, 1990; Getliffe et al., 2007). Advances in technology "have led to absorbent products that are designed to contain large quantities of urine and to protect the skin from the effects of incontinence" (Palmer, 2008, p.439). Hu et al. (1990) added that the staff use the disposable under pads to lift and reposition residents by pulling on the product. This practice results in tearing of the product, and thus leaking of urine contributes to odour. The use of absorbent products and pads should be based primarily on residents' assessments, requirements, and preferences and not for staff convenience (Palmer, 2008).

Mitteness (1990) cited that healthcare providers were informing the elderly that nothing could be done for their UI as it was just considered as a normal part of aging. This message was considered to support residents by providing a protective effect on one's self-esteem

(Herzog et al., 1989). Physicians perceived UI as a nursing task and often avoid dealing with the issue, thus ignoring the effect of UI on self-esteem of elderly women, while nurses often inappropriately focused on the management of soiling rather than on the management of incontinence (Mitteness, 1990). Staff in nursing homes reported finding UI care frustrating, time-consuming and aesthetically unpleasant, leading to staff burnout, and poor morale (Yu & Kaltreider, 1987). Notably, if caregivers view UI negatively, rather than a QoL concern, elderly women who are physically and psychologically devastated by the effects of UI are rendered helpless (Mitteness, 1990).

A study conducted by Birgersson et al. (1993) of six elderly women with a mean age of 80.5 years, living in a Swedish nursing home, identified that a decrease in self-esteem was closely linked with the manner in which nurses assisted them in changing their incontinence products. Elderly women were in a state of vulnerability regarding their intrinsic value and autonomy as a result of having UI and wearing an incontinence product. These authors send a powerful message to healthcare providers concerning UI in elderly women. The need to treat women who have UI with respect, support, and include them in decisions-making and choices regarding their UI is essential.

The implementation of fluid management and voiding schedules are strategies employed by some nursing staff in LTC as an attempt to reduce or eliminate UI (Brink, 1990). Nursing staff will often restrict fluids in the evening in order to reduce night-time toileting or wetting (Brink, 1990). However, imposing such a strategy as a policy for all residents is excessive and places individuals at risk for dehydration. The goal for creating such a policy raises the question of quality of care. By trying to control UI in elderly women, nursing staff may, in fact, be attempting to minimize their workload associated with UI. Little data was found to document the outcome of these shortages on overall care and resident's well-being.

Routine voiding schedules are considered habit training procedures that will avoid incontinence by having the resident empty their bladder regularly (Earthy & Nativ, 2009; Klusch, 2003). Voiding schedules are usually indicated for many residents living in LTC, yet too often voiding schedules become a regular regime to control incontinence (Palmer, 2008; Resnick 1992). Imposing such a strategy on a competent elderly woman, capable of making informed decisions regarding her UI has ramifications for self-esteem and QoL. A simple request to go to the washroom to void could be denied by the staff, because it is not her scheduled bathroom time. Additionally, these women who do not need to void, are forced to toilet. If voiding schedules are to assist residents in maintaining comfort and decreasing the number of incontinent episodes, they must be individualized (Birgersson et al., 1993). By providing individualized care, nurses may enable elderly women experiencing UI to increase their autonomy and self-esteem and ultimately their QoL.

Freundl and Dugan (1992) examined the relationships between attitudes, knowledge, and institutional culture in relation to management of UI in the elderly. The Incontinence Stress Questionnaire-Staff Reaction (ISQ-SR) was used to measure staff attitudes towards UI in the elderly. The participants were 336 nursing personnel from 16 different LTC agencies accrued by convenience sampling. Prevalence of UI was calculated at 72%, however written protocols were not always apparent. Also, over 50% of the agencies acknowledged to using catheters as a management strategy for UI, and almost all of the agencies used incontinence products. With regards to education, findings indicated that few of the agencies reported having no training in the management of UI. However, most of the education was agency in-services, followed by classroom instruction in a school of nursing. Notably, less than half the participants acknowledged having formal clinical educational in the management of UI. According to the study, LTC facilities generally have positive attitudes toward UI in the elderly, but they have a limited knowledge regarding application to specific clinical situations or insight into the current research relating to UI. This lack of knowledge has dramatically impacted the manner in which UI care is provided to the elderly in LTC.

Vinsnes et al (2001) completed a study to understand Norwegian nurse's attitudes towards clients with UI by place of work, age, and educational levels of staff. Five hundred thirty-five responded to the questionnaire including five nursing facilities, three home care districts and medical surgical wards at a university hospital. Findings reported that staff members working in the long- term care were older than staff working in acute care units. Further, most of the registered nurses worked in the acute care, while most of the nursing assistants worked in long- term care. Findings also indicated that working on a medical surgical unit predicted more negative reactions and feeling towards UI than working in a nursing home. Also, nursing assistants working in medical units were more positive towards UI than registered nurses in LTC. Overall, the study indicated that attitudes toward UI were positive, but did not address how this translated to practice.

5.4 Elderly women managing UI in LTC

The literature suggests that elderly women practice a multitude of psychological and behavioural strategies to manage UI in long- term care. Many elderly women view UI as an inevitable part of aging, and often develop their own coping strategies rather than seeking help for their incontinence (Beji et al., 2010; MacDonald & Butler, 2007; Porrett & Cox, 2008; Stewart, 2010; Zeznock et al., 2009). Even earlier on, Skoner and Haylor (1993) suggested that elderly women prefer to normalize UI into their daily routines in an attempt to maintain their self-esteem. Time is measured in intervals between trips to the toilet in an attempt to minimize negative social sanctions from others due to visible soiling or smell thus, preventing shame and embarrassment (Mitteness, 1990). Psychological management strategies often include secrecy and social isolation (MacDonald & Butler, 2007). Elderly women keep incontinence a secret to minimize social ostracism or gossip, which in turn leads to social isolation (Mitteness, 1990; MacDonald & Butler, 2007). Some behavioural management strategies practiced by elderly women were reported to include; reducing fluid intake, voiding frequently, modifying activities that cause urine leakage, using pads and incontinent products, wearing perfume and deodorants to hide scents of urine, and altering clothing (Brink, 1990; Dowd, 1991; Hagglund & Ahlstrom, 2007; Hu et al., 1990; Mitteness, 1990; Skoner & Haylor, 1993; Whyman et al., 1987; Wilson, 2003; Zeznock et al., 2009). In addition to behavioural management, it has also been documented that the elderly implement dietary and environmental managements as a way to cope with UI (Wilson, 2003).

Routines in LTC facilities may not be supportive in assisting incontinent elderly women to practice their psychological and behavioural strategies (MacDonald & Butler, 2007). Maintaining social isolation and secrecy is very difficult as residents share dining areas and attend the same social activities. Scent free policies in long term-care facilities as previously mentioned present challenges for elderly women by preventing the use of fragrances such as powders and perfumes to disguise the scent of urine. The lack of opportunity by women to implement the psychological and behavioural strategies they desire contribute to decreased self-esteem and further social isolation (Dowd, 1991). Consequently, it becomes imperative that healthcare providers in LTC shift their thinking of UI as a health and QoL issue, and to understand why elderly women use particular strategies to cope with UI.

5.5 The effects of UI on the QoL from the elderly women's lived experiences in LTC

There is limited literature pertaining to the impact of UI on the QoL of elderly women experiencing UI in LTC from their lived experiences. O'Dell et al. (2008) in a descriptive qualitative study interviewed 25 women aged 65-96 with pelvic floor dysfunction, to increase understanding of the views of frail elderly women in residential care related to QOL, values, and preferences for pelvic floor care. Study findings suggested that pelvic floor dysfunction was not reported to play a central role in general QOL in these elderly women with multiple co- morbidities. The women discussed the value of comfort, containment, restful sleep, and making do, and were opposed to evaluation or interventions or citing risks of discomfort and ineffectiveness. Further, these elderly women living in LTC may prefer to live with pelvic floor dysfunction, than to access evaluation and treatment, even though it is available in their LTC facility. The authors concluded that residents in LTC ought to be part of planning care if improved QoL is the primary goal.

Another qualitative study using one-to-one interviewing by MacDonald & Butler (2007), explored the experiences of elderly women living in LTC with UI. Findings revealed that UI had a dramatic impact on the QoL of elderly women residing in LTC. There existed physical costs of UI that included; skin irritation and breakdown, bladder inflammation, physical discomfort, and feelings of being wet and soggy. Women expressed feelings of being dependant on staff for care and therefore, felt like they were losing control of their body, losing dignity, losing their independence, and losing the ability to maintain active lives, which directly impacted their QoL. The study suggested opportunities for improving healthcare education related to QoL of women who experience UI, and the need to make the UI experience more visible and openly discussed as a healthcare issue. Therefore, more research studies need to be conducted to determine the effects of UI on the QoL of elderly women in LTC from their lived experiences.

6. Implications for clinical practice

6.1 A comprehensive UI assessment

Given that UI can result from a multitude of interwoven contextual origins "including anatomic, physiologic, pathologic, and external factors" (Parker, 2007, p.70), a comprehensive UI assessment is essential for quality and holistic care for elderly women in LTC experiencing UI. The importance of conducting a comprehensive UI assessment comprised of history taking and physical examination, medication review, fluid intake patterns, a voiding diary, details about UI such as voiding patterns, use of urinary bladder stimulants or irritants, environmental factors, type of UI experienced, and responding to questions about UI is evident in the literature (Benne, 2008; Borrie et al., 2002; Bucci, 2007; Parker, 2007). A voiding and intake diary is an example of one tool that is considered useful in assessing an individual's frequency, time of urination, fluid intake, and number of incontinent episodes (Nitti, 2001). The outcome of this tool supported staff in long- term care to better understand and manage UI.

A thorough and comprehensive assessment of the underlying contributing factors of UI, and the identification of the type of UI experienced are pivotal in determining appropriate interventions and treatment modalities for those experiencing UI (Benne, 2008; Borrie et al., 2002). Possible outcomes of a thorough comprehensive UI assessment may include individualized targeted interventions and approaches that can lead to improved bladder control, and subsequently, a decrease in the frequency of UI (Benne, 2008). An individualized UI care approach, using multiple interventions is recommended that can assist in improving the QoL of elderly women experiencing UI in LTC (Benne, 2008; Borrieet al., 2002; Bucci, 2007; MacDonald & Butler, 2007).

6.2 Individualizing UI care

It was apparent from the literature that continence care is comprised of rituals and routines evidenced by scheduled toileting regimes, quotas of incontinent products and procedures for changing of incontinent products. These findings suggested the need for individualized and sensitive continent care for women living in LTC. Individualized care embodies "an interdisciplinary approach which acknowledges elders as unique persons and is practiced through consistent caring relationships" (Happ et al, 1996, p.7). Individualized care also encompasses the principles that all behaviour has meaning, that individual needs are best met when behaviour is understood by the care provider, and that the best manner in which to respond to behaviour is by assessment, intervention, and evaluation (Sullivan-Marx and Strumpf, 1996). According to Bucci (2007) for individualized continence care comprehensive identification, assessment, and diagnosis are necessary. The author supports the implementation of the CHAMMP (Continence, History, Assessment, Medications, Mobility, Plan) Tool, which is a comprehensive evaluation tool to assist in developing individualized care plans for those experiencing UI in LTC. The implementation of care plans that are individualized also provides continuity among staff providing continence care to achieve the desired and shared goal of continence for their residents (MacDonald & Butler, 2007). By implementing approaches in care that are matched with the individual's preferences, needs, and capacities, then overall QoL can be improved (Newman, 2000).

6.3 Empowering women experiencing UI in LTC

As cited previously, studies have reported that women experiencing UI attempt to normalize UI into their daily lives by employing self-treatment strategies as opposed to seeking medical attention (Beji et al, 2010; Hagglund & Ahlstrom 2007; Milne & Moore, 2006; Skoner & Haylor, 1993). UI is commonly concealed to preserve a women's sense of identity, and accepted as a normal part of ageing and being a woman (Bradway et al., 2010; Bush et al., 2001; Stewart, 2010). Frequently, elderly women lack knowledge of treatments that are available and are not often presented with opportunities to discuss or explain their UI with healthcare providers (Mardon et al, 2006; Zeznock et al, 2009; Dugan et al, 2001). Dugan et al. (2001) reported that almost 70% of older adults experiencing UI were not asked by their healthcare provider about their UI. Gaps in healthcare providers' knowledge about UI and UI management, discomfort in discussing the topic and attitudes towards UI directly impact upon the quality of continence care elderly women receive in LTC (Du Beau, 2006; Palmer, 2008). Empowering elderly women to regain UI requires education and a shift from providing task related care to incorporating holistic care and opportunities to dialogue with healthcare providers (Lekan-Rutledge, 2004). Empowerment is the practice of assisting individuals to establish control over factors that impact their health (Lau, 2002). Empowerment implies that individuals will assert control over their lives, thus optimizing independence with the support of healthcare providers serving as advocates (Jones & Meleis, 1993). Empowering women to actively participate in their care may lead to managing incontinence more efficiently and effectively (Roe, 2000).

There is a need for educating the public and healthcare providers to dispel the myths and taboos that UI is a normal part of aging, and that the implementation of incontinent products is not the only option or successful solution for UI (Stewart, 2010; Shamliyan et al., 2008). Knowledge regarding alternatives to incontinent products such as habit training, regaining mobility, Kegel exercises, self-management strategies, medications or medical management maybe considered is critical for healthcare providers working in long- term care. Sharing information about possible health promoting interventions and management strategies with women experiencing UI in LTC may provide them with hope for trying alternative methods to incontinence products, while empowering them to make choices and inform decision-making about their continence care. There are too few healthcare providers communicating to the public that UI is treatable, controllable, or preventable (Du Moulin et al., 2009; Zeznock et al., 2009). If more public education and awareness were provided, individuals entering facilities such as long- term care would be better able to manage and understand UI, which in turn potentially may assist in dispelling ageism and ageist practices in LTC.

6.4 Dispelling ageism in LTC

Ageism is a form of discrimination against the elderly causing labelling and stereotyping as a consequence of chronological age (Ward, 2000). Ageism impedes self-esteem and independence, which can lead to marginalization and unsubstantiated assumptions concerning the elderly. Ageism can be manifested by the attitudes of the staff, language used by the staff, lack of decision-making power by women, and lack of decision-making choice by women regarding their incontinent care, such as types of products worn, toileting times, or changing of incontinent products (MacDonald & Butler, 2007). Healthcare providers need to be attentive and reflect on their own attitudes, beliefs, and feelings towards the elderly (Zeznock et al., 2009), given that it dramatically impacts the provision of care, and consequently the self-esteem and psychosocial aspects of the elderly individual (Palmer, 2008). In addition, healthcare providers should be cognisant of their non-verbal and verbal communication, which potentially reinforces ageism. Implementing active therapeutic communication skills are vital for advocating the needs of women experiencing UI in LTC. There exists a lack of knowledge in healthcare providers' perspectives regarding the unique needs of elderly, especially with regards to the provision of individualized and sensitive incontinent care (DuBeau et al., 2007; Zeznock et al., 2009).

Managers are responsible to ensure that their staff is educated about ageism, and it's manifestations in the work place. Managers could also foster a work environment whereby nurses and other healthcare providers can bring forth institutional ageist practices, and injustices without fear of reprisal. Healthcare professional licensing bodies must lobby governments and public policy-makers to incorporate positive awareness of the aging in developing health policies and the allocating of resources to caring for elderly with UI in LTC. Further, nurses and other healthcare providers should actively lobby governments for more healthcare programs and funding for LTC facilities, so that staffing and supplies are adequate to ensure provision of individualized, competent incontinent care. Existing national and provincial continence organizations need to be more vocally active about practice continence care guidelines, which in turn could assist in dispelling myths about incontinence, and potentially decrease ageist attitudes. Healthcare providers must be encouraged to participate in continence care committees within the LTC facilities locally, provincially, and internationally in order to attain knowledge about current evidenced-based continence care practices.

7. Implications for education

Nurses, physicians, and other healthcare providers must be educated about the implications of UI on the QoL of elderly women, a topic that is still rarely discussed, poorly understood, and considered taboo in some cultural groups. Lack of knowledge regarding UI, and the elderly perpetuates ageist attitudes of healthcare providers and consequently, negatively impacts the provision of quality and sensitive continence care. It was evident from research that healthcare providers lacked knowledge regarding assessment of UI, provision of individualized continent care, and physical and psychosocial implications of UI. Furthermore, there was little knowledge regarding assisting elderly women with UI or the influence of staff on the UI experience. Therefore, it is imperative to incorporate knowledge regarding UI into core curriculum of Nursing Undergraduate and Graduate programs, LPN programs, PCW programs, Medical Schools, and other health care professionals' education. This would help dispel the myth that UI is a normal part of ageing, while assisting healthcare providers to reflect on their own beliefs and bias regarding the elderly and UI. Furthermore, healthcare providers must be educated to initiate conversations and be confident in dialoguing about UI with elderly women, as it is a sensitive topic rarely discussed by the individual experiencing UI. While dialoguing about UI, healthcare providers should be cognisant of the ageist terminology that maybe barriers to communication and empowering women. Healthcare providers ought to be advocates and educate elderly women in LTC that experiencing UI is not normal, and there are treatment options and methods to assist in controlling UI other than incontinent products.

It is essential that mandatory continence care programs be incorporated into the orientation of new staff to LTC facilities, as nurses are often the first contact of elderly experiencing incontinent problems. A continence care program could include tools to assess, implement, and evaluate continence care and include strategies to prevent episodes of incontinence that are individualized. Another component of the educational program for healthcare providers in LTC could involve role playing, whereby each of the staff must wear an incontinent product that has been saturated with water over gym clothing, or have them lying in a bed with another staff member changing their incontinent product. Role playing is a unique interactive learning method whereby staff may appreciate what it is like to experience UI first hand. Additionally, management in LTC facilities must form partnerships with the staff in planning, implementing, and evaluating such a program for it to be successful (Palmer, 1995). Administrators, managers, and owners of LTC facilities must be educated about the negative implications that short staffing and budgeting has on elderly women's experiences with UI in LTC. It is fundamental that management and staff attend educational conferences and in-services pertaining to UI to ensure that their knowledge is current, evidence-based and without bias from incontinent companies seeking considerable profits.

Staff and managers of LTC facilities must lobby governments to formalize initiatives to educate and recruit new staff to the field of Gerontology and long-term care, so that caring for the elderly will be viewed as a valuable and a respected place for employment. Advanced Nursing Practice in Gerontology and nurse-led continence clinics must be encouraged, and financially supported to optimize health promotion and standards of care for the elderly living in LTC (Borrie et al., 2002).

8. Implications for future research

Research is required to improve and advance evidence-based continence care practices. From the literature it is evident there are areas where further research is recommended. One potential area for further research is the impact of culture, economic and social factors associated with elderly women's experiences and perceptions of UI in LTC. This research would provide healthcare providers with the knowledge to understand the implications of UI on the QoL of elderly women, and assist in implementation strategies to ensure individualized continent care. With regards to cultural factors affecting women's perceptions of UI, it would be interesting to complete a research study with extended families where long- term care would not be considered an option, and to explore how significant an impact ageism has on a women's experience with UI. Also, to complete a comparative study of for profit and non-profit LTC facilities to determine differences and similarities in the experiences women have with UI. Further, conduct research on the prevention of UI in elderly women, design and test interventions that are based on evidence, and research that supports the implementation of nurse-led continence clinics that are cost-effective. More research that improves the diagnosis, treatments and management strategies, and outcomes is necessary to guide evidenced-based clinical practice for elderly women with UI in LTCis needed (Borrie et al., 2002; MacDonald & Butler, 2007; Du Moulin et al., 2009). Du Beau et al (2007) suggested that more research is required that determines residents' and families' definitions and values of "quality" UI care and how to incorporate them into quality improvement strategies. More research that address nurses' attitudes, and their cultural and ethnic perspectives about UI are imperative to advancing continence care practices (Zeznock et al., 2009).

A comparative study to explore similarities and differences between younger women experiencing UI and older women experiencing UI in LTC could be conducted. The knowledge attained from this type of study would be fundamental to care of all women experiencing UI in LTC. This research could assist healthcare providers to understand the impact of ageing, which potentially may optimize the quality of incontinent care. Also, a research study that developed and implemented an individualized continence care program in LTC is essential given the current state of knowledge about continence care. Such a study could combine quantitative and qualitative methods. Further, more research that considers gender is essential to understanding the impact of UI on elderly women's QoL, and research that addresses the psychological, social, economic, and/or physical implications and contexts of UI, is crucial to developing and implementing holistic and quality continence care programs.

9. Conclusion

The minimal literature on such a specialized topic as UI in elderly women in LTC necessitates the use of literature that may be considered by some to be a little outdated. However, the relevance of this valuable research and insights into the topic continues to offer support in the absence of more recent research contributions. A review of the literature on UI in elderly women indicates that much of research has concentrated on the medicalization of UI, as evidenced by the predominance of diagnostic and surgical treatment regimes. Many of the studies found were quantitative, employing convenience samples of elderly women in treatment facilities or in the community, with wide age variances. Thus, these studies were not representative of the larger population of incontinent elderly women, who according to the literature, tend to harbour the secret of incontinence..Furthermore, much of the existing literature continues to explore UI from the contexts the physical and economic burdens of UI, the marginalization of elderly women experiencing UI in long- term care, and healthcare providers' attitudes, approaches, and strategies to managing UI in LTC. There is a lack of research found regarding elderly women's experiences of UI in LTC or the psychosocial impacts of UI on elderly women. Although, 80% of elderly women in one study indicated that UI was more than a minor problem, it was apparent from the literature that many healthcare providers considered UI a normal part of the aging process and a management issue, rather than a healthcare issue (Taunton et al., 2005).

Evident from the literature was the diversity in definitions and perspectives pertaining to UI, which may cause confusion and ambiguity for elderly women, healthcare providers and society. There exists a need to clearly define UI, so that there is common language to discuss UI, and common meanings about solutions and interventions for UI (Palmer, 1996; Zeznock et al., 2010). This in turn, may potentially assist in dispelling misconceptions and myths about UI, while providing elderly women with terms to foster discussions with healthcare providers about their experiences with UI.

Existing literature on elderly women's experiences with UI indicates that UI negatively impacts physical, social and emotional aspects of health, contributing to women feeling anxious, embarrassed and unwilling to participate in a wide range of activities. However, to what extent age impacts on the psychosocial effects of UI is unclear due to wide age variances in many of the study samples. Of the literature found, three of the studies (DuBeau et al, 2006; Sandvik et al., 1993; Whyman et al., 1987) quantified the psychosocial consequences of UI in elderly women, which supported the negative impact of UI. One qualitative study found described the meaning of UI to elderly women living in LTC (MacDonald & Butler, 2007). Another qualitative study by Dowd (1991) suggested that older women's UI posed a threat to their self-esteem and in order to maintain control of their lives implemented self-care strategies. However, this study neglected to discuss the self-care strategies that elderly women employed to maintain their self-esteem.

Also apparent from the literature is the importance of the physical and economic burdens of UI. Although the literature does cite the psychosocial, physical and economic burdens of UI on elderly women, few explored how these burdens impact QoL or a sense of well-being for incontinent elderly women in LTC. As well, research is needed that explores the knowledge, attitudes and behaviours of the public related to UI to develop strategies that will assist in educating the public and dispel myths and ageist perceptions about the elderly.

The research reviewed revealed that elderly women in society are marginalized by gender and age, which in turn contributes to the lack of health maintenance services for elderly women. Some literature findings reflected some healthcare providers' stereotypes of ageing further marginalized elderly women and devalued their concerns and stories, which silenced them. Yet, throughout the literature, the management of UI in LTC was emphasized. Nurses and other healthcare providers focused on the management of the soiling, and many viewed UI as a task for which incontinent products were the solution. UI care was found to be frustrating, time-consuming and comparable to a housekeeping task by healthcare professionals. The literature asserted that strategies such as pad use, fluid management, and voiding schedules were implemented by nursing staff in an attempt to reduce or eliminate UI. Unfortunately, fluid management put the elderly at risk for dehydration while voiding schedules were not individualized by nursing staff. Some literature addressed the need for comprehensive assessments and the importance of individualized continence care.

According to the research available elderly women experiencing UI practiced a number of self-management strategies; secrecy, isolation, frequent voiding, using incontinent products, reducing fluid intake, clothing changes, and wearing scents. Elderly women preferred to normalize UI into daily routines, thus preventing shame and embarrassment. Further research is required that allows elderly women to tell their stories about UI, and explore the impact of UI on women's sense of identity. By generating new knowledge, misconceptions and myths surrounding UI in elderly women can be dispelled. Knowledge will further nurses' and other healthcare providers' understanding of the meanings and effects of UI on women's QoL and sense of self, ultimately impacting healthcare practices of caring for elderly women experiencing UI in LTC.

10. Acknowledgement

I would like to acknowledge all elderly women experiencing UI in Long-term care, Dr. Lorna Butler, Dean of Nursing at the University of Saskatchewan, The Nova Scotia Gerontological Nursing Society, Atlantic Aboriginal Health Research Program (AAHRP) funding, Electa MacLennan and Margaret Cragg Scholarships, Dalhousie University, Ruby Blois Scholarship, IWK Health Centre, Halifax, Nova Scotia, Astra Zeneca Rural Scholarship, and Canadian Nurses Association.

11. References

Bayliss, V. & Salter, L. (2004). Pathways for Evidenced-based Continence Care. *Nursing Standard*, Vol.19, No.9, (November 10-16, 2004), pp. 45-52 ISSN: 0029-6570

Beji, N. K., Ozzbas, A., Aslan, E., Biligic, D. & Erkan, H. A. (2010).Overview of the Social Impact of Urinary Incontinence with a Focus on Turkish Women. *Urologic Nursing,* Vol.30, No.6, (November-December, 2010), pp.327-334, ISSN 1053-816X

Benne, J. (2008). Correct assessment is key to treatment. *Long-Term Living.* Vol. 57, No.4, (April 2008), pp. 32-34, ISSN 1940-9958

Bernard, M. (1998). Backs to the future? Reflections on women, ageing and Nursing. *Journal of Advanced Nursing,* Vol.27, No.3, (March 1998), pp. 633-640, ISSN 0309-2402

Birgersson, A. M., Hammar, V., Widerfors, G., Hallberg, I. R. & Athlin, E. (1993). Elderly Women's Feelings about Being Urinary Incontinent, Using Napkins and Being Helped by Nurses to Change Napkins. Journal of Clinical Nursing, Vol. 2, No.3,(May 1993), pp.165-171, ISSN1365-2702

Blaire, K. & White, N. (1998). Are Older Women Offered Adequate Health Care? *Journal of Gerontological Nursing,* Vol.24, No.10, (October, 1998), pp. 39-44 ISSN 0098-9134

Borrie, M. J., Bawden, M., Speechley, M. & Kloseck, M. (2002). Interventions led by Nurse Continence Advisors in the Management of Urinary Incontinence: A Randomized Controlled Trial. *Canadian Medical Association Journal,* Vol.166, No.10, (May 2002), pp.1267-1273, ISSN 0820-3946

Bradway, C., Dahlberg, B. A. & Barg, F. K. (2010). How Women Conceptualize Urinary Incontinence: A Cultural Model. *Journal of Women's Health,* Vol.19, No. 8, (December 2009), pp. 1533-1541, ISSN 1931-843X

Bradway, C.K.W. (2004) Narratives of Women with Long-term Urinary Incontinence. Nursing Dissertation. University of Pennsylvania,USA.

Brink, C. A. (1990). Absorbent Pads, Garments, and Management Strategies. *Journal of the American Geriatrics Society,* Vol.38, No.3, (March 1990), pp. 368-373, ISSN: 0002-8614

Bucci, A.T. (2007). Be a continence champion: Use the CHAMMP tool to individualize the plan of care. *Geriatric Nursing,* Vol.28, No.2, (March-April 2007), pp. 120-125, ISSN 0197-4572

Bush, T.A., Castellucci, D.Y., & Phillips, C. (2001). Exploring Women's Beliefs Regarding Urinary Incontinence. *Urologic Nursing,* Vol.21, No.3, (June 2001), pp. 211-218, ISSN 1053-816X

Coward, R., Horne, C., & Peek, C. (1995). Predicting Nursing Homes Admissions among Incontinent Older Adults: A comparison of Residential Differences across Six Years. *The Gerontologist,* Vol.35, No.6, (December 1995) pp.732- 743, ISSN 0016-9013

Day, R.A., Paul, P., Williams, B., Smeltzer, S.C. & Bare, B. (2010). *Brunner & Suddarth's textbook of medical-surgical nursing (2nd Canadian Ed).* ISBN ISBN-13: 978-0-781-799898 PA, USA.

Dowd, T. (1991). Discovering older women's experiences of urinary incontinence. *Research in Nursing and Health,* Vol.14, No.3, (September 1990), pp.179-186, ISSN1098-240X

DuBeau, C., Simon, S. E. & Morris, J. N. (2006). The Effect of Urinary Incontinence on Quality of Life in Older Nursing Home Residents. *Journal of the American Geriatrics Society,* Vol.54, No.9, (September 2006), pp. 1325-1334, ISSN 00028614

DuBeau, C. E., Ouslander, J. G. & Palmer, M. H. (2007). Knowledge and attitudes of nursing home staff and surveyors about the revised federal guidance for incontinence care. *Gerontologist,* Vol.47, No.4, (August 2007), pp. 468-479, ISSN 0016-9013

Dugan, E., Roberts, C.P., Cohen, S. J., Preisser, J. S., Davis, C. C., Bland, D. R. & Albertson, E. (2001). Why older community- dwelling adults do not discuss urinary incontinence with their primary care physicians. *Journal of the American Geriatrics Society,* Vol.49, No.4 (April 2001), pp. 462-465, ISSN 0002-8614

Du Moulin M. F. M. T., Hamers, P. P. H., Ambergen, A. W. & Halfens, R. J. G. (2009). Urinary Incontinence in Older Adults Receiving Home Care Diagnosis and Strategies. *Scandinavian Journal of Caring Sciences,* Vol.23, No.2, (June 2009), pp. 222-230, ISSN 0283-9318

Earthy, A. & Nativ, A. (2009). Incontinence. *Long-Term Living,* Vol. 58, No.3, (March 2009), pp. 24-25, ISSN 1940-9958

Edwards, D. J. (2001). Nonsurgical Options for Treating Incontinence. *Nursing Homes Long Term Care Management,* Vol.50, No.5, (May 2001), pp.40-42, ISSN 1061-4753

Freundl, M. & Dugan, J. (1992).Urinary incontinence in the elderly: Knowledge and attitude of long-term care staff. Geriatric Nursing, Vol.13, No.2, (March/April 1992), pp.70-75, ISSN 0197-4572

Gallagher, M. (1998). Urogenital distress and the psychosocial impact of urinary incontinence on elderly women. *Rehabilitation Nursing,* Vol.23, No.4, (July-August, 1998), pp. 192-197, ISSN 0278-4807

Getliffe, K, Fader, M., Cottenden, A., Jamesion, K. & Green, N. (2007). Absorbent Products for Incontinence: 'Treatment Effects' and Impact on Quality of Life. *Journal of Clinical Nursing,* Vol.16, No.10, (October 2007), pp. 1936-1945, ISSN 0962-1067

Goldstein, M., Hawthorne, M., Engeberg, S., McDowell, J., & Burgio, K. (1992). Urinary Incontinence: Why people do not seek help. *Journal of Gerontological Nursing,* Vol.18, No.4, (April 1992), pp. 15-20, ISSN 0098-9134

Hagglund, D. & Ahlstrom, G. (2007). The Meaning of Women's Experience of Living with Long-term Urinary Incontinence is Powerless. J*ournal of* clinical Nursing, Vol. 16, No.10, (October 2007), pp.1946-1954, ISSN: 0962-1067

Hagglund, D. & Wadensten, B. (2007). Fear of Humiliation Inhibits Women's Care-Seeking Behaviour for Long-term Urinary Incontinence. *Scandinavian Journal of Caring Sciences,* Vol.21, No.3, (August 2007), pp. 305-312, ISSN 0283-9318

Herzog, A., Fultz, N., Normolle, D., Brock, B., & Diokno, A. (1989). Methods used to manage urinary incontinence by older adults in the community. Journal of the American Geriatrics Society, Vol.37, No.4, (April 1989), pp. 339-347, ISSN 0002-8614

Horrocks , S, Somerset M, Stoddart H & Peters T. (2004). What prevents older people from seeking treatment for urinary incontinence? A qualitative exploration of barriers to the use of community continence services. *Family Practice,* Vol. 21, No.6, (March 2004), pp. 689–96, ISSN 0263- 2136

Howard, F. & Steggall, M. (2010). Urinary Incontinence in women: Quality of life and help-seeking. *British Journal of Nursing,* Vol.19, No.12, (June 2010), pp. 742-749, ISSN 0966-0461

Hu, T. (1990). Impact of urinary incontinence on health-care costs. *Journal of the American Geriatrics Society,* Vol.38, No. 11, (November 1990), pp. 292-295, ISSN 0002-8614

Hu, T., Kaltreider, L., & Igou, J. (1990). The cost-effectiveness of disposable versus reusable diapers: A controlled experiment in a nursing home. Journal of *Gerontological Nursing,* Vol.16, No.2, pp.19-24, ISSN 0098-9134

Huang, A. J., Brown, J. S., Kanaya, A. M., Creaseman, J. M., Ragins, A. L. Van Den Eeden, S. K. (2006). Quality-of-Life Impact and Treatment of Urinary Incontinence in Ethnically Diverse Older Women. *Archives of Internal Medicine,* Vol.166, No.18, (October 2006), pp. 2000-2006, ISSN 0003-9926

Hunskaar, S. & Vinsnes, A. (1991). The Quality of Life of Women With Urinary Incontinence as Measured by the Sickness Impact Profile. *Journal of the American Geriatrics Society,* Vol.39, No.4, (April 1991), pp.378-382, ISSN 0002-8614

International Continence Society (2011). *About the ICS.* 15.06.2010. Available from http://www.icsoffice.org/About.aspx.

Jones, P. S. & Meleis, A. I. (1993). Health is Empowerment. Advances in Nursing Science, Vol.15, No.3, (March 1993), pp.1-14, ISSN1550-5014

Klusch, L. (2003). Targeting our approach to incontinence. *Nursing Homes,* Vol.52, No.12, (December 2003), pp.28, ISSN 1061-4753

Lau, D. H. (2002). Patient empowerment—a patient-centred approach to improve care. Hong Kong Medical Journal, Vol.8, No.5, (October 2002), pp.372-374, ISSN 1024-2708

Lekan-Rutledge, D. (2004). Urinary incontinence strategies for frail elderly women. *Urologic Nursing,* Vol.24, No.4, (August 2004), pp. 281-301, ISSN 1053-816X

Lifford, K. L., Townsend, M. K., Curhan, G. C., Resnick, N. M. & Grodstein, F. (2008). The Epidemiology of Urinary Incontinence in Older Women, Incidence, Progression, and Remission. *Journal of the American Geriatrics Society,* Vol. 56, No. 7, (July 2008), pp.1191-1198, ISSN 0002-8614

Loughrey, L. (1999). Taking a Sensitive Approach to Urinary Incontinence. *Nursing,* Vol.29, No.5, (May 1999), pp. 60-61 ISSN 0360-4039

MacDonald, C., Butler, L. (2007). Silent no more: Elderly women's stories of living with urinary incontinence in long-term care. *Journal of Gerontological Nursing,* Vol.14, No.20, (January 2007), pp. 14-20, ISSN 0098-9134

Mardon, R. E., Hanlin, S., Pawlson, L. G. & Haffer, S. C. (2006). Management of Urinary Incontinence in Medicare-managed Care Beneficiaries: Results from the 2004 Medicare Health Outcomes Survey. *Archives of Internal Medicine,* Vol.166, No.10, (May 2006), pp. 1128-1133, ISSN 0003-9926

McDermott, P. (2010). Review of the Factors Influencing Continence Care. *Journal of Community Nursing,* Vol.24, No.1, (January 2010), pp. 4-7, ISSN 1462-4753

Milne, J. L., & Moore, K.N. (2006). Factors impacting self-care for urinary incontinence. *Urologic Nursing,* Vol.26, No.1, (February 2006), pp.41-51. ISSN 1053-816X

Mitteness, L. (1990). Elder care: Social aspects of urinary incontinence in the elderly. *Journal of the American Geriatrics Society,* Vol.38, No.3, (March 1990), pp. 374-378, ISSN 0002-8614

Monz, B., Chartier-Kastler. E., Hampel, C., Samsioe, G., Hunskaar, S., Espuna-Pons, M., Wagg, A., Quail, D., Castro, R. & Chinn, C. (2007). Patient characteristics associated with quality of life in European women seeking treatment for urinary incontinence: Results from PURE. *European Urology,* Vol.51, No.4, (October 2007), pp.1073-1081, ISSN 0302-2838

Newman, D. (2000). New technologies for stress urinary incontinence. *Contemporary OB/GYN,* Vol.45, (April 2000), pp. 69-83, ISSN 0090-3159

Nitti, V. W. (2001). Overactive bladder: Strategies for effective evaluation and Management. *Contemporary Urology,* Available from http://proquest.umi.com/pdq ...3&Fmt=Del =1&Mtd= 1&Idx= 3&Sid= 1&RQT=309 ISSN 1042-2250

Nix, D. & Haugen, V. (2010). Incontinence-associated Dermatitis. *Long-Term Living,* Vol.59, No.3, (March 2010), pp.32- 33, ISSN1940-9958

Norton, C. (1982). The effects of urinary incontinence in women. *International Rehabilitation Medicine,* Vol.4, No.1, pp. 9-14, ISSN 0379-0797

Norton, P. & Brubaker, L. (2006). Urinary Incontinence in Women. The Lancet, Vol. 367, No. 9504, (January, 2006), pp. 57-67, ISSN 0140-6736

O'Dell, K.K., Jacelon, C., & Morse, A.N. (2008). 'I'd rather just go on as I am'- Pelvic floor care preferences of frail, elderly women in residential care. *Urological Nursing*, Vol.28, No.1, (February 2008), pp. 36-47, ISSN1053-816X

Palmer, M. H. (1995). Nurses' knowledge and beliefs about continence interventions in long–term care. *Journal of Advanced Nursing*, Vol. 21, No. 6, (June 1995), pp. 1065-1072, ISSN: 0309-2402

Palmer, M. H. (1996). *Urinary Continence: Assessment and Promotion.* ISBN 0834207478, Gaithersburg, MD, United States of America

Palmer, M.H. (2008). Urinary incontinence quality improvement in nursing homes: Where Have we been? Where are we going? *Urologic Nursing*, Vol. 28, No. 6, (December 2008), pp.439-444, ISSN 1053-816X

Parker, K. F. (2007). The management of urinary incontinence. *Drug Topics*, Vol. 151, No. 18, (September 2007), pp. 69-76, ISSN 0012-6616

Resnick, N. (1997). Discussion: Theoretical and Practical Considerations in Modeling Outcomes in Urge Urinary Incontinence. *Urology*, Vol.50, No.6a, (December 1997), pp. 109-110 ISSN 0090-4295

Resnick, N. (1992). Urinary incontinence in older adults. *Hospital Practice*, Vol.32, No.10, (October 1992), pp. 139-184, ISSN 2154-8331

Robinson, J. P. (2000). Managing Urinary Incontinence in the Nursing Home Residents' Perspectives. *Journal of Advanced Nursing*, Vol. 31, No.1, (January, 2000), pp. 68-77, ISSN 1523-6064

Roe, B. (2000). Effective and ineffective management of incontinence: Issues around illness trajectory and health care. *Qualitative Health Research*, Vol.10, No.5, (September 2000), pp. 677-690, ISSN1049-7323

Rolls, E. .C. (1997). Night Time Sleep in a Nursing Home. Unpublished Master's Thesis, Dalhousie University, Halifax, Nova Scotia, Canada.

Romanzi, L. (2010). Vaginal Rejuvention defined. 15.05.2010, Available from www.urogynics.org/blog/2010/ vaginalrejuventiondefined

Sahyoun, N., Pratt, L., Lentzner, H., Day, A. & Robinson, K. (2001) The changing profile of nursing home residents: 1985-1997, 39.10.2004Availablefrom http://www.cdc.gov /nchs/data/agingtrends/04nursin.pdf

Sandvik, H., Kveine, E., & Hunskaar, S. (1993). Female Urinary Incontinence: Psychosocial impact, self care, and consultations. *Scandinavian Journal of Caring* Sciences, Vol.7, No.1, (May 1993), pp. 53-56, ISSN 0283-9318

Schnelle, J .F. (1991). *Managing Urinary Incontinence in the Elderly.* ISBN 0826173608, New York: United States of America

Sharpe, P. (1995). Older women and health services: Moving from Ageism Toward Empowerment. *Women and Health*, Vol.22, No.3, pp. 9-23, ISSN 0363-0242

Simons, J. (1985). Does incontinence affect your client's self concept? *Journal of Gerontological Nursing*, Vol.11, No.6, (June 1985), pp. 37-42, ISSN 0098-9134

Skoner, M. M, & Haylor, M. J. (1993). Managing incontinence: Women's normalizing strategies. *Health Care for Women International*, Vol.14, No.6, (November-December 1993), pp. 549- 560, ISSN 0739-9332

Smedley, G. (1991). Addressing sexuality in the elderly. *Rehabilitation Nursing*, Vol.16, No. 1, (January-February 1991), pp. 9-11, ISSN 0278-4807

Steinke, E. (1988). Older Adults' Knowledge and Attitudes About Sexuality and Aging. *Image: Journal of Nursing Scholarship*, Vol. 20, No.2, (June 1988), pp. 93-95, ISSN: 0743-5150

Stewart, E. (2010). Treating Urinary Incontinence in Older Women. *British Journal of Community Nursing*, Vol.15, No. 11, (November 2010), pp.526-532, ISSN 1462-4753

Sullivan-Marx, E., & Strumpt, N, (1996). Restraint -free care for acutely ill patients in the hospital, Advanced Practice in Acute and Critical Care Clinical Issues, Vol.7, No.4, (November 1996), pp. 572-578, ISSN 15597768

Taunton, R.L., Swagerty, F.D.I., Lasseter, J.A., Lee, R.H. (2005). "Continent or Incontinent? That is the question". *Journal of Gerontological Nursing*, Vol.31, No.9, (September 2005), pp. 36- 44, ISSN 0098-9134

Thakar, R. & Stanton, S. (2000). Management of Urinary Incontinence in Women. British Medical Journal, Vol.321, No.7272, (November 2000), pp.1326-1331, ISSN 0959-8138

Thom, D., Haan, M., & Van Den Eeden, S. (1997). Medically recognized urinary incontinence and risks of hospitalization, nursing home admissions and mortality. *Age and Ageing*, Vol.26, No. 5, (September 1997), pp. 367-374, ISSN: 0002-0729

Tulloch, J. (1989). The incontinency taboo. *Geriatric Nursing*, Vol.10, No.1, (January/February 1989), pp. 19, ISSN 0197-4572

Vinsnes, A. G., Harkless, G. E., Haltbakk, J., Bohm, J., & Hunskaar, S. (2001). Healthcare personnel's attitudes towards patients with urinary incontinence. *Journal of Clinical Nursing*, Vol.10, No.4, (July 2004), pp. 455-462, ISSN 0962-1067

Wagg, A., Milan, S., Lowe, D. & Potter, J., (2004). Pilot of the National Audit of Continence Care for Older People (England & Wales). Available from http://www.rcplondon.ac.uk/college/ceeu/ceeu_coop_home.htm

Ward, D (2000). Ageism and the abuse of older people in health and social work. *British Journal of Nursing*, Vol.9, No.9, (May 2003), pp. 560-563, ISSN 0966-0461

Walters, K., Iliffe, S., & Orrell, M. (2001). An exploration of help- seeking behaviour in older people with unmet needs. *Family Practice*, Vol.18, No.3, (January 2001), pp. 277-282, ISSN 0263- 2136

Watson, N.M., Brink, C.A., Zimmer, J.G. & Mayer, R.D., (2003) Use of the agency for heath care policy and research urinary incontinence guideline in nursing homes. *Journal of the American Geriatrics Society*, Vol. 51, No.12, (December 2003), pp. 1779-1786, ISSN0002-8614

Whyman, J., Harkins, S., Choi, S., Taylor, J., & Fantl, A. (1987). Psychosocial impact of urinary incontinence in women. *Obstetrics & Gynecology*, Vol.70, No.3, (September 1987), pp.378-381, ISSN 0029-7844

Wilson, M. M. G. (2003). Urinary Incontinence: Bridging the Gender Gap. *The Journals of Gerontology*, Vol.58A, No.8, (August 2003), pp.752-755, ISSN 1079-5006

Yu, H.J., Wong, W.Y., Chen, J. & Chie, W. C. (2003). Quality of Life Impact and Treatment Seeking Chinese Women with Urinary Incontinence. *Quality of Life Research*, Vol.12, No.3, (May 2003), pp. 327-333, ISSN 0962-9343

Yu, L.C., & Kaltreider, D.L. (1987). Stressed nurses dealing with incontinent patients. *Journal of Gerontological Nursing*, Vol.13, No. 1, (January 1987), pp.27-30, ISSN 0098-9134

Zeznock, D. E., Gilje, F. L. & Bradway, C. (2009). Living with Urinary Incontinence: Experiences of Women from 'The Last Frontier'. *Urologic Nursing*, Vol.29, No. 3, (May-June 2009), pp. 157-185, ISSN: 1053-816X

7

Geriatric Urinary Incontinence – Special Concerns on the Frail Elderly

Verdejo-Bravo Carlos
Servicio de Geriatría, Hospital Clínico San Carlos
Universidad Complutense, Madrid
Spain

1. Introduction

Since the last decades, the elderly population is growing significantly and the projection for the next 20-25 years is that the range of over 80 is increasing. Frailty is accepted as a syndrome of late-life decline and vulnerability that serves as a warning sign for adverse health outcomes and for mortality. The identification of vulnerable, frail, adults may allow the development of preventive interventions which help to maintain good health and high quality of life well into the 8th and 9th decade of life.

Urinary incontinence (UI) is considered one of the main giants of Geriatrics, described by Sir Bernard Isaacs in 1976, and it has also included in the list of the Geriatric syndromes. The combination of a frail elderly and UI could be very negative due to its adverse effects both in terms of health as well as on quality of life.

Nowadays, the appropriate extent of diagnostic process in the elderly incontinent is not well established. In general, healthy older patients should receive the same diagnostic scheme as younger patients. By contrast, in frail older people an individual assessment is mandatory in order to decide the step of our diagnostic intervention. In the same way, the medical management of the younger elderly patients should be very similar to the young patients. But, the frailest elderly patients should be managed individually, adapting the different levels of intervention to the complexity of the frail elderly.

As a matter of fact, the appropriate knowledge of older population, the level of vulnerability and their true possibilities of improve with our intervention is very important to decide the best way of treating this syndrome in the frailest population.

2. Frailty: Current definition and main characteristics of the frail elderly

The concept of frailty as a specific syndrome has based on the clinical experience of geriatricians and usually is clinically well recognizable. Usually it is characterized by weakness, weight loss, and low activity and is associated with adverse health outcomes (including falls, incident disability, hospitalization, and mortality) (Xue, 2011; Fedarco, 2011).

Frailty is a non-specific state of vulnerability, which reflects multisystem physiological change. These changes do not always means a disease status, so some very elderly, are frail without a specific life threatening illness. Current thinking is that, not only the physical way contributes to this syndrome, because also psychological, cognitive, and social factors take a decisive role and need to be taken into account in its definition and treatment.

Together, these signs and symptoms seem to reflect a reduced functional reserve and consequent decrease in adaptation to different type of stressors, and perhaps even in the absence of extrinsic stressors. The overall consequence is that frail elderly are at higher risk for accelerated physical and cognitive decline, disability and death. All these frailty's characteristics can easily be applied to the definition and characterization of the aging process per se, and there is little consensus in the literature concerning the physiological/biological pathways associated with or determining frailty. It is probably true to say that a consensus view would implicate heightened chronic systemic inflammation as a major contributor to frailty (Fulop et al, 2011).

Many other authors have focused on the popular definition proposed and tested in the Cardiovascular Health Study in the United States and known as the phenotypic definition of frailty. That study defined frailty by the occurrence of at least 3 of the following 5 deficits in an individual: slow walking speed, impaired grip strength, a self-report of declining activity levels, unintended weight loss, or exhaustion. In addition to the phenotypic and other approaches, frailty is considered as a risk state caused by the age-associated accumulation of deficits (Rockwood & Mitnitski, 2011).

The frailty can be considered as a complex phenomenon, with multiple links and interactions between the clinical, functional, mental and social components. In this sense, the use of the Geriatric Comprehensive Assessment (GCA) could be very useful in the detection of the frail condition of an older people. Through assessment of general health (comorbidity), function, cognition, mood and motivation, the special senses, nutrition and medications, this tool facilitates identification of health issues and the appropriate intervention and follow-up for them. As part of a comprehensive management plan, CGA also supports continued independence and improved quality of life for an individual in association with reduced medical costs (Rockwood & Mitnitski, 2011; Rosen & Reuben, 2011).

Based on these concepts, a frail elderly would be a very old person (usually more than 80-85 years), with high comorbidity, functional handicaps, cognitive impairment and also limitations in the familiar and social areas. In this group of older persons, it is expected the highest known prevalence of UI of any group of age (around 50-70%).

In frail elderly, UI constitutes a syndromic model with multiple interacting risk factors, such as age-related physiologic changes, comorbidity, and common pathways between them, in which the accumulated effects of multiple impairments increase vulnerability to situational changes (Inouye et al, 2007).

3. Aging of the urinary tract – Role of the comorbidity and the polypharmacy

With aging, the lower urinary tract undergoes to a series of morphological and/or functional changes that can lead to a different dynamic behaviour and the possibility of alterations in urine storage and bladder emptying functions. These functions as well as urinary continence are maintained due to the integrity of the lower urinary tract, the nervous system, the visceral supporting mechanism (pelvic floor) and the urine production mechanism. There must also be adequate perception and interpretation of the urge to pass urine, as well as the physical capacity to go to the toilet and to perform the activity.

The most relevant changes of lower urinary tract with aging are listed in Table 1.

Bladder	**Morphologic changes:** **↑ trabeculation** **↑ fibrosis** **↓ autonomic nerves** **Diverticula's formation** **Functional changes:** **↓ capacity** **↓ ability to put off micturition** **= ↓ contractility** **↑ involuntary contractions** **↑ post voiding residual volume**
Urethra	**Anatomical changes:** **↓ cellularity** **↑ collagen deposit** **Functional changes:** **↓ closure pressure** **↓ outflow resistance**
Prostate	**Enlargement, hyperplasia**
Vagina	**↓ cellularity** **epithelium atrophy**
Pelvic floor	**↑ collagen deposit** **↑ connective tissue ratio** **Muscle weakness**

Table 1. Lower urinary tract: main physiological changes with aging

In general, it is accepted that detrusor muscle contractility, bladder capacity and ability to put off micturition decrease in both sexes with aging. In addition, the prevalence of bladder hyperactivity increases. In women the maximum pressure of urethral closure and length of the functional urethra decreases, and post-micturition bladder residual volume increases up to 50-100 ml. Physiologically, elderly people tend to excrete more urine at night, even when there are no exacerbating factors such as heart failure, venous insufficiency, renal disease or prostatism. In men the prostate increases in volume meanwhile hypoestrogenism in women affects both the genital apparatus and urinary tract. Thus, the healthy elderly individual is much more vulnerable to suffering urinary pathological processes such as incontinence, infections, urinary retention and outflow obstruction (Verdejo, 2000).

Since the last 10-12 years, the role played by the pelvic floor in micturition dynamics and especially in the maintenance of continence has been increasingly recognised. The age related deterioration in pelvic floor functions has a multifactorial origin (physiological and pathological). With increasing age, a reduction in the muscle fibre/connective tissue ratio has been demonstrated and the connective tissue becomes more elastic with less energy needed to provoke an irreversible lesion. Some of these changes have also been described in multiparous women and in those with pelvic prolapse. As well as oestrogen deficit, other factors contributing to the deterioration of the pelvic floor include mechanical trauma, and neurological denervation. These mechanisms can modify the normal angulation of the posterior wall of the bladder and the proximal urethra, leading to stress incontinence (Verdejo, 2000; Cheng, 2007).

In fact, physiologically, the frail elderly has a high risk to suffer the loss of continence. However, the physiological circumstances of aging, the multiple diseases characteristic of the frail elderly (dementia, motor disorders, cerebrovascular disease, Parkinson's disease, malnutrition), functional deterioration (immobility, dementia) drug treatment (diuretics, psychotropic agents, anticholinergics) (Ruby CM et al, 2010) and even iatrogenic factors (catheterization, physical restriction, adverse reactions) are going to have a significant influence on the function of the lower urinary tract (Verdejo, 2004; DuBeau, 2006).

Nowadays, it is accepted that greater responsibility is given to comorbidity, functional impairment (physical and / or mental) and polypharmacy to justify the prevalence of incontinence in the frailest elderly. Table 2 presents the main medical problems more frequently associated with incontinence in the frail elderly.

Comorbidity	*** Neurological diseases: Stroke; Dementias; Parkinson's disease; spinal cord injury; autonomic and peripheral disautonomies** *** Endocrine diseases: Diabetes Mellitus** *** Cardiac diseases: Heart failure** *** Urological diseases: Benign Prostatic Hyperplasia; Infections; Neoplasms; Lithiasis; Prior Surgery.** *** Digestive diseases: chronic constipation; fecal impaction.** *** Gynaecological pathologies: pelvic floor damage; prolapses; prior surgery**
Functional impairment	**- Cognitive impairment; Dementia** **- Poor mobility; Immobility** **- Dependence on ADL's**

Table 2. Main medical and functional conditions associated with UI in the frail elderly.

However, it is very important to highlight that the pharmacologic treatment play a significant etiologic role in the loss of urinary continence, especially in the frail elderly, and it could be related to different mechanisms. Table 3 presents the main drug groups, along with its mechanism of action, most often associated with loss of continence or worsening the symptoms of incontinence.

MEDICATIONS	EFFECTS ON CONTINENCE
Diuretics	Polyuria, urgency, frequency
Hypnotics	Sedation, impaired mobility, delirium
Antipsychotics	Sedation, impaired mobility, parkinsonism, delirium
Anticholinergics	Delirium, stool impaction, urinary retention
Triciclic Antidepressants	Sedation, anticholinergic effect
Opioid analgesics	Immobility, stool impaction, delirium, urinary retention
Cholinesterase inhibitors	Increase bladder contractility, urgency
Selective Serotonin Reuptake Inhibitor	Stimulation of cholinergic bladder receptors, sedation
α-adrenergic antagonists	Decrease urethral resistance
Angiotensin Converting Enzyme inhibitors	Cough
Calcium antagonists	Constipation, stool impaction, urinary retention

Table 3. Main drugs that can be associated with UI, with their mechanism of action

4. Geriatric urinary incontinence – Main clinical types in the frail population

There are several types of UI in the frail elderly population, and more frequently than other age groups, it could presents in a mixed form (urge + stress; detrusor hyperactivity with impaired contractility).

A practical and useful approach to the frailest incontinent patient is based on its duration (acute or chronic).

4.1 Acute or transient incontinence

Acute or transient incontinence it refers to cases of short course incontinence (lasting less than four weeks), including those situations in which loss of continence is considered to be functional, without any associated structural disorder. This clinical type of UI is very common in the frail elderly, especially in the more complex elderly and with higher disability. In these cases, the medical history and physical examination will often suggest the cause. The use of mnemonic rules (DRIP or DIAPPERS), has been proposed in order to memorize the possible causes (Schröder et al, 2009; Griebling, 2009). (Table 4).

D Delirium Dementia	D Delirium/Dementia
R Restricted Mobility Retention	I Infection
I Infection Inflammation Impaction Stool	A Atrophic vaginitis
P Pharmaceutical agents Polyuria	P Pharmaceutical agents
	P Psychological causes
	E Endocrine conditions
	R Restricted mobility
	S Stool impaction

Table 4. Transient causes of urinary incontinence, based on mnemonic rules

4.2 Chronic or established incontinence

Chronic or established incontinence: it is associated with structural disorders, either in the urinary tract or outside of it, like in the nervous system. Usually the duration of this type of incontinence is over four weeks and some complementary examinations (ultrasounds, urodynamic) will be required to discover its etiology. It is important to emphasize that some transient causes of incontinence may contribute to an established form and that mixed incontinence is more common in the frail elderly population than in other groups of patients.

Mechanisms that are responsible for greater frequency of established incontinence in elderly people are:

4.2.1 Urge incontinence

Urge incontinence: this is the most common type of established incontinence in the older population. Usually underlies detrusor hyperactivity in relationship with several neurological diseases (brain ischemia, dementias, Parkinson's disease). Clinically, this type of UI presents as urgency, frequency and nocturia, and it has a higher impact on quality of life due to the bothersome and the severity of the symptoms.

4.2.2 Stress incontinence

Stress incontinence: this is most common in frail elderly women and uncommon in men, except when the external urethral sphincter has been damaged during prostatic surgery. The causes are generally related to pelvic floor weakness which produces a urethral hypermobility (multiparity, hypoestrogenism, obesity) or previous pelvic surgery (gynaecological, prostatic resection). The urine leakages will be produced with manoeuvres that cause an increase in intra-abdominal pressure (coughing, laughing, sneezing, Valsalva). Usually the length of the symptoms is long, and the impact on quality of life is lower than urge incontinence.

4.2.3 Overflow incontinence

Overflow incontinence: this appears in situations of bladder overdistension. There are two different mechanisms: bladder outlet obstruction (prostatic hyperplasia, urethral stenosis, faecal impaction) and bladder contractile impairment (spinal cord lesions, peripheral and/or autonomic neuropathy, detrusor myopathy, anticholinergic drugs). Within this subgroup of incontinence, a relatively common entity exists, especially in disabled patients, called Detrusor Hyperactivity with Impaired Contractility (DHIC). This term was coined by Resnick in 1987 when he observed a characteristic urodynamic pattern, in an incontinent and disabled elderly group, of uninhibited bladder contractions together with an inability to empty more than 50% of the bladder content (Resnick, 1996). Nowadays, DHIC is considered a subtype of bladder hyperreflexia, but the mechanism that produces bladder contractile impairment is unknown. It is proposed that it may be an evolved phase of bladder hyperreflexia, with the production of muscle failure (Smith PP, 2010). From the clinical point of view, patients may present with both irritative type urinary symptoms (urge, frequency), as well as obstructive type (incomplete voiding, urinary retention). Characteristically, post-voiding residual urine volumes are pathological. Although DHIC generally presents with urge incontinence, it may also manifest with symptoms of obstruction, stress or overflow incontinence. This form of bladder hyperactivity is the second commonest cause of incontinence in institutionalized patients. An episode of urinary retention may occur when some other factor (drugs, immobility, and fecal impaction) further alters bladder contractility (Verdejo, 2004).

4.2.4 Functional incontinence

Functional incontinence: many social and environmental factors, such as lack of carers to assist with toileting, and physical barriers, including bed-restraints, may be responsible for incontinence. However, a diagnosis of functional incontinence should only be accepted by exclusion, once other mechanisms have been ruled out.

4.2.5 Mixed incontinence

Mixed incontinence: many frail older people with chronic incontinence have a combination of different type of incontinence. A combination of urge incontinence and stress is very common. Another type of specific mixed incontinence in the frail elderly is the DHIC as previously has been exposed above.

5. Risks factors of the UI in the frail elderly

From the reports of the main epidemiological studies there have been identified several potential risk factors for UI depending of the characteristics of adult populations. However, the majority of studies have been cross-sectional in design which provides data only on risk factors for prevalent incontinence. Many of these studies are national population-based surveys on the general health of a particular population, and they are limited by the variables included in the study. Longitudinal studies incorporating multivariate analyses that provide data on the risk factors for incident incontinence are scarce. So, the data from studies which included frail population are very few.

In older women, modifiable risk factors included obesity, vaginal trauma, and vaginal prolapse. In general, the risk factors for the various types of UI (stress, urge, and mixed) also vary. Aging tends to be associated with changing risk profiles associated with UI and urge incontinence type. With limited evidence (level IIA from prospective cohort studies), appears that increased body mass index, diabetes mellitus, comorbidities, cognitive decline, and hormone therapy were associated with developing UI in community dwelling females. In men, consistent published evidence (level IIb-III) suggested that poor general health, limitation in daily activities, stroke, diabetes mellitus, and treatments for prostate cancer (mainly surgery) were associated with higher risk of UI in older men (Shamliyan et al, 2007).

Through the analysis of the studies performed in long term care (nursing homes), we know that the prevalence of UI increased with the length of stay, since 39 percent at 2 weeks to 44 percent at 1 year after admission. In that way, the majority of residents with cognitive impairment experienced UI (72 to 84 percent), and the proportion of incontinent patients increased significantly in relationship with the severity of impairment (from 60 percent in mild to 93 percent in severely demented). Physical dependency was associated with a higher prevalence of UI, from 26 percent in independent residents to 81 percent in disabled older patients (Shamliyan et al, 2007). However, few studies examined adjusted odds ratios of UI among residents in long term care independent of other confounding factors. Aging was associated with increased odds of UI by 3 percent per year to 24 percent per 5 years of age (Shamliyan et al, 2007; Offermans et al, 2009).

In addition of the medical conditions, it is very important to highlight the role of the drugs that frequently received the older patients, on the urinary continence, as previously exposed above.

In summary, a poor health status with medical problems especially in the neurological area, a high consumption of drugs (diuretics, psychotropics) and a limited functional status are main risks factors for loss of the continence in the frail elderly population.

6. Impact of urinary incontinence on the quality of life and its assessment

UI produces a wide variety of negative effects on quality of life (QOL) for patients, from medical problems (falls, urinary tract infections, pressure sores, skin's complications, kidney failure, functional decline) to psychological (anxiety, depressive symptoms, insomnia, sadness, loneliness) or social limitations (social isolation, impact on ADL, need of social resources, nursing home admission). It is considered that impact on QOL is similar as produced by Diabetes Mellitus, Stroke or Arthritis (Ko et al, 2005). The patient's perception of the impact of their UI on their lifestyle is very important, and even mild UI has a significant on a patient's QOL, including the frailest population.

Since the last 10 years, the proposal from the International Continence Society and the World Health Organization is assessing the impact of urinary symptoms have on QOL. In fact, clinicians should be aware of it and they should take consideration of the adverse effects that even mild UI has on a patient's QOL. The urinary symptoms and their impact on patient's QOL can be assessed through different ways, but only the objective assessment based on validated questionnaires is the right form (Scottish Intercollegiate Guidelines Network, 2004).

The questionnaires have been validated for measuring the severity of the symptoms and also the impact on QOL. Patterns have been developed to analyze mainly urinary symptoms and other models to know the impact on QOL. Through the urinary questionnaires we can evaluate initial symptoms as well as impact on QOL, and the further modification of the urinary symptoms and their impact on QOL with our intervention.

A list of principal urinary questionnaires is presented in the table 5, and the main combined questionnaires (urinary and QOL) in the table 6.

One of the most practical questionnaires is the Short Form of the International Consultation Incontinence (table 7), which has been validated and translated to 30 languages, and has a high level of recommendation (grade A) by the International Continence Society (Gotoh, 2007).

Urogenital Distress Inventory (UDI)
UDI-SF
Urge UDI
King's Health Questionnaire
Incontinence Severity Index (women)
International Continence Society (men)
International Continence Society male -SF
Bristol Female Lower Urinary Tract Symptoms
Danish Prostatic Symptom Score (men)

Table 5. Principal urinary questionnaires of incontinence

International Consultation on Incontinence Questionnaire (ICIQ) (men and women)
Bristol Female Lower Urinary Tract Symptoms
International Continence Society SF (men)
The Sickness Impact Profile (women)
The Quality of Life of persons with Urinary Incontinence (I-QOL) (men and women)
The Incontinence Impact Questionnaire (women)
The Urogenital Distress Inventory (women)

Table 6. Main combined urinary questionnaires (incontinence and impact on QOL)

ICIQ-SF

Initial number ☐☐ ☐☐ ☐☐☐

DAY ☐☐ MONTH ☐☐ YEAR ☐☐
Today's date

Many people leak urine some of the time. We are trying to find out how many people leak urine, and how much this bothers them. We would be grateful if you could answer the following questions, thinking about how you have been, on average, over the PAST FOUR WEEKS.

1 **Please write in your date of birth:** DAY ☐☐ MONTH ☐☐ YEAR ☐☐

2 **Are you** *(tick one)*: Female ☐ Male ☐

3 **How often do you leak urine?** *(Tick one box)*

never	☐	0
about once a week or less often	☐	1
two or three times a week	☐	2
about once a day	☐	3
several times a day	☐	4
all the time	☐	5

4 **We would like to know how much urine you think leaks.**
How much urine do you usually leak (whether you wear protection or not)? *(Tick one box)*

none	☐	0
a small amount	☐	2
a moderate amount	☐	4
a large amount	☐	6

5 **Overall, how much does leaking urine interfere with your everyday life?**
Please ring a number between 0 (not at all) and 10 (a great deal)

0 1 2 3 4 5 6 7 8 9 10

not at all … a great deal

ICIQ score: sum scores 3+4+5 ☐☐

6 **When does urine leak?** *(Please tick all that apply to you)*

never – urine does not leak	☐
leaks before you can get to the toilet	☐
leaks when you cough or sneeze	☐
leaks when you are asleep	☐
leaks when you are physically active/exercising	☐
leaks when you have finished urinating and are dressed	☐
leaks for no obvious reason	☐
leaks all the time	☐

Thank you very much for answering these questions.

Table 7. The International Consultation on Incontinence Questionnaire Short Form

7. Clinical approach of the urinary incontinence in the frail elderly

Nowadays, there are several evidences about the need of the early detection of UI in older persons, especially in the frail elderly, due to the low index consultation (about 30-50 % of patients), as well as the number of elderly people that received an effective treatment, in spite of the valid alternatives. In this sense, the Assessing Care of Vulnerable Elders, the Fourth Consultation on Incontinence, and the Guidelines on UI recently published by the European Association of Urology recommends its assessment (Grade A) (DuBeau et al, 2010).

It is very important to highlight that the extent of the clinical approach and the diagnostic process in the frail elderly incontinent is not well established. In general, healthy older persons should receive the same diagnostic schedule as younger patients. By contrast, in frail older persons an individual assessment is required, and it should include: medical and functional status; the incontinence's impact; the preferences of the patient; the life's expectancy and also the true chances to improve after a wide evaluation.

Currently, it is accepted that the clinical assessment of the elderly incontinent has two different steps, one basic and another further.

7.1 Basic step

Basic step the basic step should be done in every incontinent patient and the general practitioner can successfully do it, with several main objectives: to detect transient causes of incontinence; to exclude serious underlying diseases; to identify patients who need further evaluation and finally to decide the appropriate treatment.

Basic step has included different components of the clinical assessment, all of them very important to know the characteristics of the incontinent frail elderly.

Basic step should include:

7.1.1 Medical history

Medical history with the follow components (Abrams et al, 2010):

- A list of co-morbid conditions (neurological, cardiac, endocrine or musculoskeletal diseases, sensorial deficits) as well as the previous surgery (hysterectomy, prostatectomy), in order to detect the main risk factors for the incontinence. Also is very important to know the bowel symptoms (constipation, previous stool impaction, faecal incontinence), as well as the fluid intake (volume and the consumption of tea, coffee, alcoholic drinks).
- A review of the pharmacological treatment in order to check the use of drugs with negative effects on continence (diuretics, psychotropics)
- A practical functional evaluation (especially transfers, mobility, ability to use toilet, cognition).
- A focused urinary history assessing the onset and the length of the incontinence, and also the presence of storage symptoms (frequency, urgency, nocturia) or voiding symptoms (poor urinary stream, hesitancy) as well as the precipitants of urinary leakages (cough, exertion). In order to facilitate the assessment of the urinary symptoms, could be very practical the use of the voiding diaries, which are considered as a useful instrument in the

clinical evaluation. The information can be obtained from the patient or caregiver, and in the majority of the cases, probably a three day diary is usually sufficient. It is important to comment that in cases of high frailty, cognitive impairment or mental problems, we can use a register of the leakages and their amounts instead a formal diary. The level of recommendation of the voiding diaries is grade A.

- The impact on QOL: this area is considered very important, and the assessment should be done through a formal instrument such a valid questionnaire (as it has described above).
- The social and environmental factors: such as the access to toilets, the availability of aids.

7.1.2 Physical examination

The physical examination should include an abdominal (for excluding a distended bladder or a pelvic mass), rectal (for evaluating the sphincter tone, the prostate size, the presence of impaction faecal) a basic neurological exam (especially gait and signs of focal lesions), a genital and pelvic examinations (cough stress test, prolapse evaluation).

The International Continence Society recommends also a post-void residual volume (PVR) measurement by a non-invasive method before to start medical or surgical treatment (Grade C of recommendation), although there are no evidence-based criteria for a high volume (DuBeau et al, 2010; Abrams et al, Markland et al, 2011). In general, PVR greater than 150-200 ml is considered significant in frail older patients.

7.1.3 Basic investigations

Urine analysis should be done in all the incontinent frail patients, and it can be very useful to detect or rule out infection or hematuria. Although, -results should be interpreted with caution due to the high percentage of asymptomatic bacteriuria in the older population (at least 20%). So, it is necessary to be sure of the relation between an abnormal urine analysis and the urinary symptoms (urgency, frequency, dysuria), in order to accept the clinical diagnosis of urinary infection instead of asymptomatic bacteriuria.

Other laboratory tests (thyroid hormones, vitamin B12 or vitamin D levels) require an individualized justification.

7.2 Further step

Further step based on the findings of the basic approach we could detect some frail elderly who require further evaluation by different team of specialists (urologist, gynaecologist) or making certain techniques (ultrasounds, urodynamics) to complete the diagnostic process and provide the therapeutic alternatives.

In the table 8 are exposed the main criteria to refer a frail elderly to the specialist.

8. Diagnostic approach of the urinary incontinence in the frail elderly

In most frail older patients with incontinence, non-invasive diagnostic evaluation can be successfully done, and it will help to decide the conservative management of the patient. As previous mentioned, on the basis of basic step with its components (medical, pharmaceutical, functional, urinary diary, questionnaire of QOL, and a physical

- Surgery or irradiation involving the pelvic area
- Two or more urinary tract infections in a one-year period
- Incontinence with new-onset neurologic symptoms
- Pelvic pain associated with incontinence
- Marked pelvic prolapse on physical examination
- Difficulty passing a 14-Fr straight urinary catheter
- Post-void residual volume > 200 ml
- Abnormal prostate examination on digital rectal
- Asymptomatic microscopic or macroscopic hematuria
- Before a surgical procedure to repair urinary incontinence
- Persistent bothersome symptoms after adequate trials of behavioural or drug therapy

Table 8. Main criteria to refer a frail elderly for specialty evaluation

examination) we are able to distinguish between an acute cause or a chronic cause of incontinence, to detect the great majority of the transient causes, the main risks factors for incontinence and to recognize the clinical type of UI and its main symptoms. With this information would be possible to decide the plan of treatment and the follow-up of the older patients with incontinence.

If the basic step does not drive the physician to a conclusive diagnosis of UI type, or in cases that conservative management of the frail older patients has failed, more extensive or invasive diagnostic techniques should be planed individually. In some cases, could be necessary to practice several complementary techniques in order to discover the etiologic mechanism of the incontinence and also the status of the upper urinary tract.

The gold standard technique in diagnosis of established incontinence is Urodynamics, allowing demonstrate whether an underlying abnormality of storage or voiding is present. Nowadays, this technique is not appropriate for all older patients, and usually it is reserved for selected patients (Thirugnanasothy, 2010). Probably, the main recommendations for this technique in the frail elderly population, is the demonstration of a significant PVR and before planning a surgical procedure to repair urinary incontinence (Verdejo, 2011).

Based on the results of these techniques, especially on Urodynamics, we can obtain definitive diagnosis of UI type and organize better the complete and multidimensional plan of treatment.

9. Medical treatment of the urinary incontinence in the frail elderly

In order to decide treatment scheme, we should establish a comprehensive individualized plan of treatment, based on: the patient's characteristics (comorbidity and level of disability); the type of incontinence (urgency, at cough, mixed, overflow); the impact of incontinence; the patient's preferences and level of co-operation; the need of help by others; and also true chances of adherence to treatment (Schröder et al, 2009; Abrams et al; 2010).

It is very important to underline that the main objectives of our intervention should be: firstly, to improve the QOL; secondly, the reduction of the severity / number of leakages; and finally, if possible, the recovery of continence. In fact, the individual scheme of treatment has to be very realistic and adapted to the characteristics of each frail patient, looking more for quality of life instead of the cure of medical problem. Unfortunately, in some patients with immobility or severe dementia, the only alternative could be the use of palliative aids and general care.

9.1 Conservative management

Nowadays, the conservative treatment of UI is considered as the mainstay in its management (grade A of recommendation). There are several effective interventions such as: modification of fluid intake pattern; modification of drug treatments; type of clothes used; palliative aids; environmental manipulations; detection and correction of transient causes (especially delirium in the frailest population); and the use of behavioural procedures (Wyman et al, 2009; Imamura et al, 2010; Abrams et al, 2010; DuBeau et al, 2010).

Behavioural techniques have been demonstrated be an effective tool in the management of several types of incontinence in the elderly. The technique used depends on the individual's functional and cognitive state. In general, if the patient doesn't have cognitive impairment, pelvic floor muscle exercises and bladder training can be used successfully. For patients with cognitive impairment, the best alternative is prompted voiding (Level 1 of evidence) (Markland et al, 2011).

It is very important to highlight that all of these techniques have show to reduce the severity of urgency and stress incontinence (grade A of recommendation) (Burgio, 2009; Price et al, 2010). In cases of institutionalized older patients and cognitively impaired, scheduled and prompted voiding have demonstrated to reduce the number of leakages of urine and the severity of the incontinence. However, these techniques require many caregivers and staff in nursing home, so it is not always possible to use them in the disabled and frailest elderly patients (Thum & Wagg, 2009).

9.2 Pharmacologic management

Moreover of these general interventions, there are several effective pharmacological agents such as antimuscarinics, serotonin and noradrenaline re-uptake inhibitor (SNRI) e.g. Duloxetine or anti-diuretic homones e.g. Desmopressin.

9.2.1 Antimuscarinic drugs

At the present time, there are several available antimuscarinic drugs with a different profile based on the ability to block the muscarinic receptors. Moreover, we have to choose the antimuscarinic drug based on the safety profile. All the antimuscarinic drugs have been widely tested in randomised controlled trials and demonstrate to produce a positive effect in the treatment of urge and mixed incontinence, with about 50% reduction of leakages compared with placebo (Thirugnanasothy, 2010). According to the results of many trials of the incontinent frail elderly population, the overall efficacies of the different antimuscarinic drugs are similar, and so the initial choice of this agent should be based on its safety profile. If one antimuscarinic agent doesn't provide satisfactory relief of symptoms, an alternative antimuscarinic should be tried.

In some cases, we could decide to use antimuscarinics drugs based only on clinical symptoms (frequency, urgency, and nocturia), and also on the severity of leakages (moderate or severe), but with several requisites: the physical examination and the lab tests have to be normal. In this sense, the theoretical side effects on cognitive function must not limit its use in the elderly (Wagg et al, 2010). Furthermore, in all the cases, we must analyze the individual risks of this treatment with a close follow-up of the frailest older patients.

Table 9 shows a list of drugs with antimuscarinic action most commonly used in the treatment of incontinent frail older patients, with their level of evidence and grade of recommendation (Schröder et al, 2009; DuBeau et al, 2010).

DRUG	LEVEL	GRADE
ANTIMUSCARINICS		
Tolterodine	1	A
Trospium	1	A
Solifenacin	1	A
Fesoterodine	1	A
Darifenacin	1	A
MIXED ACTIONS		
Oxybutinin	1	A
Propiverine	1	A
Flavoxate	2	

Table 9. Antimuscarinics most commonly used in the incontinent frail elderly

9.2.2 Desmopresin

Desmopresin is a synthetic vasopressin analogue, with strong anti-diuretic effects. It could be very useful in the treatment of nocturia, but with risk of hyponatremia (between 7.6 to 10%), especially in the frail elderly patients. In addition, desmopresin should not be used in frail elderly due to the high risk of hyponatremia (level 1 of evidence) (DuBeau et al, 2010; Abrams et al; 2010).

9.2.3 Duloxetin

Duloxetin is a relative recent drug, which is useful for moderate to severe stress urinary incontinence. It has a good profile with a positive effect since the start of the treatment. Its side effects are infrequent (with mild or moderate severity), and of a short duration. Nowadays it is considered as a good alternative for the surgery of stress urinary incontinence in older females (Robinson & Cardozo, 2010).

9.2.4 Alpha-blockers

Other interesting type of drug is the group of alpha-blockers, especially in men with storage lower urinary tract symptoms and urgency, however, they should be used with caution in the frailest men due to the hemodynamic adverse effects (Schröder et al, 2009; Verdejo, 2011).

9.2.5 Catheterisation

Unfortunately, in the cases of chronic urinary retention or bladder impaired contractility in which the patient keeps a high PVR, should be considered the insertion of an urethral catheter. Intermittent catheterisation is usually safer and effective but obviously requires the patient or the carers to be able to learn and practice this technique. When intermittent catheterisation can not be possible, urethral catheter should be considered, with the secondary risks of this technique (infection, hematuria, urethral trauma, accidental removal) (Thirugnanasothy, 2010).

The main indications for long term indwelling catheterisation are exposed in the table 10.

Chronic bladder outlet obstruction and surgery is not appropriate
Patients or carers are unable to manage intermittent catheterisation
Patients with pressure sores (transient indication)
Patients severely affected by the leakages
Managing incontinence in end of life situations

Table 10. Main recommendations for using a long term indwelling catheter:

9.3 Surgical procedures

In the last years the development of surgical procedures has been very important, especially for repairing stress incontinence. Nowadays, we can obtain good results with several techniques (Way, 2009):

- The injection of bulking agents: it is a useful alternative in women with stress incontinence who have high comorbidity and high surgical risk.
- Vaginal pessaries: for treating older women with moderate or severe prolapse and with an average patient satisfaction about 50% at 12 months
- Neuromodulation (through sacral or percutaneous tibial nerve stimulation): that produces a neuromodulation at S2-S4, improving the urinary urgency, frequency and incontinence (it can be performed via a fine needle inserted percutaneously near the ankle).
- Sling procedures: well the Tension-Free Vaginal Tape (TVT) procedure (introduced in 1996) or the Trans-Obturator Tension-Free Vaginal Tape (TOT) procedure (in the year 2001 this technique was modified due a less invasive procedure with a low risk of bladder damage).
- I would like to highlight the role of Botulinum toxin because its use is increasing for patients with refractory symptoms to other treatments due to overactive bladder, with neurogenic (Grade A) as well as idiopathic type (Grade B). The technique consists in the injection of botulinum toxin by cystoscopy into the detrusor muscle. The clinical results are good, but with problems such as urinary retention and urinary tract infections. Careful and individualized patient selection is very important to ensure satisfactory response (Duthie et al, 2007; Verdejo, 2011).

10. Key points in the care of the incontinent frail elderly

- Urinary incontinence supposes the loss of a basic function, which is most prevalent in the frail and disabled elderly, and it is associated with a lot of problems.

- The frail older population have a high risk of suffer urinary incontinence, related to their medical conditions, the use of polypharmacy and the functional impairment.
- The impact on Quality of Life is very high, similar as produced by Diabetes Mellitus, Stroke or Arthritis.
- Unfortunately, and in contrast with this reality, the index consultation for UI is low, as well as the number of elderly people that received an effective treatment, in spite of the valid alternatives.
- Several conservative alternatives to manage incontinent elderly patients, including the frailest ones, are available and with high rates of effectiveness.
- Medical treatments are available (antimuscarinic drugs, duloxetine, desmopresin), and should be used knowing their characteristics and limits.
- Older patients who should be referred for further evaluation and treatment need to be identified.
- Efforts are needed to improve research in different areas, especially those related to incontinent frail elderly patients.

11. Acknowledgements

I am indebted to Dr. David Castro for his critical review and helpful suggestions.

12. References

Abrams P, Andersson KE, Birder L, Brubaker L, Cardozo L et al. Fourth International Consultation on Incontinence. Recommendations of the International Scientific Committee: Evaluation and Treatment of Urinary Incontinence, Pelvic Organ Prolapse, and Fecal Incontinence. Neurourol Urodyn 2010; 29: 213-40

Burgio KL. Behavioral treatment of urinary incontinence, voiding dysfunction, and overactive bladder. Obstet Gynecol Clin North Am 2009; 36: 475-91

Chen GD. Pelvic floor dysfunction in aging women. Taiwan J Obstet Gynecol 2007; 46: 374-8

DuBeau CE. The Aging Lower Urinary Tract. J Urol 2006; 175: S11-S15

DuBeau CE, Kuchel GA, Johnson T, Palmer MH, Wagg A. Incontinence in the frail elderly: Report from the 4th International Consultation on Incontinence. Neurourol Urodyn 2010; 29: 165-78

Duthie JB, Herbison GP, Wilson DI, Wilson D. Botulinum toxin injections for adults with overactive bladder syndrome. Cochrane Database of Systematic Reviews 2007; Issue 3. Art. Nº: CD005493. DOI: 10.1002/14651858

Fedarco NS. The biology of aging and frailty. Clin Geriatr Med 2011; 27: 27-37

Fulop T, Larbi A, Witkowski JM, McElhaney J, Loeb M, Mitnitski A, et al. Aging, frailty and age-related diseases. Biogerontology 2011: 11: 547-63

Fung CH, Spencer B, Eslami M, Crandall C. Quality indicators for the screening and care of urinary incontinence in vulnerable elders. J Am Geriatr Soc 2007; 55: S443-9

Gotoh M. Quality of life assessment for patients with urinary incontinence. Nagoya J Med Sci 2007; 69: 123-31

Griebling TL. Urinary incontinence in the elderly. Clin Geriatr Med. 2009; 25: 445-57

Imamura M, Williams K, Wells M, McGrother C. Lifestyle interventions for the treatment of urinary incontinence in adults (protocol). Cochrane Database of Systematic Reviews 2010; Issue 9: CD003505

Inouye SK, Studenski S, Tinetti ME et al: Geriatric syndromes: clinical research and policy implications of a core geriatric concept. J Am Geriatr Soc 2007; 55: 780-91

Ko Y, Lin SY, Salmon W, Bron MS. The Impact of Urinary Incontinence on Quality of Life of the Elderly Am J Manag Care 2005; 11: S103-S111

Markland AD, Vaughan CP, Johnson TM, Burgio KL, Goode P. Incontinence. Med Clin North Am 2011; 95: 539-54

Offermans MP, Du Moulin MF, Hamers JP, Dassen T, Halfens RJ. Prevalence of urinary incontinence and risk factors in nursing home residents: a systematic review. Neurourol Urodyn 2009; 28: 288-94

Price N, Dawwod R, Jackson SR. Pelvic floor exercise for urinary incontinence: a systematic literature review. Maturitas 2010; 67: 309-15

Resnick NM. Geriatric Incontinence. Urol Clin North Am 1996; 23: 55-75

Robinson D, Cardozo L. New drug treatments for urinary incontinence. Maturitas 2010; 65: 340-7

Rockwood K, Mitnitski A. Frailty Defined by Deficit Accumulation and Geriatric Medicine Defined by Frailty. Clin Geriatr Med 2011; 27:17-26

Rosen SL, Reuben DB. Comprehensive Geriatric Assessment tools. Mt Sinai J Med 2011; 78: 489-97

Schröder A, Abrams P, Andersson K-E, Artibani W, Chapple CR, Drake MJ et al. Guidelines on Urinary Incontinence. European Association of Urology. Update March 2009.

Scottish Intercollegiate Guidelines Network. Management of urinary incontinence in primary care: a national clinical guideline, 2004.

Shamliyan T, Wyman J, Bliss DZ, Kane RL, Wilt TJ. Prevention of urinary and fecal incontinence in adults. Evid Rep Technol Assess (Full report) 2007: 161: 1-379

Smith PP. Aging and the underactive detrusor: a failure of activity or activation?. Neurourol Urodyn 2010; 29: 408-12

Ruby CM, Hanlon JT, Boudreau RM, Newman AB, Simonsick EM, Shorr RI, et al. The effect of medication use on urinary incontinence in community-dwelling elderly women. Health, Aging and Body Composition Study. J Am Geriatr Soc 2010; 58:1715-20

Thirugnanasothy S. Managing urinary incontinence in older people. BMJ 2010; 341: 339-43

Thum LP, Wagg A. Management of urinary incontinence in the elderly. Aging Health 2009; 5: 647-56

Verdejo C. Aging of the urogenital system. Rev Clin Gerontol 2000; 10:315-24

Verdejo C. Urinary and fecal incontinence and dementia. Rev Clin Gerontol 2004; 14: 1-8

Verdejo C. The same patient in various European countries. Care of urinary incontinence in Spain. Eur Geriatr Med 2011 Eur Ger Med 2011; 2(5): 311-3

Wagg A., Verdejo C., Molander U. Review of cognitive impairment with antimuscarinic agents in elderly patients with overactive bladder. Int J Clin Pract 2010; 64: 1279-86

Wai CY. Surgical treatment for Stress and Urge Urinary Incontinence. Obstet Gynecol Clin North Am 2009; 36: 509-19

Wyman JF, Burgio KL, Newman DK. Practical aspects of lifestyle modifications and behavioural interventions in the treatment of OAB and urgency urinary incontinence. Int J Clin Pract 2009; 63: 1117-91

Xue Q-L. The Frailty Syndrome: Definition and Natural History. Clin Geriatr Med 2011; 27: 1-15

8

A Model of the Psychological Factors Conditioning Health Related Quality of Life in Urodynamic Stress Incontinence Patients After TVT

Mariola Bidzan[1], Leszek Bidzan[2] and Jerzy Smutek[3,4]

[1]*Department of Clinical Psychology and Neuropsychology, Institute of Psychology, University of Gdansk*

[2]*Department of Developmental Psychiatry, Psychotic Disorders and Old Age Psychiatry, Medical University of Gdansk*

[3]*Department of Obstetrics, Medical University of Gdansk*

[4]*Pro-Vita Private Medical Center for Urinary Incontinence, Gdansk*

Poland

1. Introduction

Urodynamic stress incontinence (USI) is the most common form of urinary incontinence (Thom, 1998; Lemack & Zimmern, 2000; Steciwko, 2002; Rechberger & Skorupski, 2005), accounting for about 50% of all patients with urinary incontinence (Foldspang & Mommsen, 1997; Rechberger, 2004; Rechberger & Skorupski, 2005). About 82% of USI patients are women (Kinchen et al., 2002, cited by Diokno, 2003; Rechberger, 2004; Barber et al., 2005). Approximately 63% of all women with urinary incontinence are diagnosed with USI, from 19% to 25% have urge urinary incontinence (UUI), while from 12% to 19% have a mixed form (Thom, 1998; Lemack, Zimmern, 2000; Steciwko, 2002; Rechberger, Skorupski, 2005). According to the International Continence Society, urodynamic stress incontinence is defined as the involuntary leakage of urine during increased abdominal pressure, in the absence of a detrusor contr action (Abrams et al.., 2002; , Kata & Antoniewicz, 1999; Rechberger & Skorupski, 2005; Kobashi & Kobashi, 2006). It occurs when the increased pressure inside the abdominal cavity caused by a cough or hard physical exertion is accompanied by an involuntary release of urine (Rechberger & Skorupski, 2005).

USI in women is caused by the insufficiency of the apparatus that closes the urethra, and/or hypermobility of the vesico-connection, when bladder functions are completely normal (Milart et al., 2001). This means that the reason for USI lies in the weakening of the pelvic floor muscles, whose basic task is to hold up the organs located in the pelvis, including the urinary tract. Strong pelvic muscles keep the urethra closed until a conscious decision is made to urinate. When these muscles are weakened, the result is an inability to maintain a sufficiently tight hold around the urethra, so that any pressure exerted on the bladder caused by a movement of the diaphragm (e.g. a sneeze, a cough, a sudden exertion, walking on an uneven surface) can lead to an involuntary release of urine (Dutkiewicz, 2002; Rechberger & Skorupski, 2005).

A typical feature of USI should incorporate the general similarity of symptoms in the day to day and the lack of nocturnal enuresis or nocturia. USI is thought to be caused by many different factors. Petros's Integral Theory (Petros, 2005), which is widely accepted, associates functional disturbances of the pelvic floor with structural disorders. The pelvic floor is formed by organs (the bladder with urethra, the vagina and the anus, the fascia and ligaments that bind them, the muscles). To simplify somewhat, the contracting muscles stabilize the organs in relation to the connective tissue elements, so damage to the ligaments and connective tissue can result in the lack of proper closure (manifested by urinary or fecal incontinence) or vaginal dysfunction, and the resulting symptoms and discomfort of which the patients complain.

Due to the considerable prevalence and nature of the symptoms, USI is a major medical and social problem. The intimate nature of the symptoms and their negative impact on daily functioning produces a significant mental burden for both the patients and their partners, and causes the frustration of many psychological, social and existential needs (Wyman et al., 1990; Wyman, 1994; Broome, 2003; Chiaffarino et al., 2003; Møller & Lose, 2005; Papanicolaou et al., 2005).

The scope of the psychological problems caused by the symptoms of USI is particularly large in advanced stages of the disease (Lagro-Janssen et al., 1992a; 1992b). Lalos et al. (2001) found that the life of persons with urinary incontinence changes dramatically, in respect to family life, vocational life, and social life (including the quality of life):

- The nature and style of family life is changed, sexual activity with the partner is changed(see also Norton et al., 1988), and the family budget is burdened with expenses related to treatment and mitigation of symptoms, such as sanitary pads, diaper-panties, etc.
- Career plans are changed, vocational activity is limited, and sometimes a career change is necessary, or even withdrawal from professional work.
- Social functioning is impaired and social contacts are limited (see also Brown et al., 1998; Wein & Rovner, 1999; Anders, 2000; Thom, 2000; Tołłoczko, 2002; Smutek et al., 2004; Bidzan et al., 2005a,b; Bidzan, 2008).
- It is estimated that approximately 25% of person suffering from urinary incontinence are on disability pension, where one of the main reasons for a ruling of disability is the significant extent of the incontinence and the impossibility of working because of the disease. This can cause a feeling of low self-esteem, a loss of personal dignity and social position, deterioration of mood, and social isolation, which lowers the health-related quality of life (HRQOL; Norton et al., 1988).

The lack of treatment, or the postponement of treatment until many years after the first symptoms appear, can have a major impact on the appearance of both physical and mental complications (Banach, 2004).

The problem of evaluating HRQOL in persons with urinary incontinence has been perceived by researchers and clinicians, for whom HRQOL has become in recent years an extremely important indicator of the psychological functioning of patients. An assessment of HRQOL is recommended by the International Continence Society. What is assessed with the help of HRQOL is the impact of the illness and its treatment on the patient's quality of life, not including other, non-medical aspects. Treating the patient as an active subject, rather than a passive object, plays a major role in the evaluation process, which requires taking into consideration not only the objective results of medical examinations, but also the patient's own assessment (Brown et al., 1999; Swithinbank & Abrams, 1999; Shaw, 2002; Tamanini et al., 2004).

Depending on the etiology and severity of urinary incontinence, the treatment of this condition includes both surgical procedures and conservative methods, such as kinesitherapy, behavioral therapy, physiotherapy (including biofeedback, electrostimulation, and magnetic fields), vault support, pharmacotherapy, and lifestyle modification.

Currently there are many (over 170) methods of surgical treatment of urinary incontinence. A particular surgical technique is selected individually for every given case. Patients with SUI constitute the main group qualified for the surgical treatment of urinary incontinence,. Currently, the TVT technique (tension-free vaginal tape) is a commonly used surgical intervention for SUI however there are other modificaitons of the procedure and tape that is also widely used with similar efficacy - TVTO, rectus fascial sling etc. This technique was developed in 1994 by Ulf Ulmsten from the Uppsala University Clinic, and has been practiced in Poland since 1999. TVT is a widely used method of surgical treatment thanks to its minimal invasiveness and morbidity, and particularly due to its superior recovery rate when compared to other frequently used methods (estimated at 88%) and relatively low cost (Włodarczyk et al., 2003; Konabrocka, 2006; Rechberger, 2006) These considerations, along with the fact that there is virtually no possibility of modifying this original technique (Rechberger, 2006), were the reasons for selecting patients subjected to TVT for developing a model of HRQOL determinants in USI.

The aim of this study was to create a model describing the HRQOL determinants in this group of patients.

2. Material and methods

The initial population (N = 917) consisted entirely of patients treated in the period from 2002 to 2006 in the Pro-Vita Private Medical Center for Urinary Incontinence, in Gdansk, Poland.

All these patients were subjected to a thorough diagnostic process for urinary incontinence, consistent with the standards of the International Continence Society (ICS), as follows:

1. A detailed patient history was obtained, to provide information concerning the nature of the urinary dysfunctions, possible congenital or neurological causes, history of urinary tract infections, and the course of treatment to date (drugs taken, hormone replacement therapy, surgical procedures). The history included a range of information that could have a bearing on the diagnosis of urinary incontinence, such as presenting complaint, past medical history including obstetric and surgical history, medications and social history (Abrams et al., 1988; Jensen et al., 1994; Abrams et al., 2002; Milart & Gulanowska-Gędek, 2002; Rechberger & Skorupski, 2005).
2. A detailed clinical examination was performed, which included the following elements:
   - physical examination (focusing on the evaluation of the pelvic floor support);

- self explanatory (in order to exclude urinary tract infections before treating urinary incontinence, since inflammation of the urinary tract can give symptoms of urinary incontinence);
- a cough test (to objectivize the patient's subjective complaints; the cough test is performed in the supine position immediately after micturition, while the stress cough test is performed in prone or sitting position with full bladder; the release of urine through the urethra during the cough test is considered a positive result for USI; This indicates a low leak point pressure it should be remembered, however, than in from 5% to 10% of cases the patient continues to complain of incontinence despite a negative result on this test). This should be part of the physical examination.
- measurement of residual urine volume (the volume of urine remaining in the bladder after micturition should not exceed 10-15% of its capacity, i.e. 50 ml; the measurement is done by ultrasound scan; this evaluation is essential to preclude the possibility of incontinence resulting from overfilling of the bladder;
- an evaluation of the 72hrs urination journal traditionally called a bladder diary and should be for a total of 72hrs/3 days (in which the patient writes down the number of urinations, the time interval between them, and episodes of involuntary release of urine and traditionally the amount of fluid intake);
- the 24 hour pad weight test (objectively measuring the amount of urine released involuntarily during a standard set of physical exercises performed by the patient e.g. marching, sitting, climbing stairs, by measuring the mass or the electrical resistance of the sanitary pad before and after the exercises);
- an evaluation of the mobility of the urethra, called the "Q-tip test" (a test to reveal excessive mobility of the cervix of the urinary bladder and the proximal segment of the urethra, when the change of position of a cotton swab inserted into the urethra during the valsalva maneuver is greater than 30°);
- a urodynamic examination (an objective method to confirm the previous diagnosis);
- urethral profilometry (which makes it possible to measure intratubular pressure simultaneously along the entire length of the urethra, along with intravesical pressure); Urethral pressure has now become less of a key issue in incontinence and is traditionally completed at the time of a VCMG/CMG
- an electromyogram; Not routinely used but is done in conjunction with the VCMG/CM
- ultrasound and CT imaging (in the ultrasound test a high resolution vaginal head is used to observe the dynamics of changes in spatial relations between the cervix of the urinary bladder and the urethra); Ths imaging studies should be inserted after the the physical examination but before the invasive assesments ie CMG. This is not a standard evaluation tool in incontinence and is usually only utilized in the evaluation of suspected anatomical abnormalities or suspected calculus disease or malignancy complicating the presentation
- cystoscopy (Abrams et al., 1988; Abrams et al., 2002; Milart & Gulanowska-Gędek, 2002; Rechberger & Skorupski, 2005; Waszyński, 2005).

The results of the medical examination made it possible to determine for each patient the form (type) of urinary incontinence - USI, UUI, or mixed urinary incontinence (MUI) - along with the degree of symptom intensity.

The study population is 108 patients who underwent TVT for severe SUI refractory to conservative management.

This group underwent the following:

- a structured clinical interview (developed by the authors);
- an interview conducted by a psychologist, a psychiatrist, and a neurologist;
- the NEO-FFI Personality Inventory (by Costa and McCrae), which is used to assess five basic dimensions of personality: Neurotism, Extroversion, Openness, Agreeability, and Conscientiousness;
- the King's Health Questionnaire (KHQ), used to assess the quality of life of women patients suffering from urinary incontinence;
- the Dyadic Adjustment Scale (DAS), developed by Spanier, which gives a thorough assessment of the quality of marital relations (general level, agreeability, consistency, satisfaction, emotional expression);
- the Coping Inventory for Stressful Situations (CISS), designed by Endler and Parker, which diagnoses styles of coping with stress conditioned by personality. These include the task-oriented style, the emotion-oriented style, and the avoidance-oriented style (this last style can have two variants: engaging in substitute activities and seeking social contacts).

2.1 A preliminary model of the factors conditioning HRQOL

On the basis of previous research (Bidzan, 2008) a model has been developed for the assumed relationships between HRQOL and selected psychological measures (personality traits, quality of relationship, and coping styles). The pathways analysis method was used. In the opinion of many researchers (e.g. Cwalina, 2000; Gaul & Machowski, 2004) this method is distinctly superior to both the ANOVA approach and factor analysis in testing correlational and differential accuracy on the basis of a multi-feature, multi-method matrix. Pathway analysis, unlike other methods, provides not only quantitative indices of weight (the "feature factor" and the "method factor"), but also a model of the structure of the data acquired by means of a given instrument.

The model we are proposing, which is shown in Fig. 1, takes in both the variables that directly influence the quality of life and the indirect variables.

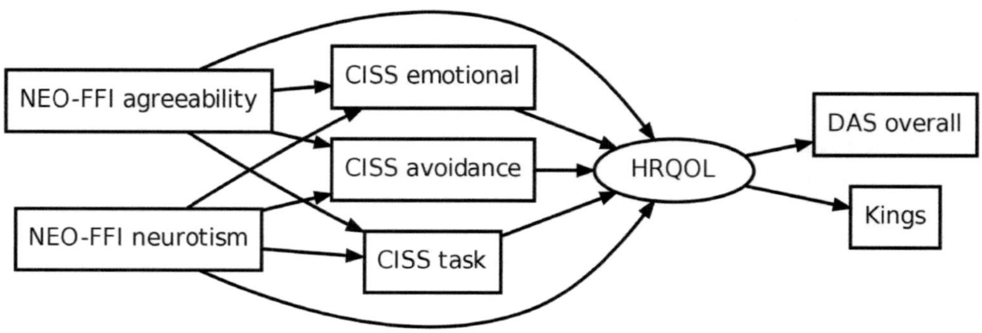

Fig. 1. Proposed model of relations between selected psychological measures and HRQOL in women patients with UUI

For purposes of the preliminary model, HRQOL was used as a latent variable. The value of this variable was indirectly observed by means of the DAS and the KHQ. It was assumed that HRQOL assumes a value on the same scale as the overall QOL score in the KHQ.

The categories incorporated in the model include two personality dimensions ("agreeability" and "neurotism") measured by the NEO-FFI Personality Inventory, the coping styles measured by the CISS, the overall QOL measured by the KHQ, and the overall quality of the marital or partner relationship, measured by the DAS.

Given the limitations of the pathways analysis method, only the foregoing variables were taken into account.

The inclusion of Neurotism in the model is justified both by the results previously obtained by the first author of the present study (Bidzan 2008), pointing to statistically significant differences in the level of Neurotism between groups of women with different forms and different intensities of urinary incontinence, and by previously published reports indicating the essential role of this trait in shaping HRQOL. To be sure, these latter reports did not deal with urinary incontinence; still, the overall regularities should be valid in this respect. The inclusion of Agreeability was also motivated by results obtained in a previous study by the first author of the present study (Bidzan 2008), indicating that this is the only personality trait besides Neurotism that differentiated the groups of women studied, with various forms of urinary incontinence (USI, MUI, UUI) and with varying degrees of intensity.

Apart from the direct impact of Agreeability and Neurotism on HRQOL, the model in question also assumes that these factors have an indirect impact, through the coping styles used by the individual. The quality of the marital or partner relationship (DAS overall) is associated with overall HRQOL according to King's Health Questionnaire.

2.2 Verification of the preliminary model of factors conditioning HRQOL - pathways analysis

The proposed model was then verified. The structural equations modeling technique was used. This makes it possible to ascertain dependencies, in terms of direction and strength, between the observed variables.

As mentioned above, the preliminary model used the latent variable "HRQOL," whose value was indirectly observed using the DAS and the KHQ. It was assumed that HRQOL takes on a value on the same scale[1] as the QOL score on the KHQ. The connection between HRQOL thus defined and the DAS is also statistically significant (see the model). For the purposes of the model, then, the results for HRQOL were negatived, so that higher scores would mean a higher HRQOL, which makes it possible to make comparisons with results from other methods, especially the DAS.

Two dimensions from the NEO-FFI are incorporated in the model (Neurotism and Agreeability), since, as indicated by previous research, these have the greatest impact on the psychological functioning of patients with urinary incontinence, including the decision to undergo treatment, which can guarantee a change in HRQOL. These two

---

[1] The linear regression coefficient for the variable HRQOL and the overall score from the KHQ equals 1.

dimensions from the NEO-FFI are the only two exogenous variables in the model. The variance of these exogenous variables is assumed to be 1 (standardized sizes). In addition to the personality variables, the model also incorporates three coping styles from the CISS: task-oriented, emotion-oriented, and avoidance. These coping styles have not previously been studied in women with urinary incontinence, though the literature refers to other kinds of strategies used by patients with urinary incontinence, such as making a toilet map, urinating "in advance," etc. The manner of coping in the face of a difficult situation depends, among other things, on previous experiences and personality traits. Health, in turn, is largely dependent on the process of coping (Makowska & Poprawa, 2001), which can also affect HRQOL.

In the course of further analysis the model has been modified in such a way as to maximize the agreement of the correlation matrix reproduced in the model with the correlation matrix observed in research. The calculations were done using the R statistical environment (www.r-project.org) and the SEM package for this environment (Structural Equations Modeling). From the diagrams we can read out the following parameters of the model thus obtained:

1. unidirectional arrows: beta coefficients for linear regression equations;
2. bidirectional arrows: covariance of variables;
3. "reversed" bidirectional arrows: variance of error (additional variance of the variable not explained by the model).

The following factors were used to evaluate the compatibility of the model:

1. The value of the chi-squared statistic for the model. It was assumed that this value should not be statistically significant (i.e. the model does not differ significantly from a model that would fit the data ideally).
2. The Goodness of Fit Index (GFI), in the range from 0 to 1. Values greater than 0.95 are regarded as indicative of a good fit.
3. The Adjusted Goodness of Fit index (AGFI). A value of at last 0.9 indicates a good fit.
4. The Root Mean Square Error of Approximation (RMSEA). A value below 0.05 indicates a good fit.
5. The Bentler-Bonett Normed Fit Index (NFI). Values above 0.90 are acceptable.
6. The Trucker-Lewis Non-Normed Fit Index (NNFI). Values above 0.95 are acceptable.
7. The Bentler Comparative Fit Index (CFI).A value of 0.9 is acceptable.

The value can be interpreted as the percentage of the observed covariance that the model explains.

The proposed model displays a significant fit to the data.

In order to test the proposed model for the factors conditioning HRQOL in a group of USI patients who have undergone TVT - that is, to check whether and how much it reflects the actual dependencies between the variables, to specify the causal effects, and to specify the degree to which it explains the variance in HRQOL, a pathways analysis was performed (Dolińska-Zygmunt, 2000). The results are presented below in tables. The results of the analysis indicate that the model is correctly constructed, i.e. it accurately reflects the dependencies between variables.

3. Results

3.1 Verification of the preliminary model of factors conditioning HRQOL for the research group

Tables 1 - 4 present the results of our pathways analysis, the coefficients of the model, the covariance matrices observed in the sample, and the matrices reflected by the model.

Coefficient	Value
GFI (Goodness-of -fit-index)	0.96
AGFI (Adjusted goodness-of-fit -index)	0.88
RMSEA index	0
NFI (Bentler-Bonnett)	0.95
NNF (Tucker-Lewis)	1.38
CFI (Bentler)	1
Chi squared = 3.03 df= 9 Pr (>chsq)= 0.96	

Table 1. Results of pathway analysis for factors conditioning HRQOL in the study population

	Coefficient	SD	z value	*Compatibility*
CISS emotion←NEO.FFI agree	-0.30	0.13	-2.40	**0.02**
CISS avoid ←NEO.FFI agree	-0.47	0.20	-2.37	**0.02**
CISS task ←NEO.FFI agree	0.06	0.20	0.28	0.78
CISS emotion ←-NEO.FFI neuro	0.65	0.13	5.16	**0.0000002**
CISS avoid ←NEO.FFI neuro	-0.14	0.20	-0.72	0.47
CISS task ←NEO.FFI neuro	-0.38	0.20	-1.89	**0.05**
NEO.FFI agree←→ NEO.FFI neuro	-0.39	0.16	-2.38	**0.02**
HRQOL← NEO.FFI Agree	0.28	0.20	1.41	0.16
HRQOL← NEO.FFI neuro	-0.01	0.26	-0.05	0.96
HRQOL ← CISS task	-0.40	0.18	-2.25	**0.02**
HRQOL←CISS emotion	-0.28	0.26	-1.06	0.29

	Coefficient	SD	z value	*Compatibility*
HRQOL ← CISS avoid	0.27	0.18	1.51	0.13
CISS emotion←→ CISS task	0.12	0.11	1.11	0.27
DAS overall ←HRQOL	0.71	0.41	1.71	0.09
CISS task←→ CISS task	0.83	0.24	3.46	**0.001**
CISS emotion←→ CISS emotion	0.33	0.09	3.46	**0.001**
CISS avoid←→CISS avoid	0.81	0.23	3.46	**0.001**
DAS overall←→ DAS overall	0.84	0.25	3.41	**0.001**
KHQ←→KHQ	0.68	0.20	3.41	**0.001**

Table 2. Coefficients for the model

Observed covariance matrix	NEO.FFI Agree	CISS emotion	CISS avoid	CISS task	NEO.FFI Neuro	DAS overall	KHQ
NEO.FFI agree	1.00	-0.56	-0.42	0.20	-0.39	0.21	0.23
CISS emotion	-0.56	1.00	0.25	-0.20	0.77	-0.35	-0.22
CISS avoid	-0.42	0.25	1.00	-0.12	0.04	-0.03	0.21
CISS task	0.20	-0.20	-0.12	1.00	-0.40	-0.19	-0.33
NEO.FFI neuro	-0.39	0.77	0.04	-0.40	1.00	-0.18	-0.13
DAS overall	0.21	-0.35	-0.03	-0.19	-0.18	1.00	0.18
KHQ	0.23	-0.22	0.21	-0.33	-0.13	0.18	1.00

Table 3. Observed covariance matrix

Covariance matrix replicated by the model	NEO.FFI agree	CISS emotion	CISS avoid	CISS. task	NEO.FFI neuro	DAS overall	KHQ
NEO.FFI agree	1.00	-0.56	-0.42	0.20	-0.39	0.18	0.25
CISS emotion	-0.56	1.00	0.15	-0.20	0.77	-0.23	-0.32
CISS avoid	-0.42	0.15	1.00	-0.04	0.04	0.09	0.13
CISS task	0.20	-0.20	-0.04	1.00	-0.40	-0.21	-0.29
NEO.FFI neuro	-0.39	0.77	0.04	-0.40	1.00	-0.12	-0.17
DAS overall	0.18	-0.23	0.09	-0.21	-0.12	1.00	0.22
KHQ	0.25	-0.32	0.13	-0.29	-0.17	0.22	1.00

Table 4. Covariance matrix replicated by the model

These results made it possible to construct a model (see Fig. 2) of the factors conditioning HRQOL for these patients.

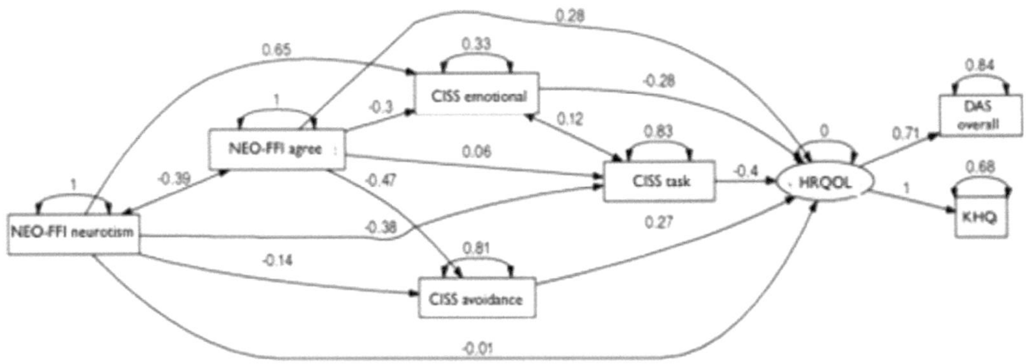

Fig. 2. A model of relations between selected psychological dimensions and HRQOL in women patients with UUI

In this model developed for patients who have undergone TVT surgery, one indirect sequence influencing the quality of life is observed: Neurotism - task-oriented style - quality of life. Neurotism has a negative effect on the selection of the CISS task-oriented style, and this determines a low level of HRQOL. The observed association with the task-oriented style may possibly be the result of dealing with the symptoms, whose severity decreased markedly in the patients' opinion following TVT surgery. Moreover, a direct positive influence of Neurotism is observed for the selection of the CISS emotion-oriented coping style. Additionally, Neurotism promoted a decrease in Agreeability (and therefore supported a confrontational attitude), hence activating emotion-oriented and avoidance-oriented styles. These latter findings, however, are not directly associated with the quality of life.

4. Discussion

In the model we developed for this group of women who had undergone TVT there is one indirect sequence of influences affecting HRQOL: Neurotism (-) - CISS task style (-) - HRQOL; that is, a lower level of Neurotism leads to the choice of the task-oriented style, and the less preference for this style, the higher the evaluation of HRQOL.

According to the assumptions of McCrea and Costa (2005), Neurotism is a personality dimension that reflects the level of emotional adaptation: the higher the score, the greater the susceptibility to experiencing such negative emotions as fear, anger, guilt, the higher the sensitivity to psychological stress, and by the same token the harder it is to cope with a difficult situation, which can have an impact on the subjective lowering of HRQOL. The impact of negative emotions on the possibility of adaptation has been confirmed in many studies.

The indirect influence that our model shows Neurotism exerting on HRQOL is consistent with the findings of other researchers (cf. Ferrie et al., 1984; Norton et al., 1990), who have reported that those women with USI function better who are characterized by a lower level of Neurotism, and with research results indicating that USI patients with low Neurotism scores show better outcomes after surgical treatment (Berglund et al., 1997). It is reasonable to assume that improved psychological functioning has a positive effect on HRQOL.

The model also shows a relationship between HRQOL and the task-oriented coping style, which may result from the possibility of overcoming the symptoms, which are much less in subjective evaluation after TVT. At the same time, the model shows a relationship between less frequent use of the task-oriented style and a higher level of HRQOL. It may seem that this dependence should be rather the reverse, since, in the opinion of many researchers (Janssen et al., 2001) coping with the symptoms of urinary incontinence requires a task-oriented approach.

In the literature the most effective methods of coping with the symptoms of urinary incontinence are thought to include a restriction in the intake of fluids, very regular urination, making toilet maps (e.g. on the road from work to home), using single-use sanitary pads and napkins, and keeping a log of urination (Kinn & Zaar, 1998; Fitzerald et al., 2001; Janssen et al., 2001). These techniques correspond, interestingly enough, with both a task-oriented approach and an avoidance approach (all forms of restriction, such as avoiding fluids), though this is seldom stated directly. This may be at least a partial explanation of the dependency we found. It should also be emphasized that many researchers (e.g. Czapiński, 1994; Bidzan et al., 2004b) emphasize the advantages gained from combining styles of coping with the problem, e.g. task-oriented with emotion, since in this case the patient begins to take some action: to undergo treatment, to comply with physician's orders, to search for their own ways of coping with the problem (using also support networks), or finally to decide on surgery. In other words, they cope more effectively with the disease (cf. Shaw, 2001), which can have a favorable impact on their evaluation of HRQOL. The task-oriented approach alone, though it seems more efficient, is not optimal, and when it is the only strategy used, it can lower HRQOL.

5. Conclusions

1. There is one indirect sequence of factors influencing HRQOL in USI patients who have undergone TVT: Neurotism - task style - HRQOL.
2. The relation between HRQOL and the task-oriented style may be associated with the possibility of overcoming the symptoms, which are significantly less in the evaluation of patients after TVT.
3. Our results point to the necessity for interdisciplinary cooperation between physicians and psychologists to develop effective interventions for genuine stress incontinence patients, and broader cooperation in the sphere of HRQOL.

6. References

Abrams, P.; Bliavas, J.G.; Stanton, S.L. & Andersen, J.T. (1988). Standarization of terminology of lower urinary tract function. *Neurourology and Urodynamics*, vol. 7, pp. 403-428

Abrams, P.; Cardozo, L.; Fall, M.; Griffiths, D.; Rosier, P.; Ulmsten, U.; van Kerrebroeck, P.; Victor, P. & Wein, A. (2002). ICS standarization of terminology of lower urinary tract function. *Neurourology and Urodynamics*, vol. 21, pp. 167-178

Anders, K. (2000). Coping strategies for women with urinary incontinence. *Best Practice & Research in Clinical Obstetrics & Gynaecology*, vol. 2, pp. 355-61

Banach, R. (2004). Wytyczne postępowania w nietrzymaniu moczu u kobiet. *Medycyna Rodzinna*, DOA 6 September 2011, Available from:

http://www.czytelniamedyczna.pl/553,wytyczne-postepowania-w-nietrzymaniu-moczu-u-kobiet.html

Barber, M.D.; Mullen, K.J.; Dowsett S.A. & Viktrupl L. (2005). The impact of stress urinary incontinence on sexual activity in women. *Cleveland Clinic Journal of Medicine*, vol. 3, pp. 225-32

Berglund, A.L.; Eisemann, M.; Lalos, A. & Lalos, O. (1997). Predictive factors of the outcome of primary surgical treatment of stress incontinence in women. *Scandinavian Journal of Urology and Nephrology*, vol. 1, pp. 49-55

Bidzan, M. (2008). *Jakość życia pacjentek z różnym stopniem nasilenia wysiłkowego nietrzymania moczu*, Oficyna Wyd. "Impuls", Kraków, Poland

Bidzan, M.; Dwurznik, J. & Smutek, J. (2005a). Jakość związku partnerskiego a poziom seksualnego funkcjonowania kobiet leczonych z powodu nietrzymania moczu w świetle wyników badania Skalą Jakości Związku DAS Spaniera oraz Kwestionariusza Zdrowia Kingsa, *Annales Universitas Mariae Curie -Skłodowska*, Vol. LX, Supl. XVI, 28, Sectio D, pp. 122 - 128

Bidzan, M.; Smutek, J. & Bidzan, L. (2005b). Nietrzymanie moczu - stygmatyzacją? Czy ostatnim tabu XXI wieku? *Annales Universitas Mariae Curie -Skłodowska*, Vol. LX, Supl. XVI., 29, Sectio D , pp. 129 -132

Broome, B.A.S. (2003). The impact of urinary incontinence on self-efficacy and quality of life. *Health and Quality of Life Outcomes*, vol. 1, pp. 35-40

Brown, J.S.; Subak, L.L.; Gras, J.; Brown, B.A.; Kuppermann, M. & Posner, S.F. (1998). Urge incontinence: the patient's perspective. *Journal of Women's Health*, vol. 7, pp. 1263-9

Brown, J.S.; Posner, S. & Stewart, A.L. (1999a). Urge incontinence: new health-related quality of life measures. *Journal of the American Geriatric Society*, vol. 47, pp. 980-8

Brown, J.S.; Grady, D.; Ouslander, J.G.; Herzog, A.R.; Varner, R.E. & Posner, S.F. (1999b). Prevalence of urinary incontinence and associated risk factors in postmenopausal women. *Obstetrics and Gynecology*, vol. 94, pp. 66-70

Chiaffarino, F.; Parazzini, F.; Lavezzari, M. & Giambanco, V. (2003). Impact of urinary incontinence and overactive bladder on quality of life. *European Urology*, vol. 43, pp. 535-8

Cwalina, W. (2000). *Zastosowanie modelowania równań strukturalnych w naukach społecznych*, StatSoft Polska, Kraków, Poland

Czapiński, J. (1994). *Psychologia szczęścia. Przegląd badań i zarys teorii cebulowej*, Pracownia Testów Psychologicznych PTP, Warsaw

Diokno, A.C. (2003). The Incidence and Prevalence of Stress Urinary Incontinence, *Proceedings of the symposium "Stress Urinary Incontinence: Expanding the Treatment Options"*, Chicago, Illinois, USA, 25 April 2003

Dolińska-Zygmunt, G. (2000). *Podmiotowe uwarunkowania zachowań promujących zdrowie*, Wydawnictwo Instytutu Psychologii PAN, Warsaw

Dutkiewicz, S. (2002). Leczenie wysiłkowego nietrzymania moczu u kobiet, *Medycyna Rodzinna*, DOA 6 September 2011, Available from: http://www.czytelniamedyczna.pl/731,leczenie-wysilkowego-nietrzymania-moczu-u-kobiet.html

Ferrie, B.G.; Smith, J.S.; Logan, D.; Lyle, R. & Paterson, P.J. (1984). Experience with bladder training in 65 patents. *British Journal of Urology*, vol. 56, pp. 482-484

Fitzgerald, S.T.; Palmer, M.H.; Berry, S.J. & Hart, K. (2000). Urinary Incontinence: Impact on Working Women. *Journal of the American Association of Occupational Health Nurses*, vol. 3, pp. 112-8

Fitzgerald, S.T.; Palmer, M.H.; Kirkland, V.L. & Robinson, L. (2001). The Impact of Urinary Incontinence on Working Women: A Study in a Production Facility. *Women & Health*, vol. 1, pp. 1-16

Gaul, M. & Machowski, A. (2004). Wprowadzenie do analizy ścieżek, In: *Metodologia badań psychologicznych. Wybór tekstów*, J. Brzeziński, pp. 362-390, Wyd. Naukowe PWN, Warsaw

Janssen, C.C.; Lagro-Janssen, A.L. & Felling, A.J. (2001). The effects of physiotherapy for female urinary incontinence: individual compared with group treatment. *British Journal of Urology International*, vol. 3, pp. 201-6

Jensen, J.K.; Nielsen, F.J. & Ostergard, D.R.(1994). The role of patient history in the diagnosis of urinary incontinence. *Obstetrics and Gynecology*, vol. 83, pp. 904-10

Kata, S.G. & Antoniewicz, A.A. (1999). Współczesne możliwości leczenia wysiłkowego nietrzymania moczu u kobiet. *Nowa Medycyna*, DOA 6 September 2011, Available from: http://www.czytelniamedyczna.pl/1172,wspolczesne-mozliwosci-leczenia-wysilkowego-nietrzymania-moczu-u-kobiet.html

Kinn, A.C. & Zaar, A. (1998). Quality of life and urinary incontinence pad use in women. *International Urogynecology Journal and Pelvic Floor Dysfunction*, vol. 2, pp. 83-7

Kobashi, K.C. & Kobashi, L.I. (2006). Female stress urinary incontinence: review of the current literature. *Minerva Ginecologica*, vol. 4, pp. 265-82

Konabrocka, J. (2006). Polski rynek leczenia operacyjnego. *Kwartalnik NTM*, vol. 4, pp. 4-5

Lagro-Janssen, T.; Smits, A. & Van-Weel, C. (1992a). Urinary incontinence in women and the effects on their lives. *Scandinavian Journal of Primary Health Care*, vol. 3, pp. 211-216

Lagro-Janssen, T.; Debruyne, F.M. & Van-Weel, C. (1992b). Psychological aspects of female urinary incontinence in general practice. *British Journal of Urology*, vol. 5, pp.499-502

Lalos, O.; Berglund, A.L. & Lalos, A. (2001). Impact of urinary and climacteric symptoms on social and sexual life after surgical treatment of stress urinary incontinence in women: a long-term outcome. *Journal of Advanced Nursing*, vol. 3, pp. 316- 27

Lemack, G.E. & Zimmern, P.E. (2000). Sexual function after vaginal surgery for stress incontinence: results of a mailed questionnaire. *Urology*, vol. 2, pp. 223 - 227

McCrae, R. & Costa, P.T. (2005). *Osobowość dorosłego człowieka*, Wydawnictwo WAM, Kraków, Poland

Milart, P.; Adamiak, A.; Skorupski, P.; Sikorski, R.; Jakowicki, J. & Rechberger T. (2001). Występowanie objawów naglącego nietrzymana moczu po operacjach TVT. *Nowa Medycyna*, DOA 6 September 2011, Available from: http://www.czytelniamedyczna.pl/1635,wystepowanie-objawow-naglacego-nietrzymania-moczu-po-operacjach-tvt.html

Milart, P. & Gulanowska-Gędek, B. (2002). Nietrzymanie moczu u kobiet w okresie pomenopauzalnym. *Nowa Medycyna - Hormonalna Terapia Zastępcza* (wydanie specjalne), vol. 9, pp. 31-36

Møller, L.A. & Lose, G. (2005). Sexual activity and lower urinary tract symptoms. *International Urogynecology Journal and Pelvic Floor Dysfunction*, vol. 17, pp. 18-21

Norton, P.A.; MacDonald, L.D.; Sedgwick, P.M. & Stanton, S.L. (1988). Distress and delay associated with urinary incontinence, frequency and urgency in women. *British Medical Journal*, vol. 297, pp. 1187-1189

Norton, K.R.W.; Bhat, A.V. & Stanton, S.L. (1990). Psychiatric aspect of urinary incontinence in women attending an outpatient urodynamic clinic. *British Medical Journal*, vol. 301, pp. 271-272

Papanicolaou, S.; Hunskaar, S.; Lose, G. & Sykes, D. (2005). Assessment of bothersomeness and impact on quality of life of urinary incontinence in women in France, Germany, Spain and the UK. *British Journal of Urology International*, vol. 96, pp. 831-38

Petros, P. (2005). Teoria Integralna - fizjologia I patologia aparatu stabilizującego narządy miednicy mniejszej kobiet, In: *Nietrzymanie moczu u kobiet. Diagnostyka i leczenie,* T. Rechberger & J. Jakowicki, pp. 69-76, Wyd. BiFOLIUM, Lublin, Poland

Rechberger, T. (2004). Wysilkowe nietrzymanie moczu u kobiet. Jak leczyć skutecznie? *Kwartalnik NTM*, vol. 1, pp. 4-5

Rechberger, T. & Skorupski, P. (2005). Nietrzymanie moczu - problem medyczny, socjalny i społeczny, In: *Nietrzymanie moczu u kobiet. Diagnostyka i leczenie,* T. Rechberger & J. Jakowicki, pp. 29-38, Wyd. BiFOLIUM, Lublin, Poland

Rechberger, T. (2006). Skuteczność taśm w leczeniu wysiłkowego nietrzymania moczu. *Kwartalnik NTM*, vol. 3, pp. 8-9

Shaw, C. (2002). A systematic review of the literature the prevalence of sexual impairment in women with urinary incontinence and the prevalence of urinary leakage during sexual activity. *European Urology*, vol. 42, pp. 432-440

Smutek, J.; Grzybowska, M.; Bidzan, M. & Płoszyński, A. (2004). Nietrzymanie moczu u kobiet. Strategie radzenia sobie z problemem gubienia moczu w czasie współżycia, *Annales Universitas Mariae Curie -Skłodowska*, Vol.LIX, Supl. XIV, Sectio D, pp. 180-186

Steciwko, A. (2002). *Wybrane zagadnienia z praktyki lekarza rodzinnego.* Tom 4: *Nietrzymanie moczu – problem interdyscyplinarny, choroby gruczołu krokowego*, Wyd. Continuo, Wrocław

Swithinbank, L.V. & Abrams, P. (1999). The impact of urinary incontinence on the quality of life of women. *World Journal of Urology*, vol. 17, pp. 225-229

Tamanini, J.T.N.; Dambros, M.; D'Ancona, C.L.; Palma, P.C.R.; Botega, N.J.; Rios, L.A.S.; Gomes, C.M.; Baracat, F.; Bezerra, C.A. & Netto, N.R. Jr. (2004). Concurrent validity, internal consistency and responsiveness of the Portuguese version of the King's Health Questionnaire in women after stress urinary incontinence surgery. *International Brazilian Journal of Urology*, vol. 6, pp. 479-486

Thom, D.H. (1998). Variation in estimates of urinary incontinence prevalence in community: effects of differences in definition, population characteristics, and study type. *Journal of the American Geriatrics Society*, vol. 4, pp. 473-480

Thom, D.H. (2000). Overactive bladder: epidemiology and impact on quality of life. *Patient Care*, Winter Suppl., pp. 6-14

Tołłoczko, T. (2002). Nietrzymanie moczu - problem społeczny i kliniczny. *Terapia*, vol. 4, pp. 4-6

Waszyński, E. (2005). Historia uroginekologii, In: *Nietrzymanie moczu u kobiet. Diagnostyka i leczenie,* T. Rechberger & J. Jakowicki, pp. 23-27, Wyd. BiFOLIUM, Lublin, Poland

Wein, A.J. & Rovner, E.S. (1999). The overactive bladder: An overview for primary care health providers. *International Journal of Fertility*, vol. 44, pp. 56-66

Włodarczyk, B.; Szyłło, K.; Kamer-Bartosińska, A. & Lewy, J. (2003). Zastosowanie taśmy TVT w leczeniu wysiłkowego nietrzymania moczu u kobiet. *Ginekologia Polska*, vol. 10, pp. 1421-1426

Wyman, F.J. (1994). The psychiatric and emotional impact of female pelvic floor dysfunction. *Current Opinion in Obstetrics and Gynecology*, vol. 4, pp. 336-339

Wyman, F.J.; Harkins, S.W. & Fantl, J.A. (1990). Psychosocial impact of urinary incontinence in the community-dwelling population. *Journal of the American Geriatrics Society*, vol. 38, pp. 282-288

The Concept and Pathophysiology of Urinary Incontinence

Abdel Karim M. El Hemaly*, Laila A. Mousa and Ibrahim M. Kandil
FRCS-MRCOG, Ob/Gyn
Al Azhar University, Cairo,
Egypt

1. Introduction

We put forward a novel concept on the Pathophysiology of micturition, urinary continence and urinary incontinence 1-7. Urinary continence depends on two main factors, one inherent and one acquired.

The inherent factor is the presence of an intact and strong internal urethral sphincter (IUS). The IUS is a collagen-muscular tissue cylinder that extends from the bladder neck down to the perineal membrane. It gets its nerve supply from the alpha sympathetic nerves from the hypogastric plexus T10-L2. The collagen sheet, being the strongest tissue in the body, is to give the IUS its high wall tension necessary to create in the urethra the high urethral pressure. The muscle fibers lie on, intermingle with the collagen fibers in the middle of the cylinder thickness, and are responsible for closure and opening of the urethra in response to alpha sympathetic tone.

The functions of the IUS are 1- to keep the urethra closed and empty all the time due to the high alpha sympathetic tone gained by learning and training early in childhood. 2- On relaxation to open the urethra to allow voiding. In women, the IUS is intimately lying on the anterior vaginal wall.

The acquired factor is an acquired behavior gained by learning and training in early childhood how to maintain a high alpha sympathetic tone at the IUS to keep it closed and empty all the time until there is a desire or a need to void.

2. Micturition

Micturition develops in two stages. First stage is uncontrolled reflex, which then gets central control in the second stage.

First stage of micturition: 2,

As the urinary bladder fills afferent sensations travel along the pelvic parasympathetic nerves (S. 2, 3 & 4) to the spinal cord. When it is full efferent pelvic parasympathetic nerve

---

* Corresponding Author

impulses induce detrusor muscle contraction; as urine enters the urethra it leads to relaxation of the external urethral sphincter (EUS) which is a skeletal muscle innervated by the somatic nerve supply, and thus micturition occurs irrespective of time and place.

Second Stage of micturition: (figure 1) 2,

At the age of about 18-24 months, the mother starts to teach her child how to hold up him self until she puts him on a ban. This is gained by building up and having high alpha sympathetic tone, (T 10- L 2) at the IUS keeping the urethra closed and empty all the time until voiding is needed and/or desired and the social circumstances allow (time and proper place are available).

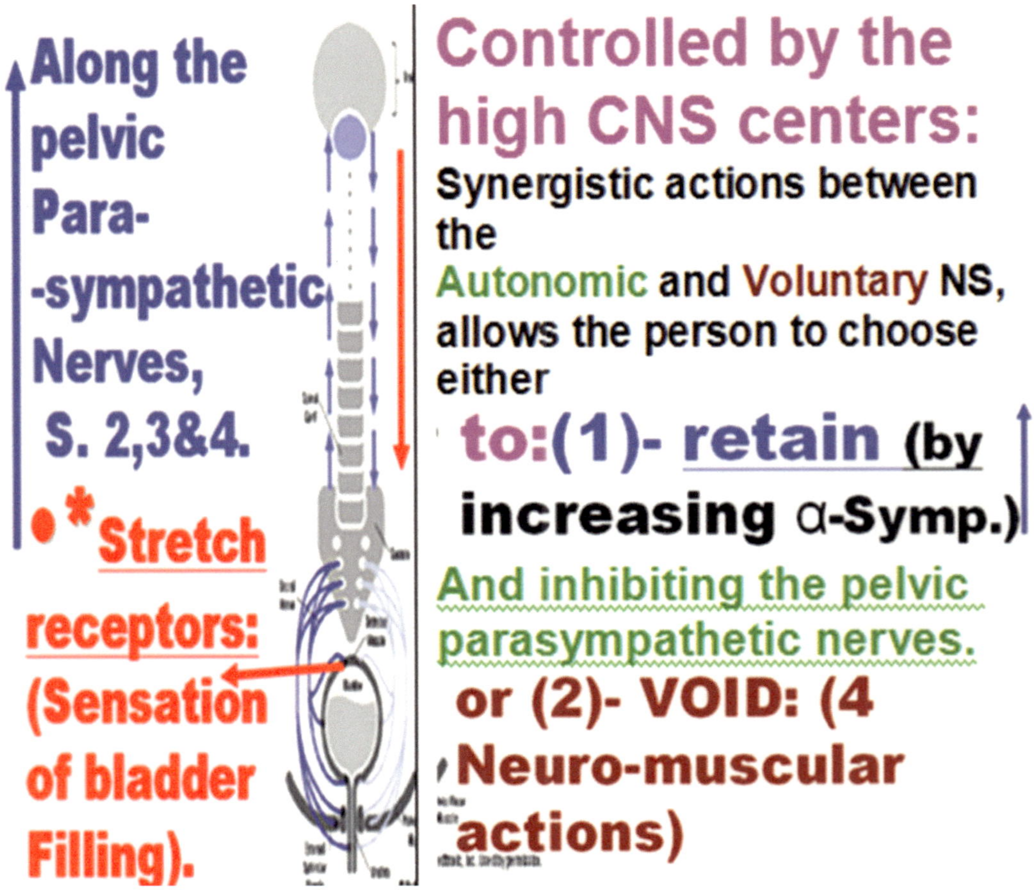

Fig. 1. Diagram that shows the CNS control of the steps taken in the second step of micturition. Sensations of bladder filling travels along the pelvic parasympathetic nerves S.2, 3 &4. Controlled by the CNS, depending on the social circumstances, synergistic neuromuscular actions take place. If time and place do not allow voiding, the person will increase the alpha sympathetic tone at the IUS. He will also inhibit the pelvic parasympathetic preventing detrusor contractions. In addition, he will confirm closure of the external urethral sphincter (EUS).

Sensations of bladder distension travel along the pelvic parasympathetic (S. 2, 3 & 4) to the central nervous system (CNS). Controlled by the high CNS, sensations of desire to void and bladder fullness, allows the person to choose either to retain the urine to a later time or to void according to the social circumstances available. If he chooses to retain the urine then three neuro-muscular actions take place: 1- He increases the alpha sympathetic tone to the IUS confirming its closure. 2- He inhibits the parasympathetic impulses to the detrusor muscle inhibiting its contractions. 3- He increases the tone of the EUS which is a skeletal muscle innervated by voluntary nervous system. When, appropriate time and place are available, then, controlled by the CNS, synergistic actions between the somatic and the autonomic nervous systems four neuro-muscular actions take place. (1) He will lower the high alpha sympathetic tone at the IUS relaxing the sphincter and opening the urethra, (2) he relaxes the EUS which is a striated muscle innervated by somatic nerve supply, (3) he activates the pelvic parasympathetic nerves to induce contraction of the detrusor muscle and empty the urinary bladder.

(4) The external urethral sphincter (Compressor Urethrae) acts to propagate and propel the stream of urine and at the end to squeeze the urethra to expel the last drops of urine in the urethra to keep the urethra closed and empty as it should be.

When social circumstances allow, he will inhibit the high alpha sympathetic tone at the IUS, thus opening the urethra. He will activate the pelvic parasympathetic inducing detrusor contractions. He will relax the EUS thus allowing voiding. The EUS tone increase to allow propulsion and ejection of the stream of urine and at the end of micturition to squeeze the urethra from the last few amount of urine. The grey drawing is from the scientific net pages on micturition, www.obgyn.net

In addition, we described the structure of the vagina in a novel way 1 & 7. The vagina is composed of collagen-muscular-elastic layer. The collagen layer is the tough layer that give the vaginal walls their strength and to keep the vagina in its upward position. Childbirth, especially prolonged, difficult, repeated & frequent and instrumental vaginal deliveries cause overstretching of the vagina with subsequent rupture of it collagen sheet. The rupture of the vagina affects mainly its transverse axis leading to flabby redundant vaginal walls with subsequent vaginal prolapse. The same trauma will affects the intimately overlying IUS leading to rupture of its collagen layer. The torn weak IUS will not stand sudden increase of abdominal pressure as coughing, jumping, sneezing, laughing and even coitus, and urine will leak involuntary, stress urinary incontinence (SUI). As soon as the woman feels wetting herself due to escape of urine, being embarrassed, reactive sympathetic activity reflex, will increase the sympathetic tone at the IUS to confirm its closure and preventing further leak of urine. This may explain the strong indications that there is a causal relationship between OAB and POP (8-18). Thus by understanding this new concept, we can explain most of the voiding troubles.

Functional disturbances, and/or structural damage of the IUS will lead to urinary incontinence, and voiding troubles 1-7.

1. Failure to acquire the second stage of micturition leads to Nocturnal Enuresis. These failures can be complete failure, (here there is a stop at the first stage of micturition), as the urinary bladder fills it empties irrespective to neither time nor place, leading to day

and night enuresis. About ten per cent of nocturnal enuresis patients suffer from diurnal enuresis as well.

The failure can be partial, during waking time as the bladder is full and there is a feeling of a desire to void, the patient will be embarrassed of wetting himself. Therefore, he increases the alpha sympathetic tone closing the IUS further preventing involuntary urination until he reaches the toilet, but on sleeping this weak partial alpha sympathetic tone will be lost and nocturnal enuresis will occur. This occurs in 90 per cent of nocturnal enuresis patients. Therefore, the treatment of nocturnal enuresis is not by giving anti-cholinergic drugs, but by giving alpha sympathomemmitc drugs 5.

2. Sympathetic over activity e.g., painful stimuli (e.g. episiotomy, abdominal or pelvic surgery), leads to retention of urine.
3. Spinal cord injury below the second lumbar neural level or spinal anesthesia, or diseases like SLE and disseminated sclerosis (DS) leads to loss of the pelvic parasympathetic sparing the thoraco-lumbar sympathetic supply will cause retention of urine or retention with overflow.
4. Sympathetic failure, like severe fear (figure 2) leads to transient urinary incontinence. Also alcohol, getting drunk (figure 3) may lead to transient UI.

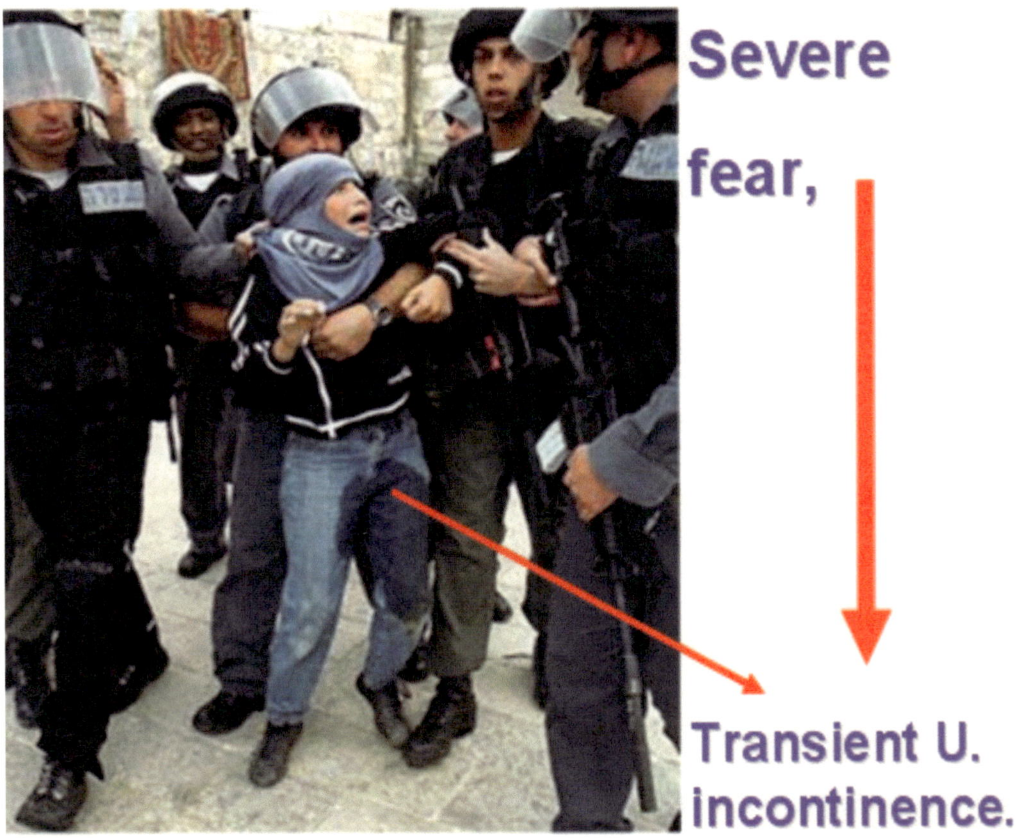

Fig. 2. Severe fear cause transient urinary incontinence.

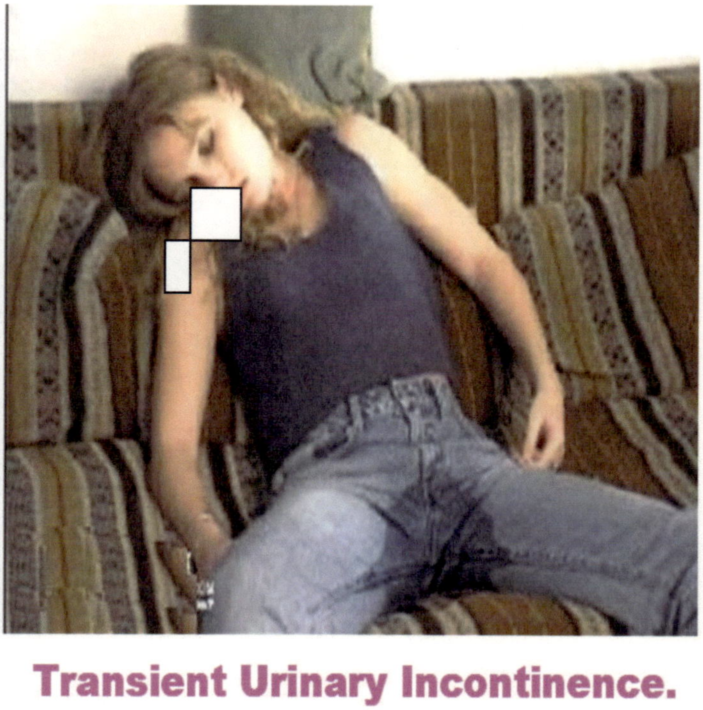

Fig. 3. Sympathetic failure due to getting drunk, leads to transient urinary incontinence.

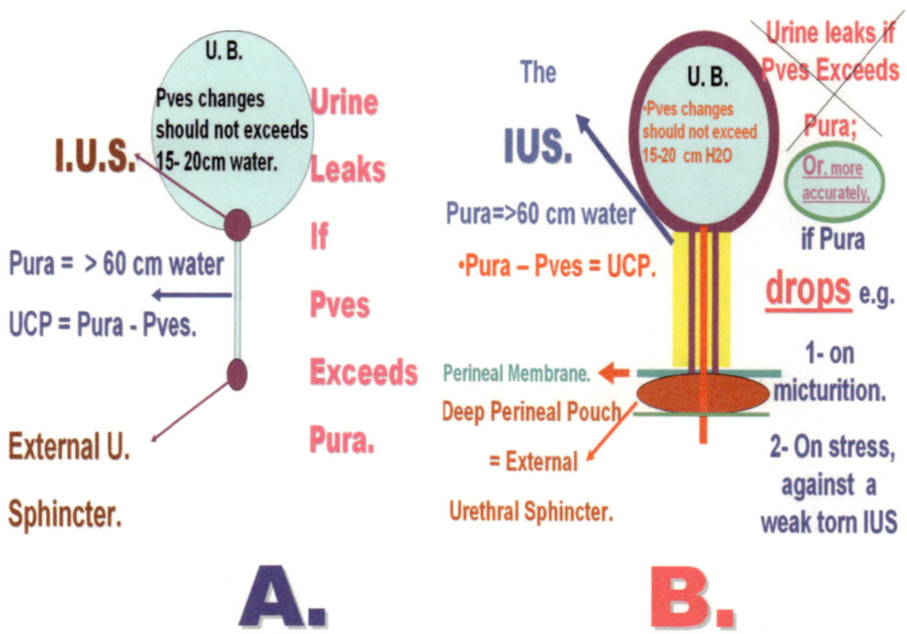

Fig. 4. A diagram to explain the site, extent and structure of the IUS and the EUS. On the left, (A) the IUS is a muscular ring at the bladder neck as described classically, on the right (B), the IUS as described in the new way.

The IUS is described by the new concept and as is seen by imaging (by three dimension ultrasound 3DUS and magnetic resonance MRI) is a cylinder that extends from the bladder neck to the urogenital diaphragm and is not a muscular ring at the bladder neck. (Figures 5, 6, 7, 8 & 9)

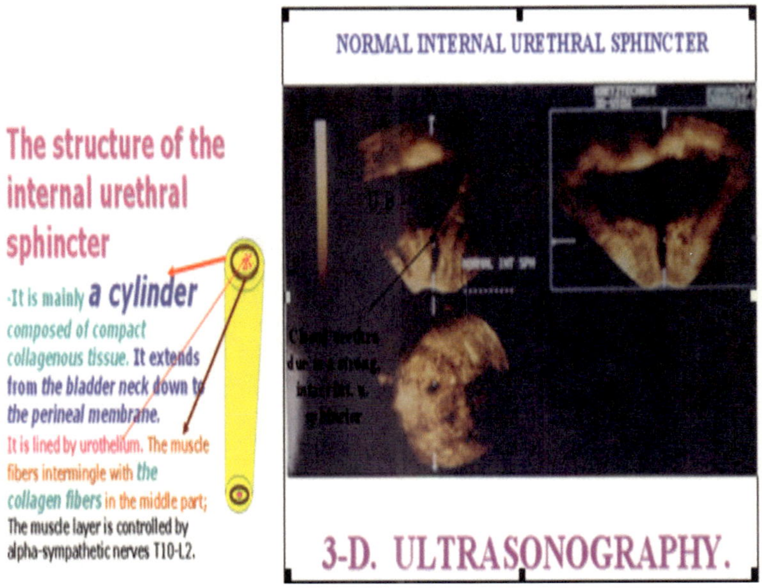

Fig. 5. On the left a diagram of the IUS as a cylinder of collagen-muscular tissue cylinder lined by urothelium is shown. On the right 3DUS image of a normal continent woman with the IUS seen as a cylinder that extends from the urinary bladder neck downwards with 2 echoes overlying each other, and a closed urethra.

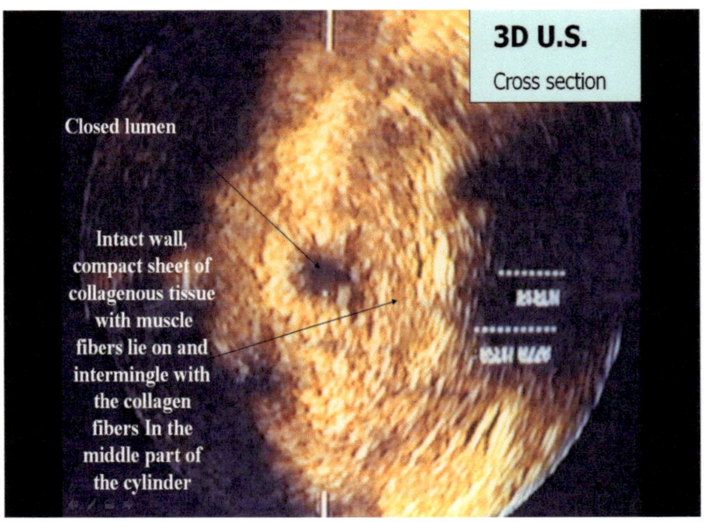

Fig. 6. Cross section of the IUS as seen by 3DUS image, it shows a closed urethral lumen, surrounded by a cylinder of collagen with superimposed muscle on top and intermingling with the collagen fibers in the mid thickness of the cylinder.

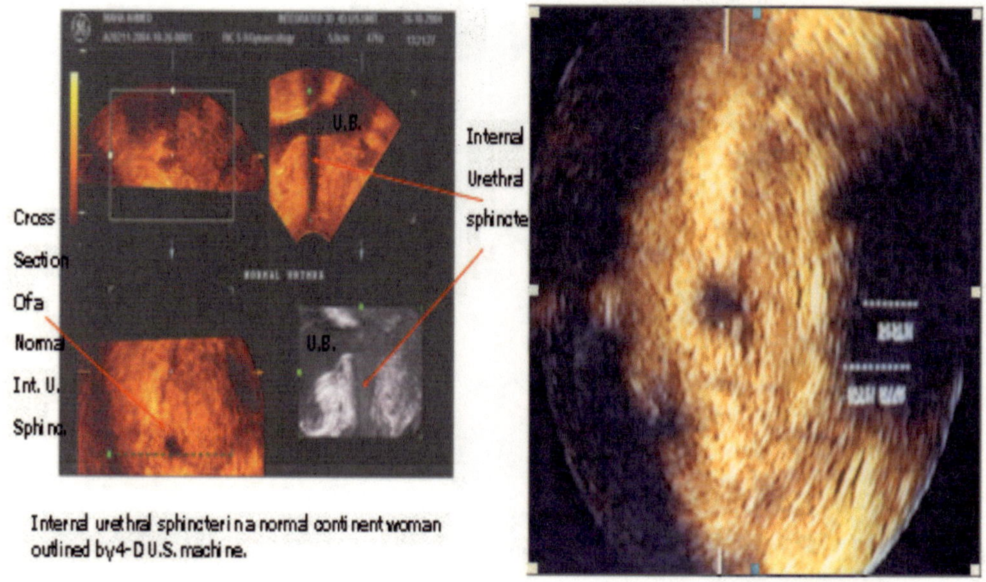

Fig. 7. Images by 3DUS and 4DUS of a normal healthy intact IUS.

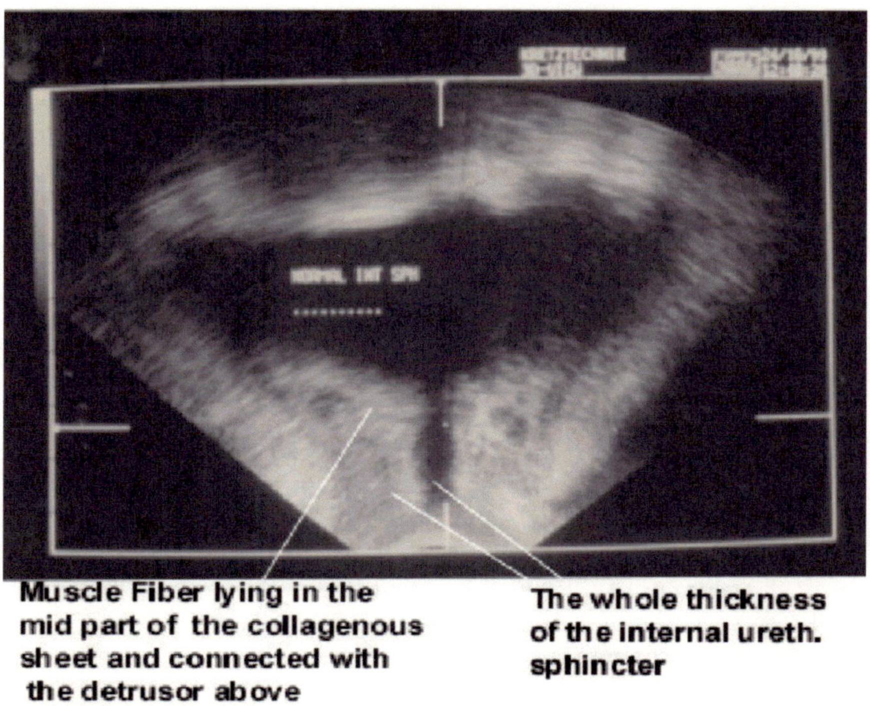

Fig. 8. Coronal section of the urinary bladder and the IUS as seen by 3DUS imaging showing uniform thickness of the intact IUS extending from the bladder neck downwards. You can kindly notice the muscle lying on the collagen cylinder and has a connection above with the detrusor muscle.

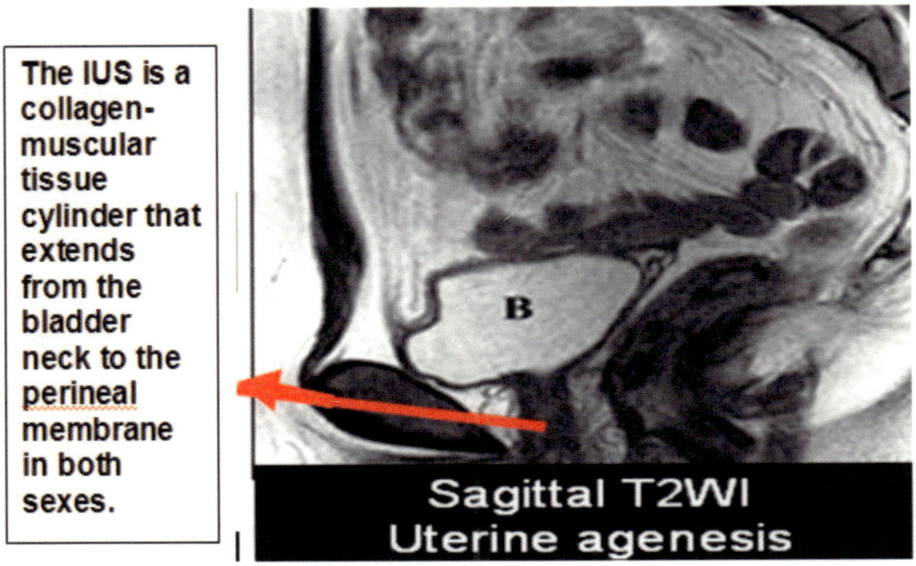

Fig. 9. MRI picture of a patient with Mullerian duct agensis (absent uterus and vagina) that shows the IUS as a thick tissue cylinder that extends from the bladder neck downwards to the perineal membrane.

The level and the extent of the lacerations along the cylinder of the IUS will determine the type and severity of SUI, and the morphological shape seen on imaging the IUS with 3DUS and MRI. When the damage affects mainly in the upper part of the IUS, DO (over active bladder, OAB) will ensue. If the damage is mainly in the lower part, then genuine, urodynamic, SUI ensues. If the damage affects the entire length of the IUS, mixed type of UI is the result.

A tough and a strong anterior vaginal wall (figures 10 & 11) is an essential support for keeping the vagina in its upward position, and is a major support for the intimately overlying IUS and the lower part of the posterior wall of the urinary bladder on filling. A weak overstretched and flabby anterior vaginal wall will fall down (prolapse), with its overlying damaged IUS and lower part of the posterior wall of the urinary bladder on filling. The strength and the toughness of the vaginal wall depend on its rich compact collagen sheet. The compact tough collagen bundles are essential elements of keeping the vagina in its normal upward position without descending or falling down. As an example, a hardcover book will stand upright on a shelf, while a paper-cover book will fall down.

Childbirth trauma causes over stretching of the vagina with attenuation, split and actual lacerations of the collagen bundles in the vagina leading to weakness and laxity of the vaginal wall. The weakness and rupture of the vaginal collagen sheet will manifest itself mostly in the transverse axis of the vagina.

Clinically and on imaging (figure 11) will demonstrate this:

1. At first, there will be loss of the nulliparous H-shape vagina, which changes into a transverse slit in parous women.
2. Then, further weakness, will lead to loss of vaginal rugae; the vaginal wall will be smooth without folds as can be seen clinically.

3. Further weakness and rupture of the vaginal collagen will induce vaginal wall redundancy and descent.

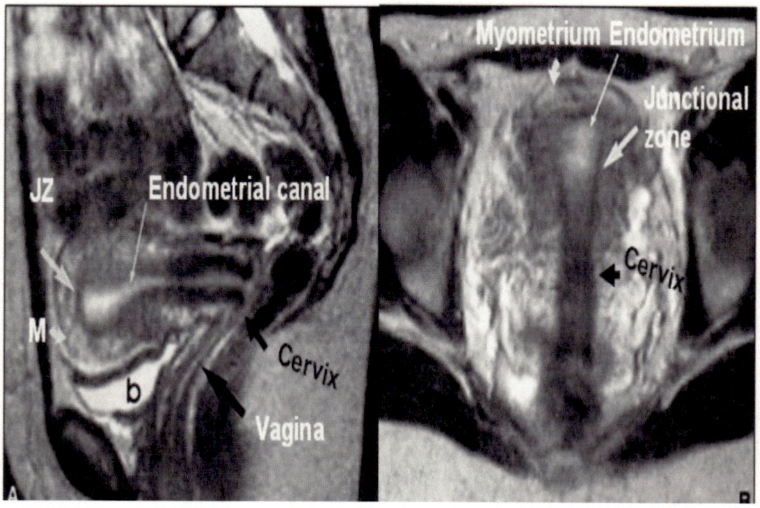

Fig. 10. MRI pictures of Normal tough vagina, which is standing up because of its tough collagen sheet.

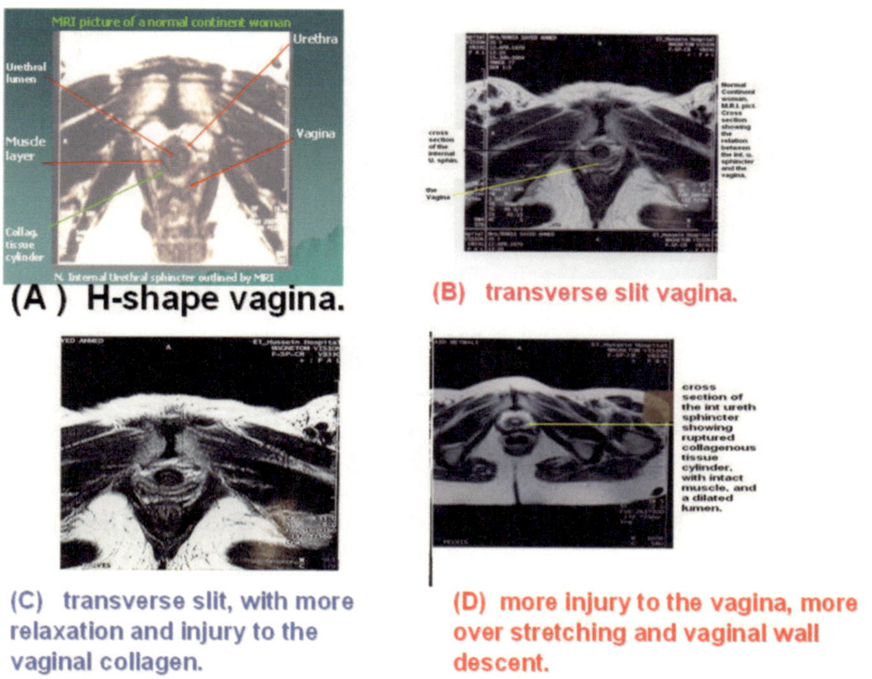

Fig. 11. MRI pictures, cross sections, (A) the vagina is seen H-shape in nulliparous woman with intact IUS. (B) Vaginal delivery transform the vagina is into transverse slit, the IUS is intact. (C) The vagina is more lax, the IUS is intact. (D) The vagina is torn and prolapsed; also, the IUS is torn.

In patients suffering SUI, the IUS is torn and disrupted with echo-lucent areas in 3DUS images (Figures 12-19). Depending on the level and extent of the damage along the cylinder there are different morphological and functional changes. When the damage affects mainly the upper part there will be funneling of the urinary bladder neck with loss of the urethro-vesical angle and apparent descent of the bladder neck and shortening of the urethra. Urine will enter the upper part of the urethra on sudden increase of intra-vesical pressure giving sensation of sudden desire to void, DO. When the damage affects mainly the lower part there will be a flask-shape appearance, and genuine SUI ensues. When the damage affects the entire length there will be collapse of the urethra, with apparent shortening and mixed type of urinary incontinence.

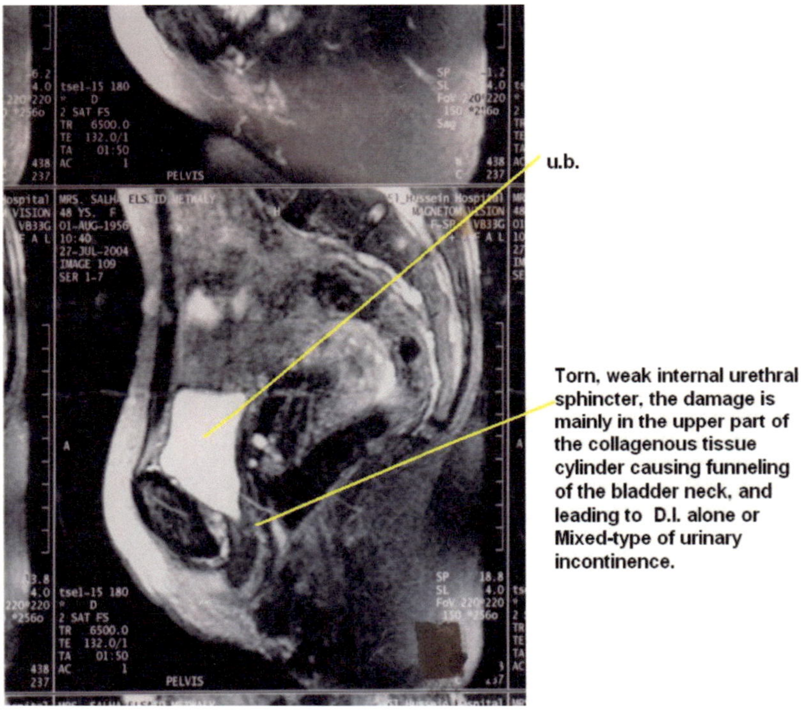

Fig. 12. Sagittal section of MRI picture showing the IUS seen as a cylinder that extends from the bladder neck to the perineal membrane. Rupture of the IUS is mainly in the upper part causing funneling of the bladder neck (leading to DO).

The torn weak IUS with a lower UCP will, on sudden increases of abdominal pressure, intra- vesical pressure, give way, with resultant leakage of urine. Leakage of urine will induce a rapid reactive sympathetic activity that will increase the sympathetic tone at the IUS preventing further loss of urine (10, 11, 12, 13, 14 &15).

In some patients suffering from SUI, the urodynamic studies show high UCP at rest. Cases where there is just splitting of the compact collagen tissue cylinder, without any observable defective rupture in this compact layer, leaving the IUS with high wall tension. However, on stress the split weak wall yields leading to leakage of urine. 3DUS and MR imaging can better assess the defect. Weakness of the IUS leads to SUI, DO and mixed type of UI. The weakness is mostly due to traumatic injury of the IUS causing rupture, and/or split of the collagen tissue cylinder, the essential constituent of the IUS. Nevertheless, weakness of the pelvic collagen (collagen of the IUS and the collagen of the vagina) can be caused by, or exaggerated, by other causes e.g. (1) hormone deficiency particularly after menopause. (2) Chronic or repeated genito-urinary infections may lead to degeneration of the pelvic collagen and its weakness. (3) Congenital collagen weakness.

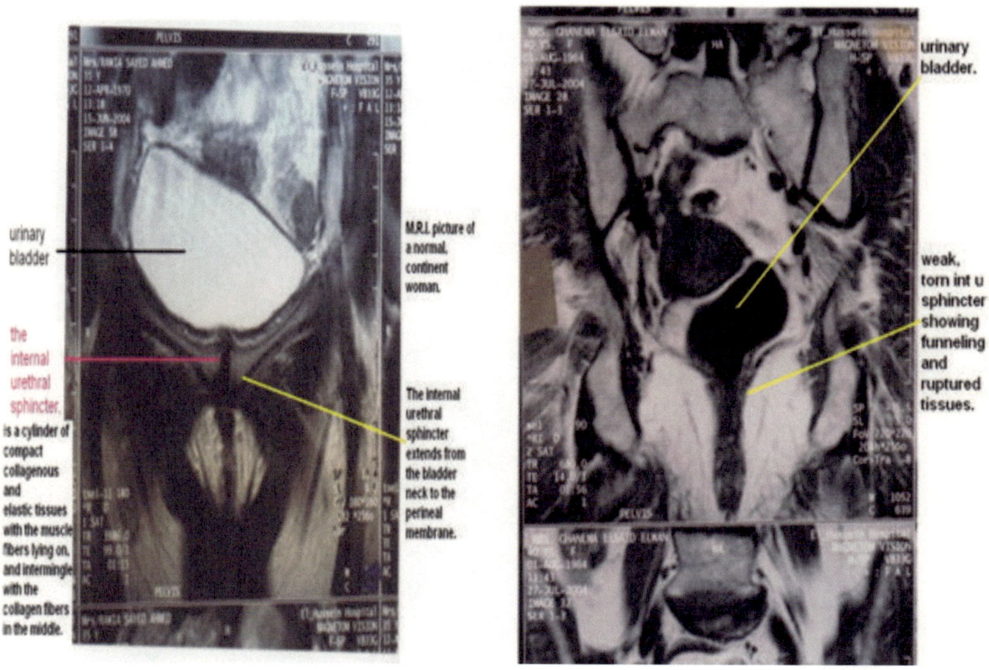

Fig. 13. Coronal sections of MRI pictures of a normal continent woman on the left showing healthy uniform cylinder compared to torn IUS on the right, the whole length is torn, showing funneling in the upper part and flak-shape appearance in the lower part (the woman is complaining of Mixed type of UI).

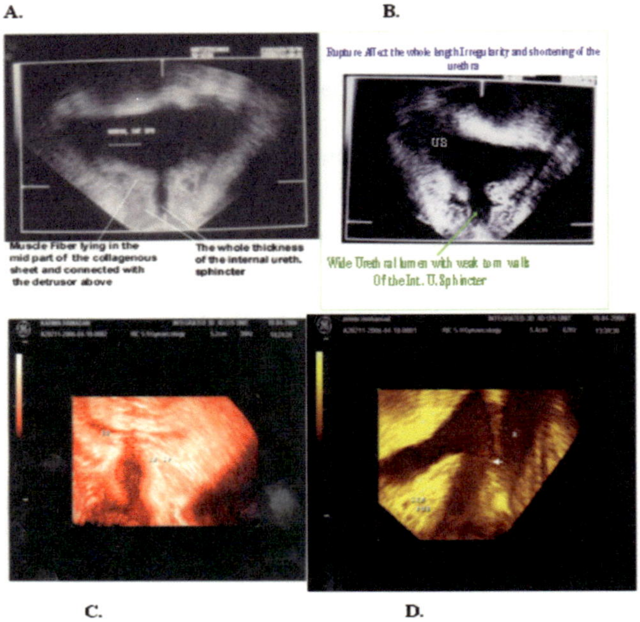

Fig. 14. Images by 3DUS, picture (A) a normal IUS, compared to torn IUS (B, C & D). The whole length is torn in (B); the rupture is mainly in the lower part in (C) leading to genuine SUI and flask-shape appearance. There is a loss of Posterior U-V angle in (D) with widely open urethra.

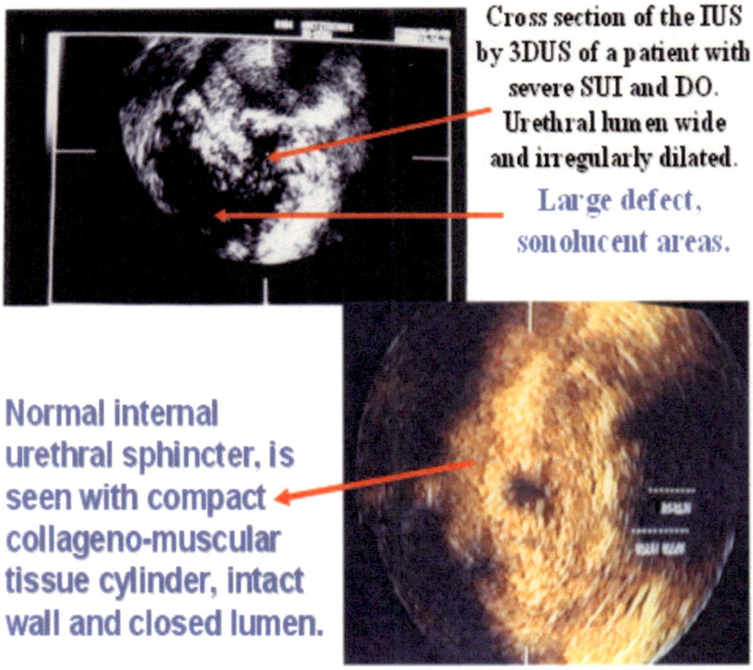

Fig. 15. Cross sections of 3DUS images of torn IUS compared to normal IUS.

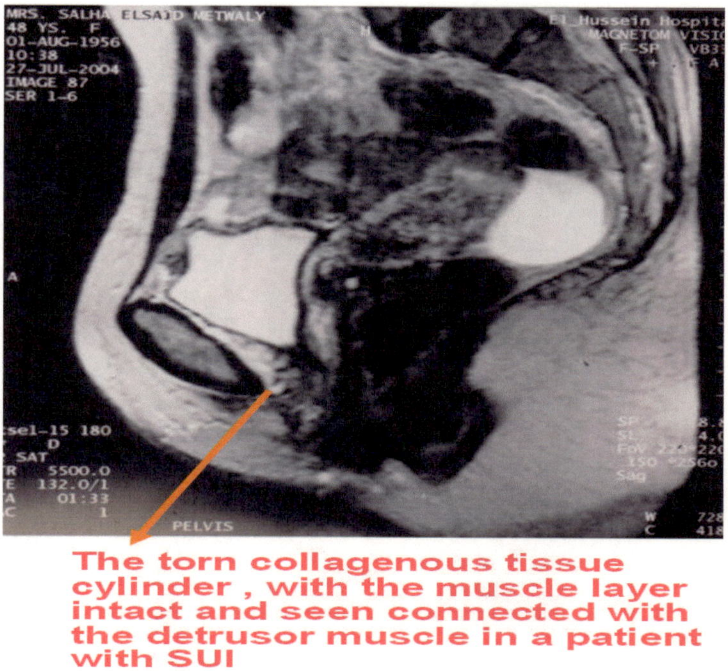

Fig. 16. MRI picture sagittal view, there is rupture of the IUS. The rupture is in the collagenous sheet; the muscle layer is intact and has a connection above with the detrusor muscle. In addition to the rupture of the collagen sheet of the IUS, hormone deficiency, (the patient is post menopause) is causing atrophy of the collagen sheet.

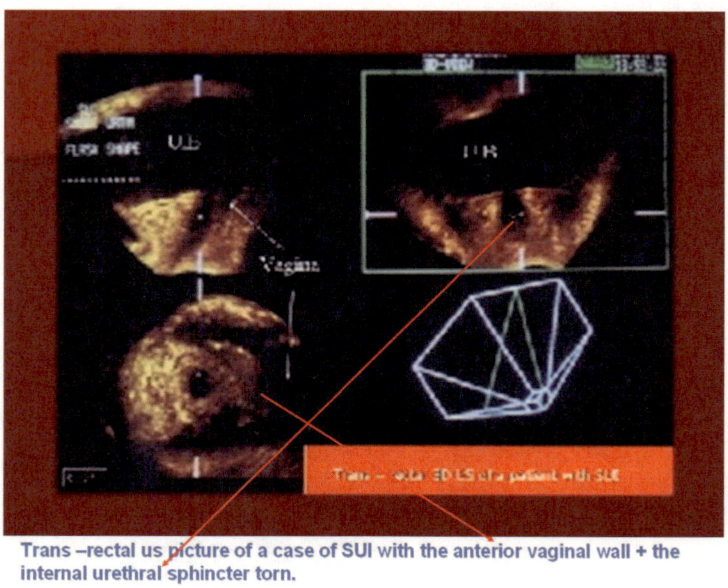

Fig. 17. Trans-rectal 3DUS image of the IUS and the anterior vaginal wall that shows torn posterior wall of the IUS together with the anterior vaginal wall. The symphsis pubis is protecting the anterior wall of the IUS.

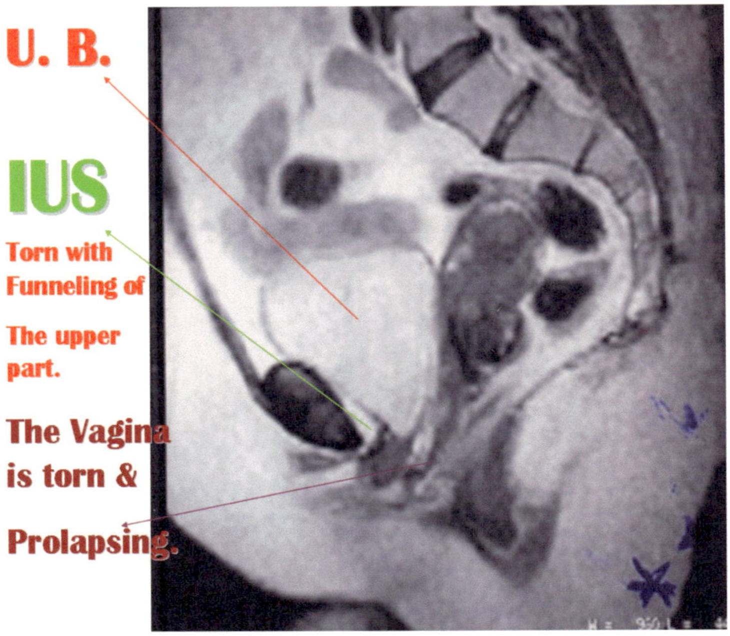

Fig. 18. MRI, sagittal view of a patient with DO that shows torn upper part of the IUS with funneling. The IUS is seen clearly as a compact tissue cylinder that extends from the bladder neck downwards.

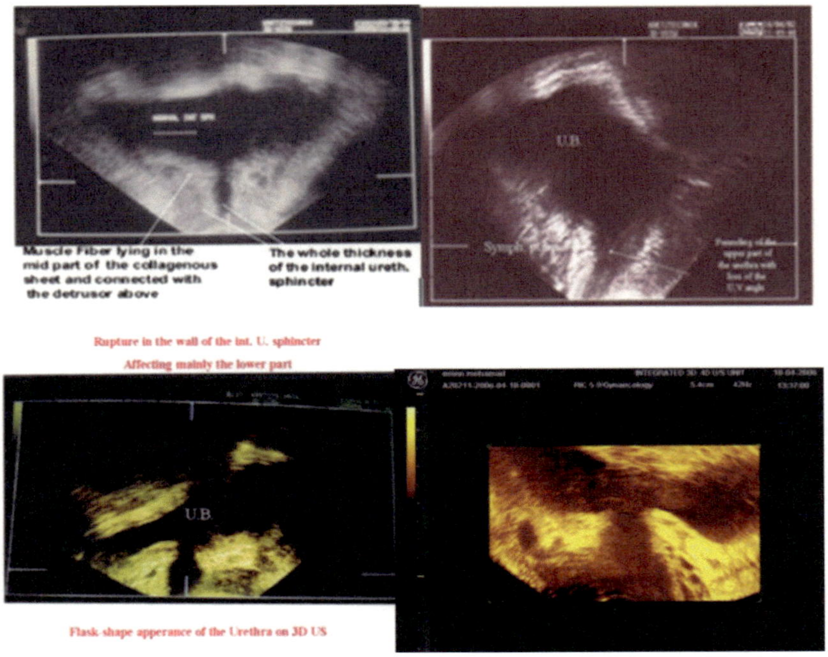

Fig. 19. 3DUS images of normal intact IUS on the upper left corner compared to a nice funnel on the upper right, the lower 2 images show torn the whole length with funneling of the upper part and flask-shape in the lower part.

3. References

[1] Abdel Karim M. El Hemaly*, Ibrahim M. Kandil, Asim Kurjak, Ahmad G. Serour, Laila A. S. Mousa, Amr M. Zaied, Khalid Z. El Sheikha. Imaging the Internal Urethral Sphincter and the Vagina in Normal Women and Women Suffering from Stress Urinary Incontinence and Vaginal Prolapse. Gynaecologia Et Perinatologia, Vol18, No 4; 169-286 October-December 2009.

[2] El Hemaly AKMA, Mousa L.A. Micturition and Urinary Continence. Int J Gynecol Obstet 1996; 42: 291-2.

[3] Abdel Karim M. El Hemaly*, Laila A. S. Mousa Ibrahim M. Kandil, Fatma S. El Sokkary, Ahmad G. Serour, Hossam Hussein. Surgical Treatment of Stress Urinary Incontinence, Fecal Incontinence and Vaginal Prolapse By A Novel Operation "Urethro-Ano-Vaginoplasty" Gynaecologia Et Perinatologia, Vol19, No 3; 129-188 July-September 2010.

[4] El Hemaly AKMA, Mousa L.A.E. Stress Urinary Incontinence, a New Concept. Eur J Obstet Gynecol Reprod Biol 1996; 68: 129-35.

[5] El Hemaly AKMA. Nocturnal Enuresis: Pathogenesis and Treatment. Int Urogynecol J Pelvic Floor Dysfunct 1998;9: 129-31.

[6] Ibrahim M. Kandil, Abdel Karim M. El Hemaly, Mohamad M. Radwan: Ultrasonic Assessment of the Internal Urethral Sphincter in Stress Urinary Incontinence. *The Internet Journal of Gynecology and Obstetrics.* 2003. Volume 2 Number 1.

[7] Abdel Karim M. El Hemaly, Ibrahim M. Kandil, Asim Kujak, Laila ASE Mousa, Hossam H. Kamel, Ahmad G. Serour. Ultrasonic Assessment of the Urethra and the Vagina in Normal Women and Women Suffering from Stress Urinary Incontinence and Vaginal Prolapse. Donald School Journal of Ultrasound in Obstetrics and Gynecology. October-December 2011, Vol 5, No 4; 330-338.

[8] .A. de Boer, S. Salvatore, L. Cardozo, C. Chapple, C. Kelleher, van Kerrebroeck, M.G. Kirby, Koelbl, Espuna-Pons, Milsom,Tubaro,Wagg, and M.E. Vierhout. Pelvic Organ Prolapse and Overactive Bladder, REVIEW ARTICLE Neurourology and Urodynamics 29:30–39 (2010)

[9] Bernard T. Haylen,y, Dirk de Ridder, Robert M. Freeman, Steven E. Swift, Bary Berghmans, Joseph Lee, Ash Monga, Eckhard Petri, Diaa E. Rizk, Peter K. Sand, and Gabriel N. Schaer. An International Urogynecological Association (IUGA)/International Continence Society (ICS) Joint Report on the Terminology for Female Pelvic Floor Dysfunction, REVIEW ARTICLE, Neurourology and Urodynamics 29:4–20 (2010)

[10] Dupont M.C., Albo ME and Raz S: Diagnosis of stress urinary incontinence: An overview. Urologic clinic of North America Urodynamic II. 1996; 23(3), 407-415.

[11] Burgio K, Diokno AC, Herzog AR, Hjalmas K, Lapitan MC. Epidemiology and natural history of urinary incontinence. In: Abrams P, Cardozo L, Khoury S, Wein A, eds. *Incontinence*. Plymouth, UK: Health Publication Ltd; 2002; 165-201.

[12] McGuire E J, Cespedes D and O'Connell H E: Leak-point pressures. Urologic clinics of North America. 1996; 23, (2), 253-262.

[13] DuBeau C, Kuchel G, Johnson T, Palmer M, Wagg A. Incontinence in the frail elderly. In: P. Abrams P, Cardozo L, Khoury S, Wein A, editors. Incontinence. 4th International Consultation on Incontinence. . 4th ed. Plymouth, UK: Health Publications Ltd.; 2009.

[14] Abrams P, Cardozo L, Fall M, Griffiths D, Rosier P, Ulmsten U, et al. The standardisation of terminology in lower urinary tract function: report from the standardisation sub-committee of the International Continence Society. Urology 2003 Jan; 61(1):37-49.
[15] Fowler, C.J., D. Griffiths, and W.C. de Groat, The neural control of micturition. Nat Rev Neurosci, 2008. 9(6): p. 453-466.
[16] Benarroch, E.E., Neural control of the bladder. Neurology, 2010. 75(20): 1839-1846.
[17] Miller J, Hoffman E. The causes and consequences of overactive bladder. *J Womens Health* 2006; 15 (3): 251–60.
[18] Wein AJ, Rackley RR. Overactive bladder: a better understanding of pathophysiology, diagnosis sand management. J Urol 2006; 175: S5–10

Part 2

The Overactive Bladder

10

Diagnosis and Treatment of Overactive Bladder

Howard A. Shaw[1,2] and Julia A. Shaw[2]
[1]*Hospital of Saint Raphael*
[2]*Yale University School of Medicine*
USA

1. Introduction

Overactive bladder (OAB) is a disturbance of filling/storage and has been defined by the International Continence Society as "a symptom syndrome consisting of urgency with or without urge urinary incontinence, often associated with urinary frequency and nocturia." (Abrams et al., 2002) OAB has been divided into OAB without urinary incontinence (OAB_{dry}) and OAB with urinary incontinence (OAB_{wet}). The reported prevalence of OAB in women varies between 7.7 and 31.3%, and increases with age. (Irwin et al., 2006a; McGother et al., 2006;Milsom, et al., 2001; Stewart et al., 2003; Wagg et al., 2007)

The symptoms of OAB include urinary urgency, urinary frequency, nocturia, and urinary urge incontinence. These symptoms often remain undetected and undertreated by both the woman and her providers, despite the substantial impact on a woman's quality of life. (Griffiths et al., 2006; Mardon et al., 2006) In a multiethnic survey, only 45 percent of women who reported weekly urinary incontinence sought care for their incontinence symptoms. (Harris et al., 2007) This leaves incontinent women with psychological morbidity and a diminished quality of life. (Irwin et al., 2006b)

2. Etiology

2.1 Normal micturition

The normal micturition cycle includes inhibition and contraction of detrusor smooth muscle, afferent signaling from the urothelium, contraction and relaxation of the smooth and striated sphincter muscles, and the central, peripheral, and autonomic nervous systems.

Urine storage occurs secondary to afferent signals stimulated by bladder filling. These afferent signals activate sympathetic pathways in the hypogastric and pudendal nerves, which lead to contraction of the smooth and striated sphincters, and at the same time inhibit detrusor contraction. In addition, high cortical centers are activated, (Griffiths et al, 2007), and stimulate the storage center in the pons. (Fowler et al, 2008) When further bladder filling leads to increased afferent signaling from the bladder, spinobulbospinal reflex pathways are carried via the pelvic nerve and spinal cord to the pontine micturition center, which activates parasympathetic pathways that cause bladder contraction and inhibit sympathetic and pudendal contraction of the sphincter (Fowler et al, 2008)

For coordinated micturition to occur, parasympathetic stimulation of the detrusor occurs via cholinergic muscarinic receptors. Urethral smooth muscle contraction occurs chiefly by stimulation of alpha-adrenerigic receptors. (Fowler et al, 2008) In addition, a variety of neurotransmitter systems in the urothelial lining of the bladder and in bladder interstitial cells likely play a role in mediating bladder contraction and relaxation via afferent signaling. (Andersson, 2002) This complex interplay results in socially appropriate and effective voiding. Any disruption in this pathway can lead to storage and/or emptying disorders. Bladder overactivity may be related to neurogenic, myogenic, or idiopathic origins.

2.2 OAB etiology

The presumed etiology of OAB is uninhibited bladder contractions, but overactivity is not sufficient to cause incontinence (e.g. OAB_{dry}). In addition, leakage symptoms may be due to factors outside of the lower urinary tract such as failure of compensatory mechanisms in the lower urinary tract (e.g. fascial and muscular urethral support "hammock" that compresses the urethra when there is increased abdominal pressure or when the pelvic muscles are contracted) , and functional impairments in some patients.

2.2.1 Neurogenic etiologies

2.2.1.1 Suprapontine lesions

Patients with suprapontine lesions such as cerebrovascular disease and Parkinson's disease can present with detrusor overactivity. These patients lose voluntary inhibition of micturition most likely secondary to uninhibited detrusor contractions. (Fall, et al, 1989) (Fall, et al, 1995) The cerebral cortex and the basal ganglia are theorized to suppress the micturition reflex. Therefore, damage to the brain results in bladder overactivity by reducing suprapontine inhibition. (Koelbl et al, 2009)

2.2.1.2 Spinal cord lesions

Spinal cord disruption below the level of the pons leads to unsustained and uncoordinated detrusor contractions. (Koelbl et al, 2009) Impairment or loss of bladder sensation usually occurs. Patients with spinal cord lesions above the lumbosacral level lose voluntary and supraspinal control of micturition. Bladder overactivity in these patients is mediated by spinal reflex pathways (deGroat et al, 1993) (Bros & Comarr,1971)

2.2.2 Non-neurogenic etiologies

2.2.2.1 Outflow obstruction

Outflow obstruction is associated with detrusor overactivity. (Koelbl et al, 2009) Up to 50% of patients with symptomatic benign prostatic enlargement exhibit bladder outlet obstruction. (de Nunzio et al, 2003) However, OAB symptoms can occur independently of bladder outlet obstruction. One hypothesis that has been proposed to explain how outflow obstruction causes OAB and detrusor overactivity includes partial denervation.

Denervation injury has been shown to increase detrusor supersensitivity to acetylcholine. (Harrison et al, 1987) This may be the basis of unstable bladder activity. However, it is not clear how denervation develops in patients with outflow obstruction. It is possible that there is a reduction of blood flow due to increased intravesical pressure during voiding or the increased tissue pressure of hypertrophied bladder wall during filling. (Azadzoi et al, 1996) (Greenland & Brading, 2001)

2.2.2.2 Aging

The prevalence of OAB in both men and women increases with age. In addition, storage symptom scores increase with age while bladder compliance decreases. (Koelbl et al, 2009) This implies that bladder function in both sexes has age related alterations. (Araki et al, 2003) There can be difficulty however, in determining in the elderly, the difference between neurogenic and non-neurogenic causes.

2.2.2.3 Estrogen deficiency

Menopause and estrogen deficiency have been implicated in the etiology of OAB symptoms. (Koelbl et al, 2009) Estrogen receptors (ERs) have been identified in the bladder and urethra. (Blakeman et al, 2000) The effect estrogen has on bladder contractility has yet to be elucidated.

However, it has been shown that estrogen replacement therapy can significantly improve the symptoms of frequency, urgency and urge incontinence. (Eriksen & Rasmussen,1992) In addition, a metaanalysis of the effects of estrogen therapy on symptoms of OAB in postmenopausal women showed that estrogen therapy was associated with significant improvements in all symptoms of OAB. (Cardoza et al, 2004b) Thus it appears that menopause plays role in the development of bladder overactivity and OAB symptoms in women.

2.2.3 Idiopathic etiologies

Idiopathic detrusor overactivity is a diagnosis of exclusion of all other known causes. Mechanisms that have been proposed for idiopathic detrusor overactivity include myogenic, urothelial and muscarinic.

2.2.3.1 Myogenic

Mills et al, noted that denervation is consistently found in detrusor biopsies from patients with non-neurogenic detrusor overactivity. (Mills et al, 2000) They hypothesize that partial denervation of the detrusor alters the properties of smooth muscle, which leads to increased excitability and increased coupling between cells. Thus, myogenic changes in the bladder increase contractility locally.

2.2.3.2 Urothelial

Another mechanism that has garnered interest in idiopathic detrusor overactivity is the roles of the urothelium and suburothelial myofibroblasts in afferent activation. The C-fiber afferents have endings in the suburothelial layer of the bladder wall, and may reach the urothelium. (Koelbl et al, 2009) Upon bladder distention ATP has been shown to be released from the urothelium. (Ferguson et al, 1997) ATP receptors on afferent nerve terminals are stimulated by ATP release to evoke a neural discharge. It has been proposed that there is up-regulation of the afferent activation mechanisms(eg. an increased generation/release of ATP increased sensitivity of afferent nerves to mediators, increased number of afferent nerves) can cause the symptoms of OAB. (Koelbl et al, 2009)

2.2.3.3 Muscarinic

As stated above, muscarinic receptors play a significant role in OAB. ATP, Acetylcholine (Ach) and other "signaling molecules, interact with the afferent nerve fibers under the urothelium. Bladder distention presumably causes release of Ach (and other molecules) to stimulate muscarinic receptors on myofibroblasts(predominantly M2). (Mansfield et al 2005) It appears that an increase in Ach release from the urothelium and/or upregulation of muscarinic receptors in the urothelium as well as in suburothelial myofibroblasts may increase afferent nerve activity and contribute to the development of detrusor overactivity. (Koelbl et al, 2009)

3. Clinical presentation

Women with OAB may experience urinary urgency at inconvenient and unpredictable times. Urgency is the complaint of a sudden compelling desire to pass urine which is difficult to defer. In addition, patients may experience increased 24-hour frequency defined as the total number of daytime voids and episodes of nocturia during a specified 24 hours period. Daytime frequency is defined as the number of voids recorded during waking hours and includes the last void before sleep and the first void after waking and rising in the morning. Both frequency and urgency may occur and urine leakage may occur prior to reaching a toilet. These symptoms interfere with work, activities of daily life, intimacy, and sexual function, and they can also cause embarrassment and diminished self-esteem. (Shaw & Burrows, 2011) Many patients with OAB have symptoms that wake them up at night. Nocturia is the complaint that the individual has to wake at night one or more times to void.

4. Diagnosis

The presumptive diagnosis of OAB can usually be made in the primary care provider's office. Patients who present with the symptoms of urinary urgency and frequency can be evaluated utilizing standardized questionnaires, bladder diaries, a thorough history and physical examination, and simple laboratory tests. Those patients with more complex presentations may require urodynamic studies to confirm the diagnosis of OAB or detrusor overactivity.

4.1 Symptom and quality of life questionnaires

One of the most important aspects of the patient's history is to establish the impact of symptoms on their lives. This will guide the rest of the evaluation and subsequent treatment decisions. Most of the currently used symptom scales focus on patient-perceived frequency of symptoms and how much bother the symptoms cause. (Basra et al., 2007; Coyne et al., 2005a; Coyne et al., 2005b) Some newer validated scales have been developed which target more specific aspects of OAB. One of these, the OAB symptom score, is a 7-item questionnaire that records all the symptoms of OAB using consistent terminology. (Blaivas et al., 2007) Additionally, the International Continence Society (ICS) have established questionnaires (eg International Consultation on Incontinence Modular Questionnaire (ICIQ)) (Abrams et al, 2009))

4.2 Bladder diaries

Bladder diaries are an excellent tool that can be utilized to assess the frequency of daytime and nighttime voiding, as well as the timing of incontinence episodes and pad usage. Recently, bladder diaries have been developed that reliably assess the rate and severity of urinary urgency and are readily available. (Abrams et al, 2009) Despite some limitations, bladder diaries do provide a baseline with which to compare treatment efficacy.

4.3 History

A thorough history should inquire about the onset, duration, severity, and bother of lower urinary tract symptoms. In addition, a medical, surgical, gynecological, and obstetrical history should be obtained. Inquire about current medications which affect bladder function, particularly diuretics, alcohol, caffeine, narcotics, and calcium channel blockers.

4.4 Physical Examination

The physical examination should be focused on the abdominal and genitourinary examinations. The pelvic examination is used to evaluate the strength of the muscles of the pelvic floor and to assess for pelvic organ prolapse, urethral mobility, and stress urinary incontinence. The rectal examination is used to assess for any masses and to evaluate for constipation and anal tone. A simple, focused neurologic examination to evaluate pelvic reflexes, innervation of the lower extremities, and the patient's mental status completes the physical examination.

4.5 Urinalysis

Because some patients who present with acute symptoms of frequency and urgency have a urinary tract infection, a urinalysis (UA) is performed. In addition a UA will detect hematuria or glucosuria.

4.6 Postvoid residual

A post-void residual (PVR) is performed as a rough evaluation of as a measurement of the efficiency of evacuation of the bladder. This can be measured by bladder ultrasonography or post-void catheterization. Although there is no universally accepted definition of an abnormally elevated PVR, a high post-void residual (greater than 100 cc) may be cause for further, more complex testing. In addition, patients with high PVR's are at high risk for urinary retention, especially when anticholinergic medications are prescribed.

4.7 Urodynamic studies

Urodynamic studies can provide additional insight into bladder pathophysiology and can be a key to making the diagnosis of OAB and destrusor overactivity. Urodynamic studies are a series of clinical tests, such as flow studies, filling cystometry, pressure-flow studies and/or urethral function measurements. These can be combined with electromyography (EMG) recording and/or imaging by either X-rays or ultrasound. (Abrams et al, 2009)

The goal of urodynamic studies is to reproduce the symptom(s) of the patient under controlled and measurable conditions. According to the 4th International Consultation on Continence (Abrams et al, 2009) the role of urodynamic studies can be:

- To identify or to rule out factors contributing to the lower urinary tract(LUT) dysfunction To obtain information about other aspects of LUT dysfunction
- To predict the consequences of LUT dysfunction for the upper urinary tract
- To predict the outcome, including undesirable side effects, of a contemplated treatment
- To confirm the effects of intervention or understand the mode of action of a particular type of treatment
- To understand the reasons for failure of previous treatments for urinary incontinence, or for LUT dysfunction in general.

In addition to recommending the role of urodynamic studies, The International Continence Society (ICS) has provided standards for urodynamic terminology and techniques (Abrams, 2002) For example, urodynamic detrusor overactivity is defined by the ICS as "Loss of urine as a result incontinence of involuntary detrusor activity during the storage phase of urodynamic testing.

Following is a brief description of the most commonly used urodynamic studies.

4.7.1 Uroflowometry

Uroflowometry is a non-invasive measurement of urine flow rate. The patient urinates into a flow meter in private. (Schafer,2002) The flow rate is measured and displayed graphically. The volume voided, shape of the curve and the maximum flow rate are automatically graphed. These parameters determine if the patient is emptying their bladder normally. When an abnormal recording is obtained, it is best to repeat the assessment for reproducibility.

4.7.2 Filling cystometry

Filling cystometry is an invasive measurement of the pressure inside the bladder to assess its storage capabilities. It involves placing a pressure sensor into the bladder and another pressure sensor rectally or vaginally to measure abdominal pressure. A computer subtracts the abdominal pressure from the bladder pressure to provide the clinician with a graphic representation of pressure changes due to the true detrusor muscle. The bladder is usually filled with normal saline through the transurethral filling channel of a dual lumen catheter. The filling rate is usually controlled by a computer and the intravesical abdominal and detrusor pressure are monitored graphically. The storage ability of the bladder is assessed and presented graphically in terms of the volumes required to elicit various bladder sensations from the patient, its capacity, its compliance and its stability. The filling (storage) phase of cystometry is also the only method of demonstrating urodynamic stress incontinence (USI). (Abrams et al, 2009)

4.7.3 Pressure-flow studies (Voiding cystometry)

Voiding cystometry is a measurement of the mechanics of micturition. Generally this study is performed after bladder filling during cystometry is complete. While monitoring intravesical, abdominal and detrusor pressures, the patient is allowed to void and empties their bladder on a flow meter. Measurement of both flow rate and pressure allows voiding to be assessed. In patients whose bladder emptying is poor, it may determine if poor flow is due to outflow obstruction or poor detrusor contractility.

4.7.4 Urethral pressure profilometry

Urethral pressure profilometry is a test that measures the urethra's ability to maintain pressure along its length. This test is performed by placing a pressure sensor transurethrally into the bladder and usually withdrawing it along the urethra by a mechanical puller at a constant rate. The pressure along the length of the urethra is measured and graphically represented. The maximum pressure measured in the urethra gives an indication of the closure function of the urethra.

4.7.5 Abdominal leak point pressure

Similar to urethral pressure profilometry, abdominal leak point pressure is used as a measure of the urethra's ability to act as a valve to store urine. Intravesical or abdominal pressure is assessed while the patient is asked to increase their abdominal pressure by valsalva or by coughing. The abdominal pressure at which the patient leaks urine gives a measure of the closure pressure of the urethra. The greater the pressure required to produce leakage, the better the closure function of the urethra.

5. Management

The most commonly used measure of urinary incontinence (UI) treatment efficacy is a reduction in urinary incontinence episodes. Generally, this is recorded as the reduction in mean number of daily episodes, percent reduction from baseline, or reduction in leakage volume. Other outcome measures commonly used for OAB are urinary frequency (total number of daytime and nighttime voids) and frequency of urgency symptoms (with or without leakage). Cure is usually defined as complete absence of urinary incontinence. (Abrams, 2009)

One of the most important measures from the patient's perspective is quality of life. In the literature, many investigations measure patient perception of improvement of OAB, general satisfaction questions, and urinary incontinence-specific quality of life measures. The ICS recommends using patient reported outcome questionnaires that have been rigorously evaluated. (Koelbl et al, 2009)

5.1 Conservative therapies

Once the diagnosis of OAB has been made, the combination of dietary and lifestyle modification, bladder training, pelvic floor muscle training (PFMT), and biofeedback should be recommended as the initial intervention for OAB. (Burgio, 2002) The Agency for Health Care Policy and Research as well as the Third International Consultation on Incontinence recommends behavioral therapy as first-line therapy. (Wilson et al., 2005) The advantages of behavioral methods include avoidance of surgery, improved central control of bladder function and no adverse drug reactions.

5.1.1 Dietary and lifestyle modification

A common sense approach to the treatment of patients with OAB should include counseling patients on dietary and lifestyle modification that may improve their symptoms and quality of life. In general, patients should increase awareness of amounts and types of fluids consumed, especially as it relates to their symptoms. Although not well studied some foods and beverages are believe to increase detrusor activity and symptoms of OAB. The authors recommend that patient's begin to eliminate one food or beverage at a time from the following list:

- Beverages
  - Alcoholic
  - Caffeinated (Coffee, Tea)
  - Carbonated
- Foods
  - Tomatoes and tomato-based products
  - Spicy foods
  - Citrus juice and fruits
  - Artificial sweeteners
  - Chocolate
  - Corn syrup
  - Sugar
  - Honey

In one study patients with caffeine intake > 400 mg/day were shown to be 2.4 times more likely to have detrusor overactivity. (Arya, et al., 2000) In addition, limiting fluid intake has been shown to reduce frequency and urgency as well as improve quality of life in patients with OAB. (Milne, 2008 and Swithinbank et al., 2005)

Although weight loss is a good lifestyle modification, in general, it has been shown to significantly improve only stress urinary incontinence symptoms, but not OAB symptoms. A large randomized trial of overweight and obese women with urinary incontinence symptoms underwent an intensive 6 month weight loss program compared to a group with a structured education program. (Subak et al., 2009) Mean weight loss was 8 percent (7.8 kg) and 1.6 percent (1.5 kg) in the intervention and control groups, respectively. The authors found that weekly incontinence episodes decreased by 47 percent in the intervention group compared to only 28 percent in the control group. Of note, is that these patients had a significant decrease in stress incontinence, but not urge incontinence episodes.

5.1.2 Bladder retraining

Bladder training involves patient education and scheduled voiding in which the voiding interval is progressively increased. This method is based upon frequent voluntary voiding which keeps the bladder volume low and training the central nervous system on pelvic floor musculature to inhibit urgency. Utilizing the patient's bladder diary, the initial frequency of timed voiding is based on the smallest time interval between voids. The goals of bladder training are to normalize urinary frequency, to improve control over bladder urgency, to increase bladder capacity, to decrease incontinence episodes, to prolong voiding intervals, and to improve the patient's confidence in bladder control. It is safe and may be beneficial. (Wallace et al., 2004) Bladder training requires compliant and motivated patients and may not be suitable for those with cognitive impairment. It can be time-consuming and is primarily effective during waking hours. (Ouslander et al., 2001)

Patients can be instructed to follow the steps listed below for bladder training :(Modified from DuBeau, 2011):

- Go to the toilet and try to pass urine every two hours while you are awake.
  - You do not have to get up during the night!
- You must try to pass urine whether you feel the need or not
- You must try to pass urine even if you have just been incontinent.
- If you get a strong urge to go to the bathroom before your scheduled time:
  - Stop, don't run to the bathroom!
  - Stand still or sit down if you can.
  - RELAX. Take a deep breath and let it out slowly.
  - Concentrate on making the urge decrease or even go away, anyway you can.
  - When you feel in control of your bladder, walk slowly to the bathroom, and then go.
- Keep this schedule until you can go two days without urine leakage.
  - Then, increase the time between scheduled trips to the toilet by one hour
  - When you can go two days without urine leakage, extend the time between trips again.
- Keep this up until you can go four hours between trips to the toilet, or until you are comfortable.
  - This may take several weeks.
  - DON'T GET DISCOURAGED! Bladder training takes time and effort, but it is an effective way to get rid of incontinence without medication or surgery

A review in 2009 found that bladder training may be helpful for the treatment of urinary incontinence, but definitive research is needed to support that conclusion. (Wallace et al., 2004) However, there is very little downside to this therapy.

5.1.3 Pelvic floor muscle training (PFMT)

PFMT involves exercises designed to improve the function of the pelvic floor muscles. Using PFMT to treat OAB is based on the theory that contraction of the levator ani muscles can reflexively inhibit contraction of the detrusor muscle. PFMT is defined as any program of repeated voluntary pelvic floor muscle contractions (VPFMC) taught by a trained healthcare professional. (Wilson et al., 2005) Patients are taught to squeeze the pelvic floor with three sets of 8 to 12 slow velocity contractions held for six to eight seconds each. These exercises should be performed at least three or four times a week and continued for at least 15 to 20 weeks. (Hay-Smith et al., 2009)

There is increasing evidence to support the use of PFMT for OAB. Patients with detrusor overactivity who completed a PFMT program experienced a clinically and statistically significant reduction in daily UI episodes. (Ba & Berghmans, 2000 and Nygaard et al., 1996) These investigators also reported a significant decrease in urge score. This urge score was defined as the frequency of leakage (0 = never to 4 = always) during 9 activities that can trigger urge incontinence.

5.1.4 Weighted vaginal cones

Patients may have additional improvement in learning to appropriately do PFMT with the use of vaginal weighted cones. These cones are inserted in the vagina by the patient and she learns to contract the pelvic floor muscles to hold the cone in place.

5.1.5 Biofeedback

Biofeedback is used to teach patients how to control normal physiologic responses of the bladder and pelvic floor muscles that mediate urinary incontinence. Biofeedback for OAB consists of bladder-pressure biofeedback as well as the pelvic floor's muscular activity feedback. (Burgio et al., 1985)

5.1.6 Limitations of behavioral therapy

Behavioral therapy requires the active participation of motivated patients and a practitioner well-trained in behavioral therapy. Behavioral therapy does not cause permanent changes in bladder function; therefore, regular adherence and long-term compliance are needed for effectiveness.

5.2 Pharmacological agents

Traditionally, drug therapy is commenced at the same time as behavioral therapy. Drug treatment plays an important role in the management of women with OAB, although many drugs currently in use have not been subjected to controlled clinical trials in the treatment of OAB. From a review of the literature, it is clear that there is no ideal drug. (Hay-Smith et al., 2005) Current pharmacological approaches to improving the treatment of OAB include delayed release formulations of existing oral agents, new pharmaceutical agents with greater specificity/selectivity, and alternative routes of administration. New generation pharmacological treatments provide better or comparable efficacy with fewer adverse drug events. (Shaw & Burrows, 2011)

5.2.1 Antimuscarinic (anticholinergic) drugs

There are many different antimuscarinic compounds licensed for use for patients with OAB. Oxybutynin was the first drug of this class used specifically to treat the symptoms of OAB. This class of drugs has been considered the "gold standard" in the treatment of OAB for many years. However, there is little or no evidence to help clinicians choose between particular anticholinergic drugs. To add to the difficulty with studying this class of drugs, compliance with antimuscarinics is generally poor. (Brubaker et al., 2010)

Traditionally, it was thought that these drugs act by blocking the muscarinic receptors on the detrusor muscle. This resulted in decreased bladder contractions and thus reduced the symptoms of OAB. However, it appears that antimuscarinic drugs act primarily during the storage phase of the micturition cycle, decreasing urgency and increasing bladder capacity.

During this phase, there is normally no parasympathetic input to the LUT. (Abrams & Andersson, 2007)

A recent Cochrane review assessed the various anticholinergics available for the treatment of OAB in adults. The conclusions of this review were when the prescribing choice is between oral immediate-release oxybutynin and tolterodine, tolterodine might be preferred due to a reduced risk of dry mouth. In addition, they concluded that if extended-release preparations of either drug are available, they would be preferred to the immediate-release preparations because of the decreased risk of dry mouth and better compliance. There were insufficient data from trials of other anticholinergic drugs to draw any conclusions. (Hay-Smith et al., 2005) The most commonly prescribed anticholinergic drugs and their dosages in the treatment of OAB are listed in Table 1. (Shaw & Burrows, 2011)

5.2.1.1 Oxybutynin

As mentioned above, oxybutynin was the first anticholinergic widely used for the treatment of OAB. It is an anticholinergic agent that has antimuscarinic, antispasmodic, and potential local anesthetic effects. Oxybutynin has been shown to have a high affinity for the M1 & M3 receptors and much less affinity for the M2 receptor. (Hughes et al., 1992 and Nilvebrant & Sparf, 1986) It is available in immediate release (IR), extended release (ER), transdermal patch and topical gel formulations. In general, the efficacy is similar for all formulations. The initial dosage for IR is 2.5 mg two to three times daily, followed by titration as needed up to 20 mg/day in divided doses. The ER formulation is started at 5 mg once daily and titrated up to 20 to 30 mg once daily.

The transdermal patch (equivalent to 3.9 mg/day) applied to the abdomen, hip, or buttock is changed twice a week. The topical 10% gel is applied as 1 gm (approximately 1 mL) daily to the thigh, abdomen, upper arm, or shoulder. Currently, oxybutynin IR and ER are available as generic formulation in the United States. Oxybutynin IR is associated with high rates of anticholinergic adverse effects. Dry mouth is a particularly bothersome side effect for patients that can limit therapy with oxybutynin IR. This side affect is less frequent with the ER and transdermal preparations (Anderson et al., 1999; Davila et al., 2001; Versi et al., 2000) Irritation and pruritus at the application site has been reported in approximately 15 percent of patients using transdermal oxybutynin and 5 percent using the topical gel. (Dmochowski et al., 2002)

5.2.1.2 Tolterodine

Tolterodine has been shown to be a competitive muscarinic receptor antagonist with some selectivity for bladder muscarinic receptors [59]. It is available in immediate- and extended-release forms. Tolterodine is administered at 1 to 2 mg twice a day for the IR preparation or 2 to 4 mg per day using the ER preparation. It has similar efficacy when compared to other antimuscarinics. Both formulations have shown efficacy for symptoms of OAB in a large study population (Choo et al., 2008).

One of the few "head to head" studies between anticholinergic drugs was The STAR trial. In this study the investigators directly compared solifenacin (discussed below) at a flexible 5 or 10 mg once daily dose with tolterodine extended release 4 mg once daily in a randomized controlled trial. (Chapple et al., 2005) The authors found that the flexible dose of solifenacin showed marked advantages over the single dose of tolterodine extended release. In a reanalysis comparing only the patients in the trial taking solifenacin 5 mg once daily with the patients in the tolterodine arm the authors found a more modest benefit. (Chapple et al., 2007) Solifenacin 5 mg once daily was superior for incontinence episodes and pad usage, but showed no difference in urge incontinence or dryness rates. Notably in both analyses, the main advantage for solifenacin was minimizing rates of dry mouth and constipation. However, there were slightly more withdrawals due to adverse events in the solifenacin group.

5.2.1.3 Solifenacin

Solifenacin is an antimuscarinic agent has potent selectivity for the M3 over the M2 receptor. (Chapple et al., 2006) In addition it has a higher affinity for the M3 receptor in smooth muscle than it does for the M3 receptor in the salivary gland. (Chapple et al., 2006). This M3 selectivity provides for an improved side effect profile. Solifenacin is administered at 5-10 mg daily for the treatment of OAB.

It has been proven efficacious in multiple trials in patients with OAB. (Cardozo et al., 2004; Cardozo et al., 2008; Chapple, 2005) Another recent study confirmed that solifenacin was significantly more effective in reducing the mean number of severe urgency episodes with or without incontinence per 24 hours, improved urgency symptoms and was well tolerated. Additionally, no cognitive impairment has been associated with this drug. (Kay et al., 2006)

5.2.1.4 Trospium chloride

Trospium chloride is a quaternary ammonium compound that is nonselective for the muscarinic receptor. It also has smooth muscle relaxant qualities. (Staskin et al., 2007) Trospium chloride is available in an IR formulation given 20 mg twice daily or an ER formula administered 60 mg daily. The uniqueness of this antimuscarinic is that it is renally cleared. Care should be used in the elderly and patients with renal impairment. The initial dosing in these patients she be the IR formulation 20 mg once daily. The ER formulation should not be used in patients with severe renal impairment. Because of poor bioavailability, trospium chloride must be taken on an empty stomach.

When compared to placebo, trospium chloride showed a greater decrease in the number of daily episodes of incontinence than patients who received placebo (from a mean of 2.9 to 1.0 with trospium and 1.6 with placebo). (Zinner et al., 2004) Side effects in the trospium chloride group included dry mouth (20 percent) and constipation (11 percent).

In a randomized trial utilizing the ER formulation (60 mg once daily) for patients with severe urge incontinence, patients' incontinence episodes decreased significantly compared to placebo. Adverse events were lower than reported for immediate-release trospium chloride (dry mouth 13 percent, constipation 8 percent). (Dmochowski et al., 2008)

5.2.1.5 Fesoterodine

Fesoterodine is given at a starting dose of 4 mg once daily, which can be increased to 8 mg. As with most of the anticholinergic drugs, the most common side effects are dry mouth and constipation.

Fesoterodine is metabolized to 5-hydroxymethyl tolterodine, (the active metabolite of tolterodine).

5.2.1.6 Darifenacin

Similar to solifenacin, the newer antimuscarinic drug darifenacin is more selective for M-3 muscarinic receptors in the bladder. Drifenacin is administered 7.5 mg daily and can be increased to 15 mg daily. In a randomized trial of darifenacin versus placebo, median incontinence episodes were show to significantly decrease with darifenacin. (Zinner et al., 2006) However, dry mouth and constipation rates were similar when compared to other anticholinergics (29% dry mouth and 18% constipation).

As noted above, the most common side effects associated with darifenacin are mild to moderate dry mouth and constipation. This drug has been studied in patients who were dissatisfied with prior OAB treatment with oxybutynin ER or tolterodine ER. The authors found significant improvements in OAB symptoms with darifenacin. (Zinner et al., 2008) Additionally, long-term studies have shown persistence of continuation with darifenacin therapy and well-maintained treatment benefits (over 2 years in duration). (Haab et al., 2006 & Hill et al., 2007)

Because of its' selectivity for the M3 receptor darifenacin minimizes the risk of side effects due to blockade of other muscarinic subtypes, such as M1 mediated cognitive impairment. (Foote et al., 2005) This is important in relation to the treatment of elderly populations who may be more susceptible to cognitive impairment and CNS effects.

Generic name	Brand Name	Dosage & Administration
Darifenacin hydrombromide	Enablex	7.5 to 15 mg daily
Fesoterodine	Toviaz	4 mg daily, can be increased to 8 mg daily
Oxybutynin extended release	Ditropan XL	5 mg daily, titrate up to 20-30 mg daily
Oxybutynin gel	Gelnique	Topical 10% gel applied as 1 g daily to thigh, abdomen, upper arm or shoulder
Oxybutynin immediate release	Ditropan	2.5 mg 2-3 times daily, followed by titration as needed u to 20 mg/d in divided doses
Oxybutynin transdermal	Oxytrol	Applied to abdomen, hip or buttock and changed twice per week (equivalent to 3.9 mg/d)
Solifenacin succinate	Vesicare	5-10 mg daily
Tolterodine tartrate extended release	Detrol LA	2-4 mg daily
Tolterodine tartrate immediate release	Detrol	1-2 mg twice daily
Trospium chloride extended release	Sanctura	60 mg daily
Trospium chloride immediate release	Sanctura	20 mg twice daily

Table 1. Commonly prescribed anticholinergic drugs for treatment of OAB

5.2.2 Antidepressants

5.2.2.1 Duloxetine

Duloxetine is a serotonin noradrenaline re-uptake inhibitor that is approved by the Food and Drug Administration (FDA) for depression, but not for urinary incontinence. The mechanism of action is to significantly increase sphincteric muscle activity during the filling/storage phase of micturition. Although not approved for use in patients with OAB symptoms alone, it may have some efficacy. Steers et al (Steers et al., 2007) randomized 306 women to placebo or duloxetine over 12 weeks. Duloxetine showed significant benefit in 24-hour urinary frequency and incontinence episodes. It also improved condition-specific quality of life measures. However, no significant increase was observed in mean voided volume, suggesting that the benefits were mediated through an effect at the urethral rhabdosphincter, rather than any direct effect on detrusor contractility. Thus, duloxetine may be considered as an option for patients who cannot tolerate antimuscarinic drugs. However, duloxetine's primary efficacy is in the treatment of stress urinary incontinence.

5.2.2.2 Imipramine

Imipramine, an antidepressant, is the only drug in this category that has been widely used to treat the symptoms of OAB. It has multiple pharmacological effects, including systemic antimuscarinic actions and blockade of the reuptake of serotonin and noradrenaline, but its mode of action in the treatment of OAB is not clear. (Hunsballe & Djurhuus, 2001) Imipramine has shown a favorable therapeutic effect in the treatment of nocturnal enuresis in children with a success rate of 10–70% in controlled trials. (Glazener et al., 2003; Hunsballe & Djurhuus, 2001) However, there are no good quality randomized trials that prove the efficacy of imipramine in the treatment of OAB.

5.2.3 Intravesical botulinum toxin

Botulinum toxin is a neurotoxin that inhibits the release of acetylcholine from presynaptic cholinergic nerve endings. This inhibition results in a localized reversible chemical denervation, with decreased detrusor contractility. Although it is currently not FDA-approved for the treatment of OAB, it shows promise as an addition to the treatment arsenal. The most likely place for its use is for patients who fail oral therapies. Current data primarily address only patients with refractory detrusor overactivity. In the most recent Cochrane review, randomized trials of intravesical botulinum versus placebo reported results favoring botulinum toxin. (Duthie et al., 2007) The authors noted that there was significant improvement in incontinence episodes, bladder capacity, maximum detrusor pressure and quality of life. They concluded "Botulinum toxin injections into the bladder appeared to give few side effects or complications, but there were no long-term follow-up studies, and there could be rare side effects that have not been discovered yet." (Duthie et al., 2007)

As stated above, many questions remain regarding its use, including the optimal dose and site of injection, the appropriate population, and long-term safety. To address this issue, Schurch et al (Schurch et al., 2007) randomized 59 patients with neurogenic detrusor overactivity to intravesical botulinum A (200 or 300 U) or placebo. These investigators noted significant improvements when compared to placebo using the Incontinence Quality of Life

Questionnaire. They did not discover clear differences between the two doses. Intravesical botulinum toxin has a variable duration of action, with loss of efficacy typically seen within one year. (Reitz et al., 2007) Based upon this limited data, it appears that there may be a role for the use of intravesical botulinum for patients with OAB, especially when other therapies fail. Finally, one of the bothersome adverse effects is urinary retention which can last up to three months after one injection. This, the clinician must have considerable knowledge and skill in the judicious use of botulinum toxin.

In a recent literature review (Anger et al, 2010) the authors systematically reviewed the efficacy and safety of botulinum toxin in the management of overactive bladder. Based upon this review of three small randomized placebo controlled trials they found that patients treated with botulinum toxin-A had 3.88 fewer incontinence episodes per day (95% CI -6.15, -1.62). Patients also noted significant improvements in quality of life compared with placebo. In addition they found a 9-fold increased odds of increased post-void residual after botulinum toxin-A compared with placebo (8.55; 95% CI 3.22, 22.71). They concluded that "intravesical injection of botulinum toxin resulted in improvement in medication refractory overactive bladder symptoms".

5.2.4 Combination therapies

Since most patients do not achieve complete continence with behavioral therapy or anticholinergic therapies alone, many clinicians combine these two in the treatment of OAB. A combination of anticholinergic agents and behavioral interventions have been shown to be safe and effective in many studies. (Fantl et al., 1996; Gormley, 2002; Milne & Moore, 2006) Side affect profiles of most of the drugs used for OAB make long term adherence to therapy difficult.

In a large study, Mattiasson et al (Mattiasson et al., 2003) showed additional benefit from bladder retraining when compared with tolterodine alone. Additionally, 76% of the patients on tolterodine and behavioral therapy noted improvement in their bladder symptoms compared to baseline as compared with 71% in the tolterodine group (Mattiasson et al., 2003)

Combination therapy has been shown to be associated with significantly fewer incontinent episodes, an improved quality of life, and greater treatment satisfaction when compared to non-pharmacologic intervention alone or drug treatment alone. (Wyman et al., 1998) However, the authors found that the effects of each of the interventions were similar 3 months after treatment. They concluded that the nature of the treatment may not be as important as having a structured intervention program that includes education, counseling, and frequent monitoring of the treatment. (Wyman et al., 1998)

Finally, Chancellor et al (Chancellor et al., 2008), in a more recent trial, compared the benefits of anticholinergic therapy alone against a combination of anticholinergic and behavioral therapy in 395 patients in a randomized controlled trial of flexible dose darifenacin (7.5 mg/day increased to 15 mg/day if required), with or without additional advice about dietary modification, timed voiding/bladder retraining, and pelvic floor training. No significant differences were observed between groups in OAB symptoms.

5.3 Neuromodulation

Neuromodulation can be utilized to increase pelvic muscle contraction and decrease detrusor contractions. The use of neuromodulation is assumes that OAB results from an imbalance of inhibitory and excitatory control systems of the detrusor that leads to the symptoms of OAB during the filling phase. (Fall and Lindstrom ,1991) Neuromodulation is gaining popularity because it bridges the gap between conservative treatments and highly invasive options. Currently, the methods used include sacral nerve modulation (SNM) via surgically implanted electrodes and other newer methods that deliver percutaneous stimulation of the peripheral tibial nerve.

The exact mechanism of action for neuromodulation is not well understood. However, many theories have been proposed as follows. (Al-Shaiji et al, 2011)

- Sensory input through the pudendal nerve has been shown to inhibit detrusor activity. Pudendal nerve stimulation and enhancement of external sphincter tone may serve to control bladder overactivity and facilitate urine storage. (Vodusek et al, 1986)
- The bladder responds to neural stimulation initially with rapid contraction. This is then followed by slow, longer-lasting relaxation. With recurrent, repetitive electrical stimulation, there is a downregulation of the bladder's response, thus reducing the detrusor muscle overactivity. (Appell & Boone, 2007)
- Stimulation of afferent sacral nerves in the pelvis or lower extremities has been shown to increase the inhibitory stimuli to the efferent pelvic nerve thus reducing detrusor contractility. (Fall & Lindstrom, 1991)
- Neuromodulation affects the "neuroaxis" at various levels and restores the balance between excitatory and inhibitory regulation at various locations within the peripheral and central nervous system. (Van Der Pal, 2006)

5.3.1 Noninvasive electrical stimulation

There are several devices on the market to provide noninvasive electrical stimulation to the pelvic floor. The removable device is placed in the. Its mechanism of action in the treatment of OAB is thought to be secondary to reflex inhibition of the detrusor muscle by stimulation of the pudendal nerve. There is some evidence that this therapy has some efficacy in the treatment of OAB. (Berghmans et al., 2000; Goode et al., 2003)

5.3.2 Sacral neuromodulation (SNM)

SNM uses mild electrical pulses to stimulate the sacral nerves that innervate the pelvic floor and lower urinary tract. InterStimTM therapy was developed by Medtronic (Minneapolis, Minn, USA) for use in humans. This technology utilizes an implanted unilateral lead stimulating the S3 nerve root. This electrode is attached to a small pacemaker placed within a subdermal pocket in the buttock region. It is FDA approved for refractory urge incontinence, refractory urgency frequency, and idiopathic nonobstructive urinary retention. "Off-label uses of the technology include for treatment of interstitial cystitis and pelvic pain syndrome. (Al-Shaiji et al, 2011)

Implantation of the device usually proceeds in 2 steps: a test phase and implantation or lead removal based on test response. The initial test phase can be performed in the office or operating room allowing for placement of the lead with a test period of 1 to 2 weeks; full implantation can be performed under local or general anesthesia. Response is objectively evaluated by pre- and postvoiding diaries assessing various urinary parameters.

The test phase of the procedure consists of implantation of tined quadripolar leads, under intravenous (IV) sedation, local anaesthesia, or general anaesthesia. Under fluoroscopy with a C-arm the right or left S3 foramen is identified and the permanent tined lead is passed through the foramen needle. The lead is then tested for a response. Correct placement in the S3 foramina includes bellows contraction of the pelvic floor and plantar flexion of the great toe. Once the appropriate side and position is selected, the lead is connected to an external pulse generator and taped to the skin surface. A 7- to 14-day home test period is used to determine which patients meet criteria to have the IPG implanted. Patients who respond favorably and demonstrate a 50% symptom improvement from baseline have the permanent generator implanted. (Al-Shaiji et al, 2011)

The most common adverse events include lead migration, implant site pain, bowel dysfunction, and infection. Infection usually resolves with antibiotics and the lead adverse events can usually be corrected by reprogramming, reinforcing the lead, or inserting a new lead contralaterally.

There is now convincing evidence for the success of SNM for refractory OAB. Several studies including RCTs and long-term observational studies reported fair clinical response between 64 and 88% of all patients (Leong et al, 2010).

5.3.3 Percutaneous stimulation of the tibial nerve

In addition, percutaneous stimulation of the tibial nerve (PTNS) has shown promise in the treatment of patients with refractory urge incontinence. PTNS is a minimally invasive, office-based procedure that involves percutaneous placement of a 34-gauge (ga) needle over the medial malleolus of the ankle to provide stimulation of the posterior tibial nerve. The procedure is repeated in 30-minute treatment sessions over a period of 12 weeks. PTNS in patients with OAB has been shown to significantly reduce in symptoms and improvement in health-related quality of life. (Yoong et al, 2010) However, one multicenter randomized trial of 100 patients with OAB symptoms did not show a reduced rate of urinary frequency when PTNS was compared to tolterodine extended release, 4mg daily. (Peters, 2009)

5.4 Surgery

In general most patients with OAB symptoms can be treated with medical and behavioral therapies. Generally, augmentation cystoplasty is only considered when patients have small volume bladders and are debilitated by their symptoms.

5.4.1 Augmentation cystoplasty

Augmentation cystoplasty (AC) is a surgery where a portion of the bowel is removed and patched to the bisected bladder. This procedure increases bladder capacity and decreases bladder pressure caused by unstable detrusor contractions. Considered a procedure of last resort, the risks of the surgery include recurrent UTI's, renal or bladder infections, metabolic changes and mucus production. (Khastgir et al., 2003) reviewed outcomes associated with augmentation cystoplasty. This group emphasized clinical outcomes (e.g. maximum detrusor pressure and bladder volume capacity) and patient symptoms (e.g. incontinence episodes and number of pads). Other outcomes included a questionnaire that measured quality of life, and the evaluation of complications from the surgery.

Using a definition of success as a $\geq$ 50% reduction in symptoms, one group found a 97% success rate for AC. (Blaivas et al., 2005)

5.5 Future therapies

5.5.1 Beta adrenoreceptor agonists

The human detrusor muscle contains B_2 and B_3-adrenoceptors. Both receptors are thought to be involved in detrusor relaxation. Currently, there are a number of [beta] 3-adrenoceptor selective agonists being evaluated as potential treatment for OAB, including YM178 (mirabegron). Chapple et al (Chapple et al., 2008) conducted a clinical trial with mirabegron versus tolterodine and placebo in patients with OAB. Patients in the treatment arm had a statistically significant reduction in mean micturition frequency when compared to placebo. In addition, mirabegron was superior to placebo in regard to mean volume voided per micturition, mean number of incontinence episodes, nocturia episodes, urgency incontinence episodes, and urgency episodes per 24 hours. The drug was well tolerated, and the most commonly reported adverse effects were headache and gastrointestinal adverse effects. Further randomized trials will be needed to prove efficacy.

5.5.2 Centrally acting drugs

5.5.2.1 Tramadol

Many parts of the brain are activated during storage and voiding and there is increasing interest in centrally acting drugs which modulate the micturition reflex. (Andersson & Pehrson, 2003) Tramadol is an analgesic that is a weak μ-receptor agonist; however, it is metabolized to several different compounds, which inhibit serotonin (5-HT) and noradrenaline reuptake. (Grond & Sablotzki, 2004;Safarinejad & Hosseini, 2006) Both μ-receptor agonist and amine reuptake inhibition are useful in the treatment of OAB. In a double-blind, placebo-controlled, randomized study, 76 patients were given 100 mg tramadol sustained release every 12 hours for 12 weeks. Tramadol significantly reduced the number of incontinence periods by 50% per 24 hours. The authors concluded that tramadol provided beneficial clinical and urodynamic effects.

5.5.2.2 Tachykinins

Tachykinins such as substance P, neurokinin A (NKA), and neurokinin B (NKB) may play a role in OAB. Substance P has a specific receptor (NK1) that is expressed in the dorsal horn of the spinal cord and may play an important role in detrusor overactivity. (Grond & Sablotzki, 2004; Safarinejad & Hosseini, 2006)

Aprepitant, an NK1 receptor antagonist, has been shown to significantly improve symptoms of OAB in postmenopausal women with a history of urgency incontinence or mixed incontinence in a small pilot. (Green et al., 2006) Aprepitant significantly decreased the average daily number of micturitions (−1.3 ± 1.9) compared with placebo (−0.4 ± 1.7). The average daily number of urgency episodes was significantly reduced, as were the average daily number of urgency incontinence and total urinary incontinence episodes. The authors concluded that NK1 receptor antagonism holds promise as a potential treatment approach for OAB.

6. Summary

Overactive bladder (OAB) is a common medical condition, yet often undetected and undertreated despite the substantial impact on a woman's quality of life. The etiology of OAB is unclear, but several mechanisms may interplay and interconnected in contributing to the multi-symptom condition. Despite symptoms that often interfere with work, daily life, intimacy, and also cause embarrassment and diminished self-esteem, less than half of sufferers seek treatment from a licensed provider.

A working clinical diagnosis of OAB can usually be made simply by utilizing proper urinary questionnaires, urinary diaries or a thorough medical history and physical examination. Confirmation of diagnosis is most often achieved via a post-void residual, simply cystometry or multichannel urodynamic testing.

The primary goal of treatment of OAB is simply a reduction in urinary incontinence episodes. First-line therapy for OAB should include conservative options such as timed voiding and alterations in types and amount of fluid intake. Counseling patients on dietary and lifestyle modification will often improve their acute symptoms and decrease the number of voiding episodes per day. Other non surgical first line options include pelvic floor muscle training and/or biofeedback, both of which center around exercises designed to improve the function of the pelvic floor muscles. The primary limitations of behavioral therapy is the required long term patient commitment required for effectiveness.

Antimuscarinic (anticholinergic) drugs are the cornerstone of pharmacological treatment of OAB and provide a favorable efficacy/tolerability/safety profile. These result in decreased bladder contractions and thus reduced the symptoms of OAB. For patients who are not candidates for antimuscarinic (anticholinergic) therapy or have failed previous trials of other medical therapy, noninvasive electrical stimulation to the pelvic floor via neuromodulation may increase pelvic muscle contractions and decrease detrusor contractions . More aggressive nerve modulation and stimulation therapies include, sacral nerve stimulation or peripheral nerve stimulation , which can be considered in patients with refractory urge incontinence. Lastly, surgical options, including augmentation cystoplasty and detrusor myectomy have been developed for those in which all other treatment alternatives have been exhausted.

Lastly, there are promising new receptor-specific medical alternatives emerging and future studies will determine their place in the therapeutic arsenal.

Despite the prevalence of OAB, and the patients' lack of willingness to report their life altering symptoms, screening for OAB should be part of every woman's annual well woman visit. Health care providers need not shy away from urinary incontinence questionnaires, as straightforward diagnosis and OAB treatments are available. Although the primary treatment goal of OAB is the reduction in urinary incontinence episodes, to the patient, the most important measure is quality of life.

7. References

Abrams P, Cardozo L, Fall M, et al; Standardisation Sub-committee of the International Continence Society. The standardisation of terminology of lower urinary tract function: report from the Standardisation Sub-committee of the International Continence Society. Neurourol Urodyn 2002;21:167–178.

Abrams P, Andersson KE. Muscarinic receptor antagonists for overactive bladder. BJU Int 2007;100:987–1006.

Al-Shaiji TF, Banakhar M, Hassouna MM. Pelvic Electrical Neuromodulation for the Treatment of Overactive Bladder Symptoms. Advances in Urology. Volume 2011, Article ID 757454, 7 pages. doi:10.1155/2011/757454

Anderson RU, Mobley D, Blank B, et al. Once daily controlled versus immediate release oxybutynin chloride for urge urinary incontinence. OROS Oxybutynin Study Group. J Urol 1999; 161:1809.

Anderson KE. Potential benefits of Muscarinic M3 receptor selectivity," European Urology Supplements, vol. 1, no. 4, pp. 23–28, 2002.

Andersson KE. Bladder activation: afferent mechanisms. Urology 2002; 59:43.

Andersson KE, Pehrson R. CNS involvement in overactive bladder: pathophysiology and opportunities for pharmacological intervention. Drugs 2003;63:2595–2611.

Andersson KE, Wein AJ. Pharmacology of the lower urinary tract: basis for current and future treatments of urinary incontinence. Pharmacol Rev 2004;56:581–631.

Andersson KE. LUTS treatment: future treatment options. Neurourol Urodyn 2007;26(6 suppl):934–947

Appell R, Boone TB. Surgical management of overactive bladder, Current Bladder Dysfunction Reports, vol. 2, pp. 37–45, 2007.

Arya LA, Myers DL, and Jackson ND. Dietary caffeine intake and the risk for detrusor instability: a case-control study. Obstetrics and Gynecology, vol. 96, no. 1, pp. 85–89, 2000.

Anger JT, Weinberg A, Suttorp MJ, Litwin, MS, Shekelle PG. Outcomes of intravesical botulinum toxin for idiopathic overactive bladder symptoms: a systematic review. Journal of Urology. 183(6):2258-2264, June 2010.

Araki, I., et al., Lower urinary tract symptoms in men and women without underlying disease causing micturition disorder: a cross-sectional study assessing the natural history of bladder function. J Urol, 2003. 170(5): p. 1901-4.

Azadzoi, K.M., et al., Canine bladder blood flow and oxygenation: changes induced by filling, contraction and outlet obstruction. J Urol, 1996. 155(4): p. 1459-65.

Basra R, Artibani W, Cardozo L, et al. Design and validation of a new screening instrument for lower urinary tract dysfunction: the bladder control self-assessment questionnaire (B-SAQ). Eur Urol 2007;52:230–237.

Berghmans LC, Hendriks HJ, De Bie RA, et al. Conservative treatment of urge urinary incontinence in women: a systematic review of randomized clinical trials. BJU Int 2000; 85:254.

Blakeman PJ, Hilton P,Bulmer JN. Oestrogen and progesterone receptor expression in the female lower urinary tract, with reference to oestrogen status. BJU Int, 2000.86(1): p. 32-8.

Bo K, Berghmans LCM. Nonpharmacologic treatments for overactive bladder—pelvic floor exercises. Urology, vol. 55, no. 5, supplement 1, pp. 7–11, 2000.

Bogart LM, Berry SH, Clemens JQ. Symptoms of interstitial cystitis, painful bladder syndrome and similar diseases in women: a systematic review. J Urol 2007; 177:450.

Blaivas JG, Weiss JP, Desai P, Flisser AJ, Stember DS, Stahl PJ: Longterm followup of augmentation enterocystoplasty and continent diversion in patients with benign disease. The Journal of urology 2005, 173(5):1631-1634.

Blaivas JG, Panagopoulos G, Weiss JP, et al. Validation of the overactive bladder symptom score. J Urol 2007;178:543–547; discussion 547.

Bros E, ComarrAE. Physiology of Micturition, Its Neurological Disorders and Sequelae. 1971, Baltimore: University Park Press.

Brubaker L, Fanning K, Goldberg EL, et al. Predictors of discontinuing overactive bladder medications. BJU Int 2010;105:1283–1290.

Burgio KL, Whitehead WE, Engel BT. Urinary incontinence in the elderly. Bladder-sphincter biofeedback and toileting skills training. Ann Intern Med 1985;103:507–515.

Burgio KL. Influence of behavior modification on overactive bladder. Urology 2002;60(5 suppl 1):72–76; discussion 77.

Campbell JD, Gries KS, Watanabe JH, Ravelo A, Dmochowski RR, Sullivan SD. Treatment success for overactive bladder with urinary urge incontinence refractory to oral antimuscarinics: a review of published evidence. BMC Urology 2009, 9:18.

Cardozo L, Lisec M, Millard R, et al. Randomized, double-blind placebo controlled trial of the once daily antimuscarinic agent solifenacin succinate in patients with overactive bladder. Journal of Urology, vol. 172, no. 5, part 1, pp. 1919–1924, 2004.

Cardozo, L., et al., A systematic review of the effects of estrogens for symptoms suggestive of overactive bladder. Acta Obstet Gynecol Scand, 2004. 83(10): p. 892-7.

Cardozo L, Hessdorfer E, Milani R, et al. Solifenacin in the treatment of urgency and other symptoms of overactive bladder: results from a randomized, double-blind, placebocontrolled, rising-dose trial. BJU International, vol. 102, no. 9, pp. 1120–1127, 2008.

Chapple CR, Martinez-Garcia R, Selvaggi L, et al; for the STAR study group. A comparison of the efficacy and tolerability of solifenacin succinate and extended release tolterodine at treating overactive bladder syndrome: results of the STAR trial. Eur Urol 2005;48:464–470.

Chapple CR, Cardozo L, Steers WD, Govier FE. Solifenacin significantly improves all symptoms of overactive bladder syndrome," International Journal of Clinical Practice, vol. 60, no. 8, pp. 959–966, 2006.

Chapple CR, Fianu-Jonsson A, Indig M, et al; STAR study group. Treatment outcomes in the STAR study: a subanalysis of solifenacin 5 mg and tolterodine ER 4 mg. Eur Urol 2007;52:1195–1203.

Chapple CR, Yamaguchi O, Ridder A, et al. Clinical proof of concept study (Blossom) shows novel β3 adrenoceptor agonist YM178 is effective and well tolerated in the treatment of symptoms of overactive bladder. Eur Urol Suppl 2008.

Chancellor MB, Kianifard F, Beamer E, et al. A comparison of the efficacy of darifenacin alone vs. darifenacin plus a Behavioural Modification Programme upon the symptoms of overactive bladder. Int J Clin Pract 2008;62:606–613.

Choo MS, Doo CK, Lee KS. Satisfaction with tolterodine: assessing symptom-specific patient-reported goal achievement in the treatment of overactive bladder in female patients (STARGATE study)," International Journal of Clinical Practice, vol. 62, no. 2, pp. 191–196, 2008.

Colli E, Digesu GA, Olivieri L. Overactive bladder treatments in early phase clinical trials. Expert Opin Investig Drugs 2007;16:999–1007.

Coyne KS, Zyczynski T, Margolis MK, et al. Validation of an overactive bladder awareness tool for use in primary care settings. Adv Ther 2005;22:381–394.

Coyne KS, Matza LS, Thompson CL. The responsiveness of the overactive bladder questionnaire (OAB-Q). Qual Life Res 2005;14:849–855.

Davila GW, Daugherty CA, Sanders SW, Transdermal Oxybutynin Study Group. A short-term, multicenter, randomized double-blind dose titration study of the efficacy and anticholinergic side effects of transdermal compared to immediate release oral oxybutynin treatment of patients with urge urinary incontinence. J Urol 2001; 166:140.

de Nunzio, C., et al., The evolution of detrusor overactivity after watchful waiting, medical therapy and surgery in patients with bladder outlet obstruction. J Urol, 2003. 169(2): p. 535-9.

de Groat, W.C., A.M. Booth, and N. Yoshimura, Neurophysiology of micturition and its modeification in animal models of human disease, in The Autonomic Nervous System:Nervous Control of the Urogenital System, C.A. Maggi, Editor. 1993, Harwood Academic Publishers: London. p.27-290.

de Groat WC, Yoshimura N. Pharmacology of the lower urinary tract. Annu Rev Pharmacol Toxicol 2001;41:691–721.

de Groat WC. The urothelium in overactive bladder: passive bystander or active participant? Urology 2004;64(6 suppl 1):7–11.

Dmochowski RR, Davila GW, Zinner NR, et al. Efficacy and safety of transdermal oxybutynin in patients with urge and mixed urinary incontinence. J Urol 2002; 168:580.

Dmochowski RR, Sand PK, Zinner NR, Staskin DR. Trospium 60 mg once daily (QD) for overactive bladder syndrome: results from a placebo-controlled interventional study. Urology 2008; 71:449.

DuBeau CE. (2011). Treatment of urinary incontinence, In: UpToDate, accessed 8/18/2011, Available from: http://www.uptodate.com/contents/treatment-of-urinary-incontinence?source=search_result&selectedTitle=1%7E81#H3

Duthie J, Wilson DI, Herbison GP, et al. Botulinum toxin injections for adults with overactive bladder syndrome. Cochrane Database Syst Rev 2007;3:CD005493.

Elbadawi A, Yalla SV, Resnick NM. Structural basis of geriatric voiding dysfunction. II. Aging detrusor: normal versus impaired contractility. J Urol, 1993. 150(5 Pt 2): p.1657-67.

Elbadawi A, Yalla SV, Resnick NM. Structural basis of geriatric voiding dysfunction. III. Detrusor overactivity. J Urol, 1993. 150(5 Pt 2): p. 1668-80.

Elbadawi A, Yalla SV, Resnick NM.. Structural basis of geriatric voiding dysfunction. IV. Bladder outlet obstruction. J Urol, 1993. 150(5 Pt 2): p. 1681-95.

Eriksen PS, Rasmussen H. Low-dose 17 beta-estradiol vaginal tablets in the treatment of atrophic vaginitis: a doubleblind placebo controlled study. Eur J Obstet Gynecol Reprod Biol, 1992. 44(2): p. 137-44.

Fall, M., B.L. Ohlsson, and C.A. Carlsson, The neurogenic overactive bladder. Classification based on urodynamics. Br J Urol, 1989. 64(4): p. 368-73.

Fall M, Lindstrom S, Electrical stimulation: a physiologic approach to the treatment of urinary incontinence, Urologic Clinics of North America, vol. 18, no. 2, pp. 393–407, 1991.

Fall, M., G. Geirsson, and S. Lindstrom, Toward a new classification of overactive bladders. Neurourol Urodyn, 1995. 14(6): p. 635-46.

Fantl JA, Newman DK, Colling J, et al. Urinary Incontinence in Adults: Acute and Chronic Management, Clinical

Practice Guideline no. 2, Agency for Health Care Policy and Research, Rockville,Md, USA, 1996, AHCPR publication no. 96-0682.

Ferguson DR, Kennedy I, Burton TJ. ATP is released from rabbit urinary bladder epithelial cells by hydrostatic pressure changes—a possible sensory mechanism? J Physiol, 1997. 505 (Pt 2): p. 503-11.

Foote J, Glavind K, Kralidis G, Wyndaele JJ. Treatment of overactive bladder in the older patient: pooled analysis of three phase III studies of darifenacin, an M3 selective receptor antagonist," European Urology, vol. 48, no. 3, pp. 471–477, 2005.

Fowler CJ, Griffiths D, de Groat WC. The neural control of micturition. Nat Rev Neurosci 2008; 9:453.

Glazener CM, Evans JH, Peto RE. Tricyclic and related drugs for nocturnal enuresis in children. Cochrane Database Syst Rev 2003;3:CD002117.

Goode PS, Burgio KL, Locher JL, et al. Effect of behavioral training with or without pelvic floor electrical stimulation on stress incontinence in women: a randomized controlled trial. JAMA 2003; 290:345.

Gormley EA. Biofeedback and behavioral therapy for the management of female urinary incontinence," Urologic

Clinics of North America, vol. 29, no. 3, pp. 551–557, 2002.

Green SA, Alon A, Ianus J, et al. Efficacy and safety of a neurokinin-1 receptor antagonist in postmenopausal women with overactive bladder with urge urinary incontinence. J Urol 2006;176:2535–2540.

Greenland JE,Brading AF. The effect of bladder outflow obstruction on detrusor blood flow changes during the voiding cycle in conscious pigs. J Urol, 2001. 165(1): p.245-8

Griffiths AN, Makam A, Edwards GJ. Should we actively screen for urinary and anal incontinence in the general gynaecology outpatients setting?—a prospective observational study. J Obstet Gynaecol 2006;26:442–444.

Griffiths D, Tadic SD, Schaefer W, Resnick NM. Cerebral control of the bladder in normal and urge-incontinent women. Neuroimage 2007; 37:1.

Grond S, Sablotzki A. Clinical pharmacology of tramadol. Clin Pharmacokinet 2004;43:879–923.

Haab F, Corcos J, Siami P, et al. Long-termtreatment with darifenacin for overactive bladder: results of a 2-year, open label extension study," BJU International, vol. 98, no. 5, pp. 1025–1032, 2006.

Harrison, S.C., et al., Bladder instability and denervation in patients with bladder outflow obstruction. Br J Urol, 1987. 60(6): p. 519-22.

Harris SS, Link CL, Tennstedt SL, et al. Care seeking and treatment for urinary incontinence in a diverse population. J Urol 2007;177:680–684.

Hay-Smith J, Herbison P, Ellis G, et al. Which anticholinergic drug for overactive bladder symptoms in adults. Cochrane Database Syst Rev 2005;3:CD005429.

Hay-Smith, J, Berghmans, BK, et al. Adult conservative management. In: Abrams, P, Cardozo, L, Khoury, S, Wein, A. Paris: Editions 21, for Health Publications Ltd, 2009; p.1025.

Hill S, Elhilali M, Millard RJ, et al. Long-term darifenacin treatment for overactive bladder in patients aged 65 years and older: analysis of results from a 2-year, open-label extension study. Current Medical Research and Opinion, vol.23, no. 11, pp. 2697–2704, 2007.

Homma Y. The clinical significance of the urodynamic investigation in incontinence. BJU Int 2002;90:489–497.

Hosker G, Rosier P, Gajewski J, Sand P, Szabo L, Capewell A. Dynamic testing. In:Abrams P, Cardozo L, Khoury S, Wein A. Incontinence. Health Publication Ltd 2009 Paris France.

Hughes KM, Lang JCT, Lazare R, et al. Measurement of oxybutynin and its N-desethyl metabolite in plasma, and its application to pharmacokinetic studies in young, elderly and frail elderly volunteers," Xenobiotica, vol. 22, no. 7, pp. 859–869, 1992.

Hunsballe JM, Djurhuus JC. Clinical options for imipramine in the management of urinary incontinence. Urol Res 2001;29:118–125.

International Continence Society. Available at www.ics.org. Accessed 10/14/2011.

Irwin DE, Milsom I, Hunskaar S, et al. Population-based survey of urinary incontinence, overactive bladder, and other lower urinary tract symptoms in five countries: results of the EPIC study. Eur Urol 2006;50:1306–1315.

Irwin DE, Milsom I, Kopp Z, et al. Impact of overactive bladder symptoms on employment, social interactions and emotional well-being in six European countries. BJU Int 2006;97:96–100.

Ishizuka O, Igawa Y, Lecci A, et al. Role of intrathecal tachykinins for micturition in unanaesthetized rats with and without bladder outlet obstruction. Br J Pharmacol 1994;113:111–116.

Janknegt RA, Hassouna MM, Siegel SW, et al. Long-term effectiveness of sacral nerve stimulation for refractory urge incontinence. Eur Urol 2001;39:101–106.

Kay G, Crook T, Rekeda L, et al. Differential effects of the antimuscarinic agents darifenacin and oxybutynin ER on memory in older subjects. European Urology, vol. 50, no. 2, pp. 317–326, 2006.

Khastgir J, Hamid R, Arya M, Shah N, Shah PJ: Surgical and patient reported outcomes of 'clam' augmentation ileocystoplasty in spinal cord injured patients. Eur Urol 2003, 43(3):263-269.

Koelbl H, Nitti V, Baessler K, Salvatore S, Sultan A, Yamaguchi O. Pathophysiology of Urinary Incontinence,

Faecal Incontinence and Pelvic Organ Prolapse. In:Abrams P, Cardozo L, Khoury S, Wein A. Incontinence Health Publication Ltd 2009 Paris France.

Leong RK, De Wachter SGG, Van Kerrebroeck,PEV. Current information on sacral neuromodulation and

botulinumtoxin treatment for refractory idiopathic overactive bladder syndrome: a review, Urologia Internationalis, vol. 84, no. 3, pp. 245–253, 2010.

Mansfiel, KJ et al., Muscarinic receptor subtypes in human bladder detrusor and mucosa, studied by radioligand

binding and quantitative competitive RT-PCR: changes in ageing. Br J Pharmacol, 2005. 144(8): p. 1089-99.

Mardon RE, Halim S, Pawlson LG, et al. Management of urinary incontinence in Medicare managed care beneficiaries: results from the 2004 Medicare Health Outcomes Survey. Arch Intern Med 2006;166:1128–1133.

Mattiasson A, Blaakaer J, Høye K, et al. Simplified bladder training augments the effectiveness of tolterodine in patients with an overactive bladder. BJU Int. 2003;91:54–60.

McGrother CW, Donaldson MM, Hayward T, et al; Leicestershire MRC Incontinence Study Team. Urinary storage symptoms and comorbidities: a prospective population cohort study in middle-aged and older women. Age Ageing 2006;35:16–24.

Mills IW et al., Studies of the pathophysiology of idiopathic detrusor instability: the physiological properties of the detrusor smooth muscle and its pattern of innervation. J Urol, 2000. 163(2): p. 646-51.

Milne JL and Moore KN. Factors impacting self-care for urinary incontinence," Urologic Nursing, vol. 26, no. 1, pp. 41–51, 2006.

Milne JL. Behavioral therapies for overactive bladder: making sense of the evidence. Journal of Wound, Ostomy and Continence Nursing, vol. 35, no. 1, pp. 93–101, 2008.

Milsom I, Abrams P, Cardozo L, et al. How widespread are the symptoms of an overactive bladder and how are they managed? A population-based prevalence study. BJU Int 2001;87:760–766.

Nilvebrant L, Sparf B. Dicyclomine, benzhexol, and oxybutynine distinguish between subclasses of muscarinic binding sites. European Journal of Pharmacology, vol. 123, no. 1, pp. 133–143, 1986.

Nixon A, Colman S, Sabounjian L, et al. A validated patient reported measure of urinary urgency severity in overactive bladder for use in clinical trials. J Urol 2005;174:604–607.

Nygaard IE, Kreder KJ, Lepic MM, Fountain KA, Rhomberg AT. Efficacy of pelvic floor muscle exercises in women with stress, urge, and mixed urinary incontinence. American Journal of Obstetrics and Gynecology, vol. 174, no. 1, part 1, pp. 120–125, 1996.

Ouslander JG, Ai-Samarrai N, Schnelle JF. Prompted voiding for nighttime incontinence in nursing homes: is it effective? J Am Geriatr Soc 2001;49:706–709.

Peters KM, Macdiarmid SA, Wooldridge LS, et al. Randomized trial of percutaneous tibial nerve stimulation versus extended-release tolterodine: results from the overactive bladder innovative therapy trial. J Urol 2009;182:1055–1061. Reitz A, Denys P, Fermanian C, et al. Do repeat intradetrusor botulinum toxin type A injections yield valuable results? Clinical and urodynamic results after five injections in patients with neurogenic detrusor overactivity. Eur Urol 2007;52:1729–1735.

Safarinejad MR, Hosseini SY. Safety and efficacy of tramadol in the treatment of idiopathic detrusor overactivity: a double-blind, placebo-controlled, randomized study. Br J Clin Pharmacol 2006;61:456–463.

Schafer W et al., Good urodynamic practices: uroflowmetry, filling cystometry, and pressure-flow studies. Neurourol Urodyn, 2002. 21(3): p. 261-74.

Schurch B, Denys P, Kozma CM, et al. Botulinum toxin A improves the quality of life of patients with neurogenic urinary incontinence. Eur Urol 2007;52:850–858.

Shaw HA, Burrows LJ. Etilogy and treatment of overactive bladder in women. South Med J. 2011 Jan;104(1):34-9. Review.

Staskin D, Sand P, Zinner N, Dmochowski R. Once daily trospium chloride is effective and well tolerated for the treatment of overactive bladder: results from a multicenter phase III trial. Journal of Urology, vol. 178, no. 3, pp. 978–984, 2007.

Steers WD, Herschorn S, Kreder KJ, et al; Duloxetine OAB Study Group. Duloxetine compared with placebo for treating women with symptoms of overactive bladder. BJU Int 2007;100:337–345.

Stewart WF, Van Rooyen JB, Cundiff GW, et al. Prevalence and burden of overactive bladder in the United States. World J Urol 2003;20:327–336.

Subak LL, Wing R, West DS, et al. Weight loss to treat urinary incontinence in overweight and obese women. N Engl J Med 2009; 360:481.

Swithinbank L, Hashim H, and Abrams P, "The effect of fluid intake on urinary symptoms in women," Journal of Urology, vol. 174, no. 1, pp. 187–189, 2005.

Van Der Pal F, Heesakkers JPFA, Bemelmans BLH. Current opinion on the working mechanisms of neuromodulation in the treatment of lower urinary tract dysfunction, Current Opinion in Urology, vol. 16, no. 4, pp. 261–267, 2006.

van Kerrebroeck PE, van Voskuilen AC, Heesakkers JP, et al. Results of sacral neuromodulation therapy for urinary voiding dysfunction: outcomes of a prospective, worldwide clinical study. J Urol 2007;178:2029–2034.

Versi E, Appell R, Mobley D, et al. Dry mouth with conventional and controlled-release oxybutynin in urinary incontinence. The Ditropan XL Study Group. Obstet Gynecol 2000; 95:718.

Vodusek, DB, Light JK, Libby JM. Detrusor inhibition induced by stimulation of pudendal nerve afferents. Neurourology and Urodynamics, vol. 5, no. 4, pp. 381–389, 1986.

Wagg AS, Cardozo L, Chapple C, et al. Overactive bladder syndrome in older people. BJU Int 2007;99:502–509.

Wallace SA, Roe B, Williams K, Palmer M. Bladder training for urinary incontinence in adults. Cochrane Database of Systematic Reviews 2004, Issue 1. Art. No.: CD001308. DOI: 10.1002/14651858.CD001308.pub2

Wein AJ. Pathophysiology and categorization of voiding dysfunction, in Walsh P, Retik A, Vaughan ED Jr, et al (eds): Campbell's Urology. Philadelphia, Saunders, 2002, ed 8, pp 887.

Wilson PD, Berghmans B, Hagen S, et al. Adult conservative management, in Abrams P, Cardozo L, Khoury S, et al (eds): Incontinence Management. Paris, Health Publications, 2005, pp 855–894.

Wyman JF, Fantl JA, McClish DK, Bump RC. Comparative efficacy of behavioral interventions in themanagement of female urinary incontinence. American Journal of Obstetrics and Gynecology, vol. 179, no. 4, pp. 999–1007, 1998.

Yoong W, Ridout AE, Damodaram M, Dadswell R. Neuromodulative treatment with percutaneous tibial nerve stimulation for intractable detrusor instability: outcomes following a shortened 6-week protocol, BJU International, vol. 106, no. 11, pp. 1673–1676, 2010.

Zinner N, Gittelman M, Harris R, et al. Trospium chloride improves overactive bladder symptoms: a multicenter phase III trial. J Urol 2004; 171:2311.

Zinner N, Susset J, Gittelman M, et al. Efficacy, tolerability and safety of darifenacin, an M(3) selective receptor antagonist: an investigation of warning time in patients with OAB. Int J Clin Pract 2006; 60:119.

Zinner N, Kobashi KC, Ebinger U, et al. Darifenacin treatment for overactive bladder in patients who expressed dissatisfaction with prior extended-release antimuscarinic therapy," International Journal of Clinical Practice, vol. 62, no.11, pp. 1664–1674, 2008.

Biomarkers in the Overactive Bladder Syndrome

Célia Duarte Cruz[1,2,3], Tiago Antunes Lopes[2,3,4],
Carlos Silva[2,3,4] and Francisco Cruz[2,3,4,*]
[1]*Department of Experimental Biology, Faculty of Medicine of Porto,*
[2]*IBMC – Instituto de Biologia Molecular e Celular,*
[3]*University of Porto,*
[4]*Department of Urology, Hospital de S. João, Porto,*
Portugal

1. Introduction

Overactive bladder (OAB) is a symptomatic complex affecting both men and women. The overall incidence is above 10% but may exceed 40% in the elderly population (Irwin et al., 2006; Irwin et al., 2009; Sexton et al., 2009a). OAB is defined by the International Continence Society (ICS) as a clinical syndrome characterized by urinary urgency, with or without incontinence, usually with frequency and nocturia (Abrams et al., 2002, 2003; Hashim & Abrams, 2007). Urgency, which is a storage symptom defined as a sudden compelling desire to pass urine difficult to defer, is the hallmark symptom as it is the only one that must be present in order to establish the diagnosis of OAB (Abrams et al., 2002, 2003). Several co-morbidities are very common among OAB patients, including depression, insomnia and fractures (Coyne et al., 2008; Sexton et al., 2009a; Sexton et al., 2009b). The economic costs of OAB, associated with medical consultations, therapy and diminished productivity at work, may reach billions of dollars (Irwin et al., 2009) and will certainly increase with the demographic shift of an ageing population.

The true causes of urgency/OAB remain poorly understood. The difficulty in establishing animal models that accurately represent urgency/OAB still holds. It was originally thought that the origin of OAB could be ascribed to anomalies in the neuromuscular junction and myocites. More recent data indicate a strong involvement of bladder sensory mechanisms involving the urothelium and suburothelial afferent nerves. In addition, dysfunction of central nervous system centres that control the micturition reflex, including the Periaqueductal Gray (PAG) and pontine micturition centre, has been implicated in the genesis of OAB (Fowler et al., 2008; Drake et al., 2010; Fowler & Griffiths, 2010).

No cure exists for OAB. Management is initiated by exclusion of confounding diseases and by the introduction of conservative measures, including limiting fluid intake, avoiding caffeinated, acidic and carbonated drinks, weight reduction, smoke avoidance and bladder training. If bothersome OAB symptoms persist, patients are initiated on antimuscarinic

---

* Corresponding Author

therapy, the current mainstay for pharmacological management of OAB (Henderson & Drake, 2010; Athanasopoulos & Cruz, 2011). Nevertheless, despite significant improvement, antimuscarinics still produce important side-effects that may lead patients to discontinue treatment (Andersson, 2004; Andersson et al., 2009; Gulur & Drake, 2010). Moreover, antimuscarinics are contra-indicated for patients with narrow angle, may interfere with cognitive function and aggravate constipation (Gulur & Drake, 2010), all of which commonly occur in the typical OAB age group. More recently, the administration of vanilloids and botulinum toxin have been proposed as a possible treatment for OAB but these approaches should be taken with care as they are off-label procedures (Cruz & Dinis, 2007; da Silva & Cruz, 2009).

The key symptom in OAB, urgency, may often be confounded with urge to void. Urge is a normal bladder sensation, the intensity of which is proportional to the degree of bladder filling and allows the subject to fully control bladder function. Differentiation between urge and urgency may not always be an easy task for the caregiver or patients, particularly those who are cognitively impaired by age or disease (Michel & Chapple, 2009a, b). In addition, grading urgency is a difficult task to be accomplished by the clinician, even with the use of standardized questionnaires (Nixon et al., 2005; Starkman & Dmochowski, 2008). Currently, there is no objective test to diagnose OAB although several attempts have been made in order to overcome this. Here, we will review recent data proposing new biomarkers for a better characterization of OAB patients. The value of a biomarker in medicine is considerable and lies in its ability to identify the disease, back diagnostic and therapeutic decisions and establish a valuable prognosis to the condition. In addition, it will positively influence the outcome of the condition. In OAB, investigators have focused on bladder parameters (the presence of detrusor overactivity and the thickness of the bladder wall), serum proteins (the C reactive protein) and urinary elements (prostaglandins, cytokines and neurotrophins).

2. Bladder criteria

2.1 Detrusor overactivity

Detrusor overactivity (DO) is the urodynamic observation of involuntary detrusor contractions during the filling phase of cystometry (Abrams et al., 2002).Thus, DO can only be detected by urodynamic assessment, an invasive and expensive test. It has been demonstrated that DO was present in approximately 45% of OAB-dry and 60% of OAB-wet patients (Hashim & Abrams, 2006). As the main symptoms of OAB may suggest the presence of DO, several attempts have been made in order to correlate urgency with DO. However, in a recent study it was shown that reports of urgency sensations during filling cystometry were as likely to occur before or after an episode of DO and approximately one third of the DO events recorded were not associated with urgency (Lowenstein et al., 2009). In addition, DO, may be found in healthy individuals (Heslington & Hilton, 1996; van Waalwijk van Doorn et al., 1997; Hashim & Abrams, 2006). In fact, in the study by Hashim and Abrams 36% of the OAB patients studied (1076) did not present DO and more than 30% of individuals without OAB had DO (Hashim & Abrams, 2006). In addition, DO does not predict the response of patients to antimuscarinic treatment (Malone-Lee & Al-Buheissi, 2009). Hence, the combination of the discomfort felt by patients during an urodynamic evaluation with a low predictive value both for the diagnosis and successful outcome of OAB treatment impedes the routine use of urodynamic assessment for the majority of OAB patients. In a recent study, investigators tried to identify the presence of involuntary detrusor contractions through near-infrared spectroscopy (NIRS), a non-invasive method (Farag et al., 2011a; Farag et al., 2011b). NIRS is an imaging technique that can be used to monitor haemodynamic events. As the name indicates, it uses light in the near-infrared area, which is able to penetrate the skin. It is absorbed by oxyhaemoglobin and deoxyhaemoglobin, the levels of which can reflect oxygen consumption. In those studies, investigators were able to demonstrate that detrusor contractions were accompanied by changes in those chromophores (Farag et al., 2011a; Farag et al., 2011b). The overall specificity of NIRS to detect DO was 86% when measuring oxyhaemoglobin, 80% for deoxyhaemoglobin and 72% for the sum of both chromophores. Despite obvious limitations, such as the inclusion of more men than women, results are interesting and deserve further investigation.

2.2 Bladder wall thickness/Detrusor thickness (BWT/DT)

In patients with bladder outlet obstruction, the thickness of the total bladder wall or simply the thickness of the detrusor layer was shown in several studies to be significantly increased in OAB patients when compared with healthy volunteers (Hakenberg et al., 2000; Oelke et al., 2006; Oelke et al., 2007). Hence, it was forwarded that BWT/DT could be influenced by the work overload of the bladder wall introduced by DO. Indeed, some authors have reported a trend of increasing DT associated with the severity of urgency as reported by Panayi and coworkers (Panayi et al., 2010). Khullar and co-workers analysed the total BWT via transvaginal ultrasound in a group of female patients with idiopathic DO (Khullar et al., 1996). They found that 58.7% of all analysed subjects had a mean BWT greater than 5 mm, 94% of which had DO. Only 1.6% of subjects had DO with a BWT of 3.5 mm or less. The authors proposed that the measurement of mean BWT by transvaginal ultrasound, with a cut-off of 5mm, is a suitable screening method (Khullar et al., 1996). In addition, by determining BWT also with transvaginal ultrasound, Kuhn and co-workers were able to differentiate between women suffering from stress urinary incontinence or bladder outlet obstruction (Kuhn et al., 2011). In OAB patients, DWT was reduced after anti-muscarinic treatment (Liu et al., 2009b; Kuo et al., 2010b). In addition, a positive correlation has been found between the presence of OAB and high BWT/DT(Robinson et al., 2002; Kuo, 2009).

However, the reliability of DT as a marker for DO or OAB is still debatable. BWT/DT are typically measured by ultrasound. One particular problematic issue is the well-known bias associated to the different operators of ultrasound. Another unsolved issue regards the best way to measure BWT/DT. Should the bladder be empty of filled? If filled, at which volume? Should one use an abdominal or transvaginal approach? Which are the costs? In addition, several studies failed to demonstrate significant differences between healthy controls, patients with DO, bladder outlet obstruction or with increased bladder sensation (Blatt et al., 2008). More recently, Liu et al measured the DT in normal controls and patients suffering from OAB or interstitial cystitis (Liu et al., 2009b). They found a wide variation amongst all groups of individuals with a trend of higher BWT/DT in OAB-wet patients that did not reach statistical significance. In another study, no differences in the BWT/DT were found between OAB patients and individuals with no OAB symptoms (Chung et al., 2010).

Clearly, the measurement of BWT or DT by ultrasound faces some drawbacks that are not yet overcome. Intra- and inter-operator variability in ultrasound measurements is probably the most important one. The use of different ultrasound probes, as well as in the resolutions of ultrasound-generated images (Kuo, 2009), is another limiting factor to the use of BWT/DT as a biomarker. Although clinically appealing, more studies are necessary before it becomes a tool for daily practice.

3. Urinary biomarkers

3.1 Prostaglandins

Prostanoids (prostaglandins and thromboxanes) are synthesized by cyclo-oxygenase (COX), present in several tissues including the bladder wall (Khan et al., 1998; Lecci et al., 2000; Azadzoi et al., 2003; Andersson & Wein, 2004). Two COX isoforms exist. COX-1 is expressed constitutively and participates in normal bladder function whereas COX-2 is activated during cystitis (Lecci et al., 2000; Tramontana et al., 2000). Prostanoid synthesis can be induced by physiological stimuli (for example, detrusor muscle stretching), injuries of the mucosa, nerve stimulation, ATP and inflammatory mediators such as bradykinin and the chemotactic peptide N-formyl-l-methionyl-l-leucyl-l-phenylalanine (Khan et al., 1998; Andersson & Wein, 2004).

Prostaglandin (PG) E_2 is one the most abundant prostanoid in the bladder (Jeremy et al., 1987; Khan et al., 1998). In rats, intravesical administration of PGE_2 facilitates micturition, increases basal intravesical pressure and induces bladder hyperactivity (Ishizuka et al., 1995). In the urethra, topical application of PGE_2 causes relaxation of the sphincter (Yokoyama et al., 2007). Likewise, intravesical instillation of an inhibitor of the COX-2 enzyme improved bladder function in an animal model of OAB (Jang et al., 2006). This supports a role for this prostanoid during bladder dysfunction and has justified a few inconclusive clinical trials regarding the use of non-steroidal anti-inflammatory drugs in the treatment of OAB. So, expectations were raised when Kim and co-workers found that levels of PGE_2 and $PGF_{2\alpha}$ were significantly higher in male and female OAB patients that in healthy controls (Kim et al., 2005; Kim et al., 2006). However, PG concentrations were not corrected for urine concentration. After correction for creatinine values, Liu and co-workers found no significant differences in PGE_2 content in patients with OAB wet, OAB dry and controls (Liu et al., 2010).

Thus, at this moment the role of urinary PGs, most notably PGE_2, as a putative tool for OAB diagnosis and follow-up is highly debatable. Moreover, the measuring methods rely on labour-intensive and expensive laboratory procedures. In addition, although it is relatively consensual that prostanoids participate in the mechanisms of OAB, it is not known if the recommended OAB therapies effectively reduce the PGs levels.

3.2 Urinary cytokines

The presence of cytokines in the urine has been addressed in various bladder and kidney disorders, including chronic renal disease, interstitial cystitis and vesicoureteral reflux (Ninan et al., 1999; Abdel-Mageed et al., 2003). It has been suggested that OAB may result from an underlying inflammation of the bladder, a hypothesis supported by recent studies reporting the presence of histological signs of inflammation in biopsies from OAB patients (Comperat et al., 2006; Apostolidis et al., 2008). However, confirming the presence of inflammation through biopsies is certainly an invasive procedure not exempt of morbidities. The detection of signs of inflammation in the urine of OAB patients is a more attractive alternative. Tyagi and co-workers have recently collected urine samples from patients and determined the levels of various cytokines, chemokines, growth factors and soluble receptors (Tyagi et al., 2010). Using a luminometry-based assay, they found a significant increase, when compared with controls, in the concentration of various elements, including the monocyte chemotatic protein-1 (MCP-1), the soluble fraction of the CD40 ligand, the macrophage inflammatory protein (MIP-1β) and interleukins 10, 5 and 12. Another group of researchers also analysed of urine samples from healthy individuals and OAB patients using a proteomic approach (Ghoniem et al., 2011). Interestingly, their results indicate that while the concentration of certain elements increases (such as interleukin 16), the concentration of others decreases (such as interleukin 7). Thus, the actual role of all of these cytokines in OAB is far from being well understood, undermining its utility as biomarkers.

3.3 Neurotrophins

Neurotrophins are tissue-derived trophic factors necessary for the embryonic differentiation, survival and maintenance of neuronal cells both in the peripheral and central nervous system (Pezet & McMahon, 2006). The most well studied neurotrophins are Nerve Growth Factor (NGF) and Brain Derived Neurotrophic Factor (BDNF). They exert their effects via their specific tyrosine kinase (Trk) receptors. NGF binds to TrkA while TrkB is the receptor of BDNF. Both TrkA and TrkB are present in the bladder urothelium and sensory afferents innervating the organ (Qiao & M.A. Vizzard, 2002; Murray et al., 2004).

3.3.1 Nerve Growth Factor (NGF)

NGF has attracted considerable attention in the Urology field. It is accepted that NGF is produced by detrusor muscle cells and by the urothelium (Steers et al., 1991; Steers et al., 1996; Clemow et al., 1997; Clemow et al., 2000; Steers & Tuttle, 2006). In humans and in rodents, the production of NGF in the lower urinary tract and in the neuronal circuits regulating bladder function is increased in pathological conditions, including cystitis and spinal cord injury (Lowe et al., 1997; Vizzard, 2000; Murray et al., 2004). In addition, exogenous NGF is known to induce bladder overactivity, irrespective of the route of delivery (Lamb et al., 2004; Yoshimura et al., 2006; Zvara & Vizzard, 2007). Likewise, manipulation of NGF levels improves bladder function and referred pain in rats with cystitis (Hu et al., 2005; Frias et al., 2009).

Recent studies have demonstrated the presence of NGF in the urine of OAB patients (Kim et al., 2005; Kim et al., 2006; Liu & Kuo, 2008; Liu et al., 2009a, b; Liu et al., 2009c; Jacobs et al., 2010; Liu et al., 2011a). Levels were significantly higher than in healthy individuals and subsided after successful treatment with antimuscarinics (Liu et al., 2009b) or botulinum toxin-A (Liu et al., 2009a), in parallel with a decrease in the USS score. Based on these results, some authors have forwarded the use of NGF as presumed biomarker for OAB (Kuo et al., 2010a). Nevertheless, caution should be advised as most studies have not been placebo controlled which may hamper the interpretation of results.

3.3.2 Brain Derived Neurotrophic Factor (BDNF)

The presence and role of BDNF in the bladder has been scarcely analysed and available results mostly refer to rodent models of bladder dysfunction. Like NGF, BDNF can be synthesized by bladder cells, most notably the urothelium during cystitis (Pinto et al., 2010a) or spinal cord injury (Vizzard, 2000). The expression of TrkB is also abundant in sensory neurons innervating the bladder wall (Qiao & Vizzard, 2002; Murray et al., 2004). Like in somatic tissue (Kerr et al., 1999; Thompson et al., 1999), BDNF expression in the bladder seems to be under the control of NGF (Schnegelsberg et al., 2010; Girard et al., 2011). BDNF appears to be a key participant in bladder dysfunction in an animal model of cystitis as its sequestration improved both bladder reflex activity and peripheral hypersensitivity (Frias et al., 2009; Pinto et al., 2010a).

In humans, it has been reported that urinary BDNF is elevated in patients suffering from bladder pain syndrome/interstitial cystitis (Pinto et al., 2010b). In OAB, a recent study demonstrated that urinary BDNF was also elevated and significantly decreased after therapeutic intervention (Antunes-Lopes et al., 2011). In addition, the concentration of urinary BDNF was shown to be decreased to normal values after successful OAB treatment (Antunes-Lopes et al., unpublished observations). This may indicate that, like NGF (Kuo et al., 2010a), urinary BDNF may serve as an OAB biomarker. However, further studies are necessary to fully understand the importance of BDNF in OAB, particularly how it can influence the OAB outcome.

4. Urinary proteomics

There is a considerable interest in urine as a source of biomarkers for bladder pathologies, OAB assuming one of the foremost active areas of research. Indeed, urine is one of the most versatile biofluids as it can be easily obtained in large quantities with non-invasive methods and is stable in comparison with other fluids. Several peptides and low molecular weight proteins can be found in urine. When urine is collected for analysis, most of them should have undergone physiological proteolysis as urine may stagnate for hours in the bladder before micturition occurs. This might constitute an advantage as, in contrast with blood, serum or plasma, urinary proteins and peptides will not undergo further degradation upon collection (Kolch et al., 2005; Omenn et al., 2005).

With the advent and improvement of proteomic analysis, increasing attention has been given to the description of the urinary proteome. The number of proteins identified in the human urine is still increasing and is well above 1500 (Adachi et al., 2006; Good et al., 2010). The combination of different analysis methods and sample treatment recently allowed the identification of more than 100 000 peptides, 5000 of which were present in more than 40% of the individuals analysed (Coon et al., 2008). Several methods are currently being used to analyse the urinary proteome, including two dimensional gel electrophoresis mass spectrometry (2DE-MS), liquid chromatography MS (LC-MS), surface-enhanced laser desorption/ionization (SELDI-TOF) and capillary electrophoresis MS (CE-MS). If interested in more details and the specific advantages and disadvantages of each method, the readers are advised to seek that information elsewhere (Decramer et al., 2008).

With the recent advances in urinary proteomics, researchers are becoming more aware of problems arising during storage and preparation of samples. One important issue is the stability of urine samples. Studies show that sequential freeze/thaw cycles may affect the concentration of certain proteins. Schaub and co-workers showed that there were no significant differences in the protein profile between samples analysed before freezing and after 1 to 4 freeze-thaw cycles (Schaub et al., 2004). These results have been confirmed in subsequent studies by non-related groups (Fiedler et al., 2007; Thongboonkerd, 2007). No data is available regarding the proteomic analysis of the urine of OAB patients.

5. Serum biomarkers

5.1 C- reactive protein (CRP)

CRP is a highly conserved plasma protein. It was identified in the 1930's in the sera of patients in the acute phase of pneumonia by Tillet and co-workers (Tillett & Francis, 1930; Black et al., 2004). Further studies demonstrated that the concentration of CRP in plasma is significantly increased during inflammatory states, a characteristic that has often been used for diagnostic purposes. In what concerns the urinary tract, plasma CRP has been used to monitor the progression of bladder cancer (Hilmy et al., 2006; Gakis et al., 2011a; Gakis et al., 2011b). As far as we are aware, CRP has been addressed in OAB only in a recent pilot study. Chung and co-workers observed higher levels of serum CRP in OAB patients than in controls, particularly in the group of OAB wet patients (Chung et al., 2011). Both urinary CRP and the amount of CRP mRNA present in the bladder wall were very low, indicating that the serum is the body fluid of choice to measure this protein. However, one should be aware that serum CRP would most likely reflect the presence of any inflammatory condition (Black et al., 2004), making its use as a putative biomarker in OAB is very modest.

5.2 Serum NGF

Like in urine, the presence of NGF in the serum of OAB patients has also been investigated (Liu et al., 2011b). The authors found a positive correlation between urinary and serum NGF contents. Interestingly, serum NGF remained elevated in OAB patients not responding to antimuscarinic treatment, suggesting that increased circulating NGF may be a factor in refractory OAB. This is, however, the only available study regarding serum NGF levels in OAB. It is presently not clear if the high content of NGF in the serum was strictly associated with OAB or dependent on associated comorbidities (hypertension, diabetes, coronary arterial disease, etc.) (Brown et al., 2000). More studies are needed in order to fully understand the relevance of serum NGF in OAB.

6. Conclusion

Clinicians and researchers are still far from having a tool to efficiently detect and monitor OAB. Several attempts have been made to identify specific bladder parameters, serum and urinary proteins that could fulfil such purpose. In all cases, researchers have come across issues. Due to several problems, the real clinical relevance of each proposed biomarker is still very much unclear, most of the publications reflecting more the willingness of the investigators rather than the true scientific value of findings. More studies are clearly necessary. In the near future, it is likely that some of these issues are overcome, as researchers are increasingly aware of the need to standardize methodologies and are already proposing basic protocols that could be easily adopted by most laboratories. Multicentre collaborative studies are also necessary to increase the size of the cohorts analysed and decrease the obvious bias of single centre findings. Hopefully, this area of research will arrive to a positive destiny with a beneficial impact on the diagnosis and outcome of OAB patients.

7. Acknowledgment

This work has been funded by INCOMB - FP7 Health project no. 223234.

8. References

Abdel-Mageed, A.B.; Bajwa, A.; Shenassa, B.B.; Human, L. & Ghoniem, G.M. (2003). NF-kappaB-dependent gene expression of proinflammatory cytokines in T24 cells: possible role in interstitial cystitis. *Urol Res*, Vol.31, No.5, (Oct 2003), pp. 300-305, ISSN 0300-5623 (Print) 0300-5623 (Linking)

Abrams, P.; Cardozo, L.; Fall, M.; Griffiths, D.; Rosier, P.; Ulmsten, U.; van Kerrebroeck, P.; Victor, A. & Wein, A. (2002). The standardisation of terminology of lower urinary tract function: report from the Standardisation Sub-committee of the International Continence Society. *Neurourol Urodyn*, Vol.21, No.2, (2002), pp. 167-178, ISSN 0733-2467 (Print), 0733-2467 (Linking)

Abrams, P.; Cardozo, L.; Fall, M.; Griffiths, D.; Rosier, P.; Ulmsten, U.; Van Kerrebroeck, P.; Victor, A. & Wein, A. (2003). The standardisation of terminology in lower urinary tract function: report from the standardisation sub-committee of the International Continence Society. *Urology*, Vol.61, No.1, (Jan 2003), pp. 37-49, ISSN 1527-9995 (Electronic) 0090-4295 (Linking)

Adachi, J.; Kumar, C.; Zhang, Y.; Olsen, J.V. & Mann, M. (2006). The human urinary proteome contains more than 1500 proteins, including a large proportion of membrane proteins. *Genome Biol*, Vol.7, No.9, (2006), pp. R80, ISSN 1465-6914 (Electronic) 1465-6906 (Linking)

Andersson, K.E. & Wein, A.J. (2004). Pharmacology of the lower urinary tract: basis for current and future treatments of urinary incontinence. *Pharmacol Rev*, Vol.56, No.4, (Dec 2004), pp. 581-631, ISSN 0031-6997 (Print) 0031-6997 (Linking)

Andersson, K.E.; Chapple, C.R.; Cardozo, L.; Cruz, F.; Hashim, H.; Michel, M.C.; Tannenbaum, C. & Wein, A.J. (2009). Pharmacological treatment of overactive bladder: report from the International Consultation on Incontinence. *Curr Opin Urol*, Vol.19, No.4, (Jul 2009), pp. 380-394, ISSN 1473-6586 (Electronic) 0963-0643 (Linking)

Andersson, K.E.S., A. (2004) Pharmacology of the lower urinary tract., *Textbook of the neurogenic bladder* (Corcos JS, E, ed), pp 57-72. London: Dunitz, M.

Antunes-Lopes, T.; Pinto, R.; Carvalho-Barros, S.; Diniz, P.; Martins-Silva, C.; Duarte-Cruz, C. & Cruz, F. (2011). Urinary levels of Brain Derived Neurotrophic Factor (BDNF) in women with overactive bladder (OAB) syndrome correlate with the severity of symptoms. *European Urology Supplements*, Vol.10, No.2, (Mar 2011), pp. 277-278, ISSN 1569-9056

Apostolidis, A.; Jacques, T.S.; Freeman, A. et al. (2008). Histological changes in the urothelium and suburothelium of human overactive bladder following intradetrusor injections of botulinum neurotoxin type A for the treatment of neurogenic or idiopathic detrusor overactivity. *Eur Urol*, Vol.53, No.6, (Jun 2008), pp. 1245-1253, ISSN 0302-2838 (Print) 0302-2838 (Linking)

Athanasopoulos, A. & Cruz, F. (2011). The medical treatment of overactive bladder, including current and future treatments. *Expert Opin Pharmacother*, Vol.12, No.7, (May 2011), pp. 1041-1055, ISSN 1744-7666 (Electronic) 1465-6566 (Linking)

Azadzoi, K.M.; Shinde, V.M.; Tarcan, T.; Kozlowski, R. & Siroky, M.B. (2003). Increased leukotriene and prostaglandin release, and overactivity in the chronically ischemic bladder. *J Urol*, Vol.169, No.5, (May 2003), pp. 1885-1891, ISSN 0022-5347 (Print) 0022-5347 (Linking)

Black, S.; Kushner, I. & Samols, D. (2004). C-reactive Protein. *J Biol Chem*, Vol.279, No.47, (Nov 19 2004), pp. 48487-48490, ISSN 0021-9258 (Print) 0021-9258 (Linking)

Blatt, A.H.; Titus, J. & Chan, L. (2008). Ultrasound measurement of bladder wall thickness in the assessment of voiding dysfunction. *J Urol*, Vol.179, No.6, (Jun 2008), pp. 2275-2278; discussion 2278-2279, ISSN 1527-3792 (Electronic) 0022-5347 (Linking)

Brown, J.S.; McGhan, W.F. & Chokroverty, S. (2000). Comorbidities associated with overactive bladder. *Am J Manag Care*, Vol.6, No.11 Suppl, (Jul 2000), pp. S574-579, ISSN 1088-0224 (Print) 1088-0224 (Linking)

Chung, S.D.; Chiu, B.; Kuo, H.C.; Chuang, Y.C.; Wang, C.C.; Guan, Z. & Chancellor, M.B. (2010). Transabdominal ultrasonography of detrusor wall thickness in women with overactive bladder. *BJU Int*, Vol.105, No.5, (2010 Mar 2010), pp. 668-672, ISSN 1464-410X (Electronic) 1464-4096 (Linking)

Chung, S.D.; Liu, H.T.; Lin, H. & Kuo, H.C. (2011). Elevation of serum c-reactive protein in patients with OAB and IC/BPS implies chronic inflammation in the urinary bladder. *Neurourol Urodyn*, Vol.30, No.3, (Mar 2011), pp. 417-420, ISSN 1520-6777 (Electronic) 0733-2467 (Linking)

Clemow, D.B.; McCarty, R.; Steers, W.D. & Tuttle, J.B. (1997). Efferent and afferent neuronal hypertrophy associated with micturition pathways in spontaneously hypertensive rats. *Neurourol Urodyn*, Vol.16, No.4, (1997), pp. 293-303, ISSN 0733-2467 (Print) 0733-2467 (Linking)

Clemow, D.B.; Steers, W.D. & Tuttle, J.B. (2000). Stretch-activated signaling of nerve growth factor secretion in bladder and vascular smooth muscle cells from hypertensive and hyperactive rats. *J Cell Physiol*, Vol.183, No.3, (Jun 2000), pp. 289-300, ISSN 0021-9541 (Print) 0021-9541 (Linking)

Comperat, E.; Reitz, A.; Delcourt, A.; Capron, F.; Denys, P. & Chartier-Kastler, E. (2006). Histologic features in the urinary bladder wall affected from neurogenic overactivity--a comparison of inflammation, oedema and fibrosis with and without injection of botulinum toxin type A. *Eur Urol*, Vol.50, No.5, (Nov 2006), pp. 1058-1064, ISSN 0302-2838 (Print) 0302-2838 (Linking)

Coon, J.J.; Zurbig, P.; Dakna, M. et al. (2008). CE-MS analysis of the human urinary proteome for biomarker discovery and disease diagnostics. *Proteomics Clin Appl*, Vol.2, No.7-8, (Jul 10 2008), pp. 964, ISSN 1862-8354 (Electronic) 1862-8346 (Linking)

Coyne, K.S.; Sexton, C.C.; Irwin, D.E.; Kopp, Z.S.; Kelleher, C.J. & Milsom, I. (2008). The impact of overactive bladder, incontinence and other lower urinary tract symptoms on quality of life, work productivity, sexuality and emotional well-being in men and women: results from the EPIC study. *BJU Int*, Vol.101, No.11, (Jun 2008), pp. 1388-1395, ISSN 1464-410X (Electronic) 1464-4096 (Linking)

Cruz, F. & Dinis, P. (2007). Resiniferatoxin and botulinum toxin type A for treatment of lower urinary tract symptoms. *Neurourol Urodyn*, Vol.26, No.6 Suppl, (Oct 2007), pp. 920-927, ISSN 0733-2467 (Print) 0733-2467 (Linking)

da Silva, C.M. & Cruz, F. (2009). Has botulinum toxin therapy come of age: what do we know, what do we need to know, and should we use it? *Curr Opin Urol*, Vol.19, No.4, (Jul 2009), pp. 347-352, ISSN 1473-6586 (Electronic) 0963-0643 (Linking)

Decramer, S.; Gonzalez de Peredo, A.; Breuil, B.; Mischak, H.; Monsarrat, B.; Bascands, J.L. & Schanstra, J.P. (2008). Urine in clinical proteomics. *Mol Cell Proteomics*, Vol.7, No.10, (Oct 2008), pp. 1850-1862, ISSN 1535-9484 (Electronic) 1535-9476 (Linking)

Drake, M.J.; Fowler, C.J.; Griffiths, D.; Mayer, E.; Paton, J.F. & Birder, L. (2010). Neural control of the lower urinary and gastrointestinal tracts: supraspinal CNS mechanisms. *Neurourol Urodyn*, Vol.29, No.1, (2010), pp. 119-127, ISSN 1520-6777 (Electronic) 0733-2467 (Linking)

Farag, F.F.; Martens, F.M.; D'Hauwers, K.W.; Feitz, W.F. & Heesakkers, J.P. (2011a). Near-infrared spectroscopy: a novel, noninvasive, diagnostic method for detrusor overactivity in patients with overactive bladder symptoms--a preliminary and experimental study. *Eur Urol*, Vol.59, No.5, (May 2011a), pp. 757-762, ISSN 1873-7560 (Electronic) 0302-2838 (Linking)

Farag, F.F.; Martens, F.M.; Feitz, W.F. & Heesakkers, J.P. (2011b). Feasibility of Noninvasive Near-Infrared Spectroscopy to Diagnose Detrusor Overactivity. *Urol Int*, (Aug 24 2011b), pp. ISSN 1423-0399 (Electronic) 0042-1138 (Linking)

Fiedler, G.M.; Baumann, S.; Leichtle, A.; Oltmann, A.; Kase, J.; Thiery, J. & Ceglarek, U. (2007). Standardized peptidome profiling of human urine by magnetic bead separation and matrix-assisted laser desorption/ionization time-of-flight mass spectrometry. *Clin Chem*, Vol.53, No.3, (Mar 2007), pp. 421-428, ISSN 0009-9147 (Print) 0009-9147 (Linking)

Fowler, C.J.; Griffiths, D. & de Groat, W.C. (2008). The neural control of micturition. *Nat Rev Neurosci*, Vol.9, No.6, (Jun 2008), pp. 453-466, ISSN 1471-0048 (Electronic) 1471-003X (Linking)

Fowler, C.J. & Griffiths, D.J. (2010). A decade of functional brain imaging applied to bladder control. *Neurourol Urodyn*, Vol.29, No.1, (2010), pp. 49-55, ISSN 1520-6777 (Electronic) 0733-2467 (Linking)

Frias, B.; Charrua, A.; Pinto, R.; Allen, S.; Dawbarn, D.; Cruz, F. & Cruz, C.D. (2009). Intrathecal blockade of Trk receptors and neurotrophin sequestration reduces pain and urinary frequency in an animal model of chronic bladder inflammation. *Neurourology and Urodynamics*, Vol.28, No.7, (2009 2009), pp. 708-708, ISSN 0733-2467

Gakis, G.; Todenhoefer, T.; Renninger, M.; Schilling, D.; Sievert, K.D.; Schwentner, C. & Stenzl, A. (2011a). Development of a new outcome prediction model in carcinoma invading the bladder based on preoperative serum C-reactive protein and standard pathological risk factors: the TNR-C score. *BJU Int*, (Apr 20 2011a), pp. ISSN 1464-410X (Electronic) 1464-4096 (Linking)

Gakis, G.; Todenhofer, T. & Stenzl, A. (2011b). The prognostic value of hematological and systemic inflammatory disorders in invasive bladder cancer. *Curr Opin Urol*, Vol.21, No.5, (Sep 2011b), pp. 428-433, ISSN 1473-6586 (Electronic) 0963-0643 (Linking)

Ghoniem, G.; Faruqui, N.; Elmissiry, M.; Mahdy, A.; Abdelwahab, H.; Oommen, M. & Abdel-Mageed, A.B. (2011). Differential profile analysis of urinary cytokines in patients with overactive bladder. *Int Urogynecol J*, Vol.22, No.8, (Aug 2011), pp. 953-961, ISSN 1433-3023 (Electronic) 0937-3462 (Linking)

Girard, B.M.; Malley, S.E. & Vizzard, M.A. (2011). Neurotrophin/receptor expression in urinary bladder of mice with overexpression of NGF in urothelium. *Am J Physiol Renal Physiol*, Vol.300, No.2, (Feb 2011), pp. F345-355, ISSN 1522-1466 (Electronic) 1522-1466 (Linking)

Good, D.M.; Zurbig, P.; Argiles, A. et al. (2010). Naturally occurring human urinary peptides for use in diagnosis of chronic kidney disease. *Mol Cell Proteomics*, Vol.9, No.11, (Nov 2010), pp. 2424-2437, ISSN 1535-9484 (Electronic) 1535-9476 (Linking)

Gulur, D.M. & Drake, M.J. (2010). Management of overactive bladder. *Nat Rev Urol*, Vol.7, No.10, (Oct 2010), pp. 572-582, ISSN 1759-4820 (Electronic) 1759-4812 (Linking)

Hakenberg, O.W.; Linne, C.; Manseck, A. & Wirth, M.P. (2000). Bladder wall thickness in normal adults and men with mild lower urinary tract symptoms and benign prostatic enlargement. *Neurourol Urodyn*, Vol.19, No.5, (2000), pp. 585-593, ISSN 0733-2467 (Print) 0733-2467 (Linking)

Hashim, H. & Abrams, P. (2006). Is the bladder a reliable witness for predicting detrusor overactivity? *J Urol*, Vol.175, No.1, (Jan 2006), pp. 191-194; discussion 194-195, ISSN 0022-5347 (Print) 0022-5347 (Linking)

Hashim, H. & Abrams, P. (2007). Overactive bladder: an update. *Curr Opin Urol*, Vol.17, No.4, (Jul 2007), pp. 231-236, ISSN 0963-0643 (Print) 0963-0643 (Linking)

Henderson, E. & Drake, M. (2010). Overactive bladder. *Maturitas*, Vol.66, No.3, (Jul 2010), pp. 257-262, ISSN 1873-4111 (Electronic) 0378-5122 (Linking)

Heslington, K. & Hilton, P. (1996). Ambulatory monitoring and conventional cystometry in asymptomatic female volunteers. *Br J Obstet Gynaecol*, Vol.103, No.5, (May 1996), pp. 434-441, ISSN 0306-5456 (Print) 0306-5456 (Linking)

Hilmy, M.; Campbell, R.; Bartlett, J.M.; McNicol, A.M.; Underwood, M.A. & McMillan, D.C. (2006). The relationship between the systemic inflammatory response, tumour proliferative activity, T-lymphocytic infiltration and COX-2 expression and survival in patients with transitional cell carcinoma of the urinary bladder. *Br J Cancer*, Vol.95, No.9, (Nov 6 2006), pp. 1234-1238, ISSN 0007-0920 (Print) 0007-0920 (Linking)

Hu, V.Y.; Zvara, P.; Dattilio, A.; Redman, T.L.; Allen, S.J.; Dawbarn, D.; Stroemer, R.P. & Vizzard, M.A. (2005). Decrease in bladder overactivity with REN1820 in rats with cyclophosphamide induced cystitis. *J Urol*, Vol.173, No.3, (Mar 2005), pp. 1016-1021, ISSN 0022-5347 (Print) 0022-5347 (Linking)

Irwin, D.E.; Milsom, I.; Hunskaar, S. et al. (2006). Population-based survey of urinary incontinence, overactive bladder, and other lower urinary tract symptoms in five countries: results of the EPIC study. *Eur Urol*, Vol.50, No.6, (Dec 2006), pp. 1306-1314; discussion 1314-1305, ISSN 0302-2838 (Print) 0302-2838 (Linking)

Irwin, D.E.; Milsom, I.; Kopp, Z.; Abrams, P.; Artibani, W. & Herschorn, S. (2009). Prevalence, severity, and symptom bother of lower urinary tract symptoms among men in the EPIC study: impact of overactive bladder. *Eur Urol*, Vol.56, No.1, (Jul 2009), pp. 14-20, ISSN 1873-7560 (Electronic) 0302-2838 (Linking)

Ishizuka, O.; Mattiasson, A. & Andersson, K.E. (1995). Prostaglandin E2-induced bladder hyperactivity in normal, conscious rats: involvement of tachykinins? *J Urol*, Vol.153, No.6, (Jun 1995), pp. 2034-2038, ISSN 0022-5347 (Print) 0022-5347 (Linking)

Jacobs, B.L.; Smaldone, M.C.; Tyagi, V.; Philips, B.J.; Jackman, S.V.; Leng, W.W. & Tyagi, P. (2010). Increased nerve growth factor in neurogenic overactive bladder and interstitial cystitis patients. *Can J Urol*, Vol.17, No.1, (Feb 2010), pp. 4989-4994, ISSN 1195-9479 (Print) 1195-9479 (Linking)

Jang, J.; Park, E.Y.; Seo, S.I.; Hwang, T.K. & Kim, J.C. (2006). Effects of intravesical instillation of cyclooxygenase-2 inhibitor on the expression of inducible nitric oxide synthase and nerve growth factor in cyclophosphamide-induced overactive bladder. *BJU Int*, Vol.98, No.2, (Aug 2006), pp. 435-439, ISSN 1464-4096 (Print) 1464-4096 (Linking)

Jeremy, J.Y.; Tsang, V.; Mikhailidis, D.P.; Rogers, H.; Morgan, R.J. & Dandona, P. (1987). Eicosanoid synthesis by human urinary bladder mucosa: pathological implications. *Br J Urol*, Vol.59, No.1, (Jan 1987), pp. 36-39, ISSN 0007-1331 (Print) 0007-1331 (Linking)

Kerr, B.J.; Bradbury, E.J.; Bennett, D.L.; Trivedi, P.M.; Dassan, P.; French, J.; Shelton, D.B.; McMahon, S.B. & Thompson, S.W. (1999). Brain-derived neurotrophic factor modulates nociceptive sensory inputs and NMDA-evoked responses in the rat spinal cord. *J Neurosci*, Vol.19, No.12, (Jun 15 1999), pp. 5138-5148, ISSN 1529-2401 (Electronic) 0270-6474 (Linking)

Khan, M.A.; Thompson, C.S.; Mumtaz, F.H.; Jeremy, J.Y.; Morgan, R.J. & Mikhailidis, D.P. (1998). Role of prostaglandins in the urinary bladder: an update. *Prostaglandins Leukot Essent Fatty Acids*, Vol.59, No.6, (Dec 1998), pp. 415-422, ISSN 0952-3278 (Print) 0952-3278 (Linking)

Khullar, V.; Cardozo, L.D.; Salvatore, S. & Hill, S. (1996). Ultrasound: a noninvasive screening test for detrusor instability. *Br J Obstet Gynaecol*, Vol.103, No.9, (Sep 1996), pp. 904-908, ISSN 0306-5456 (Print) 0306-5456 (Linking)

Kim, J.C.; Park, E.Y.; Hong, S.H.; Seo, S.I.; Park, Y.H. & Hwang, T.K. (2005). Changes of urinary nerve growth factor and prostaglandins in male patients with overactive bladder symptom. *Int J Urol*, Vol.12, No.10, (Oct 2005), pp. 875-880, ISSN 0919-8172 (Print) 0919-8172 (Linking)

Kim, J.C.; Park, E.Y.; Seo, S.I.; Park, Y.H. & Hwang, T.K. (2006). Nerve growth factor and prostaglandins in the urine of female patients with overactive bladder. *J Urol*, Vol.175, No.5, (May 2006), pp. 1773-1776; discussion 1776, ISSN 0022-5347 (Print) 0022-5347 (Linking)

Kolch, W.; Neususs, C.; Pelzing, M. & Mischak, H. (2005). Capillary electrophoresis-mass spectrometry as a powerful tool in clinical diagnosis and biomarker discovery. *Mass Spectrom Rev*, Vol.24, No.6, (Nov-Dec 2005), pp. 959-977, ISSN 0277-7037 (Print) 0277-7037 (Linking)

Kuhn, A.; Genoud, S.; Robinson, D.; Herrmann, G.; Gunthert, A.; Brandner, S. & Raio, L. (2011). Sonographic transvaginal bladder wall thickness: does the measurement discriminate between urodynamic diagnoses? *Neurourol Urodyn*, Vol.30, No.3, (Mar 2011), pp. 325-328, ISSN 1520-6777 (Electronic) 0733-2467 (Linking)

Kuo, H.C. (2009). Measurement of detrusor wall thickness in women with overactive bladder by transvaginal and transabdominal sonography. *Int Urogynecol J Pelvic*

Floor Dysfunct, Vol.20, No.11, (Nov 2009), pp. 1293-1299, ISSN 1433-3023 (Electronic) 0937-3462 (Linking)

Kuo, H.C.; Liu, H.T. & Chancellor, M.B. (2010a). Can urinary nerve growth factor be a biomarker for overactive bladder? *Rev Urol*, Vol.12, No.2-3, (Spring 2010a), pp. e69-77, ISSN 1523-6161 (Print) 1523-6161 (Linking)

Kuo, H.C.; Liu, H.T. & Chancellor, M.B. (2010b). Urinary nerve growth factor is a better biomarker than detrusor wall thickness for the assessment of overactive bladder with incontinence. *Neurourol Urodyn*, Vol.29, No.3, (2010 Mar 2010b), pp. 482-487, ISSN 1520-6777 (Electronic) 0733-2467 (Linking)

Lamb, K.; Gebhart, G.F. & Bielefeldt, K. (2004). Increased nerve growth factor expression triggers bladder overactivity. *J Pain*, Vol.5, No.3, (Apr 2004), pp. 150-156, ISSN 1526-5900 (Print) 1526-5900 (Linking)

Lecci, A.; Birder, L.A.; Meini, S.; Catalioto, R.M.; Tramontana, M.; Giuliani, S.; Criscuoli, M. & Maggi, C.A. (2000). Pharmacological evaluation of the role of cyclooxygenase isoenzymes on the micturition reflex following experimental cystitis in rats. *Br J Pharmacol*, Vol.130, No.2, (May 2000), pp. 331-338, ISSN 0007-1188 (Print) 0007-1188 (Linking)

Liu, H.T. & Kuo, H.C. (2008). Urinary nerve growth factor level could be a potential biomarker for diagnosis of overactive bladder. *J Urol*, Vol.179, No.6, (Jun 2008), pp. 2270-2274, ISSN 1527-3792 (Electronic) 0022-5347 (Linking)

Liu, H.T.; Chancellor, M.B. & Kuo, H.C. (2009a). Urinary nerve growth factor levels are elevated in patients with detrusor overactivity and decreased in responders to detrusor botulinum toxin-A injection. *Eur Urol*, Vol.56, No.4, (Oct 2009a), pp. 700-706, ISSN 1873-7560 (Electronic) 0302-2838 (Linking)

Liu, H.T.; Chancellor, M.B. & Kuo, H.C. (2009b). Decrease of urinary nerve growth factor levels after antimuscarinic therapy in patients with overactive bladder. *BJU Int*, Vol.103, No.12, (Jun 2009b), pp. 1668-1672, ISSN 1464-410X (Electronic) 1464-4096 (Linking)

Liu, H.T.; Liu, A.B.; Chancellor, M.B. & Kuo, H.C. (2009c). Urinary nerve growth factor level is correlated with the severity of neurological impairment in patients with cerebrovascular accident. *BJU Int*, Vol.104, No.8, (Oct 2009c), pp. 1158-1162, ISSN 1464-410X (Electronic) 1464-4096 (Linking)

Liu, H.T.; Tyagi, P.; Chancellor, M.B. & Kuo, H.C. (2010). Urinary nerve growth factor but not prostaglandin E2 increases in patients with interstitial cystitis/bladder pain syndrome and detrusor overactivity. *BJU Int*, Vol.106, No.11, (Dec 2010), pp. 1681-1685, ISSN 1464-410X (Electronic) 1464-4096 (Linking)

Liu, H.T.; Chen, C.Y. & Kuo, H.C. (2011a). Urinary nerve growth factor in women with overactive bladder syndrome. *BJU Int*, Vol.107, No.5, (Mar 2011a), pp. 799-803, ISSN 1464-410X (Electronic) 1464-4096 (Linking)

Liu, H.T.; Lin, H. & Kuo, H.C. (2011b). Increased serum nerve growth factor levels in patients with overactive bladder syndrome refractory to antimuscarinic therapy. *Neurourol Urodyn*, (Aug 8 2011b), pp. ISSN 1520-6777 (Electronic) 0733-2467 (Linking)

Lowe, E.M.; Anand, P.; Terenghi, G.; Williams-Chestnut, R.E.; Sinicropi, D.V. & Osborne, J.L. (1997). Increased nerve growth factor levels in the urinary bladder of women with idiopathic sensory urgency and interstitial cystitis. *Br J Urol*, Vol.79, No.4, (Apr 1997), pp. 572-577, ISSN 0007-1331 (Print) 0007-1331 (Linking)

Lowenstein, L.; Pham, T.; Abbasy, S. et al. (2009). Observations relating to urinary sensation during detrusor overactivity. *Neurourol Urodyn*, Vol.28, No.6, (2009), pp. 497-500, ISSN 1520-6777 (Electronic) 0733-2467 (Linking)

Malone-Lee, J.G. & Al-Buheissi, S. (2009). Does urodynamic verification of overactive bladder determine treatment success? Results from a randomized placebo-controlled study. *BJU Int*, Vol.103, No.7, (Apr 2009), pp. 931-937, ISSN 1464-410X (Electronic) 1464-4096 (Linking)

Michel, M.C. & Chapple, C.R. (2009a). Basic mechanisms of urgency: roles and benefits of pharmacotherapy. *World J Urol*, Vol.27, No.6, (Dec 2009a), pp. 705-709, ISSN 1433-8726 (Electronic) 0724-4983 (Linking)

Michel, M.C. & Chapple, C.R. (2009b). Basic mechanisms of urgency: preclinical and clinical evidence. *Eur Urol*, Vol.56, No.2, (Aug 2009b), pp. 298-307, ISSN 1873-7560 (Electronic) 0302-2838 (Linking)

Murray, E.; Malley, S.E.; Qiao, L.Y.; Hu, V.Y. & Vizzard, M.A. (2004). Cyclophosphamide induced cystitis alters neurotrophin and receptor tyrosine kinase expression in pelvic ganglia and bladder. *J Urol*, Vol.172, No.6 Pt 1, (Dec 2004), pp. 2434-2439, ISSN 0022-5347 (Print) 0022-5347 (Linking)

Ninan, G.K.; Jutley, R.S. & Eremin, O. (1999). Urinary cytokines as markers of reflux nephropathy. *J Urol*, Vol.162, No.5, (Nov 1999), pp. 1739-1742, ISSN 0022-5347 (Print) 0022-5347 (Linking)

Nixon, A.; Colman, S.; Sabounjian, L.; Sandage, B.; Schwiderski, U.E.; Staskin, D.R. & Zinner, N. (2005). A validated patient reported measure of urinary urgency severity in overactive bladder for use in clinical trials. *J Urol*, Vol.174, No.2, (Aug 2005), pp. 604-607, ISSN 0022-5347 (Print) 0022-5347 (Linking)

Oelke, M.; Hofner, K.; Jonas, U.; Ubbink, D.; de la Rosette, J. & Wijkstra, H. (2006). Ultrasound measurement of detrusor wall thickness in healthy adults. *Neurourol Urodyn*, Vol.25, No.4, (2006), pp. 308-317; discussion 318, ISSN 0733-2467 (Print) 0733-2467 (Linking)

Oelke, M.; Hofner, K.; Jonas, U.; de la Rosette, J.J.; Ubbink, D.T. & Wijkstra, H. (2007). Diagnostic accuracy of noninvasive tests to evaluate bladder outlet obstruction in men: detrusor wall thickness, uroflowmetry, postvoid residual urine, and prostate volume. *Eur Urol*, Vol.52, No.3, (Sep 2007), pp. 827-834, ISSN 0302-2838 (Print) 0302-2838 (Linking)

Omenn, G.S.; States, D.J.; Adamski, M. et al. (2005). Overview of the HUPO Plasma Proteome Project: results from the pilot phase with 35 collaborating laboratories and multiple analytical groups, generating a core dataset of 3020 proteins and a publicly-available database. *Proteomics*, Vol.5, No.13, (Aug 2005), pp. 3226-3245, ISSN 1615-9853 (Print) 1615-9853 (Linking)

Panayi, D.C.; Tekkis, P.; Fernando, R.; Hendricken, C. & Khullar, V. (2010). Ultrasound measurement of bladder wall thickness is associated with the overactive bladder syndrome. *Neurourol Urodyn*, Vol.29, No.7, (Sep 2010), pp. 1295-1298, ISSN 1520-6777 (Electronic) 0733-2467 (Linking)

Pezet, S. & McMahon, S.B. (2006). Neurotrophins: mediators and modulators of pain. *Annu Rev Neurosci*, Vol.29, (2006), pp. 507-538, ISSN 0147-006X (Print) 0147-006X (Linking)

Pinto, R.; Frias, B.; Allen, S.; Dawbarn, D.; McMahon, S.B.; Cruz, F. & Cruz, C.D. (2010a). Sequestration of brain derived nerve factor by intravenous delivery of TrkB-Ig2 reduces bladder overactivity and noxious input in animals with chronic cystitis. *Neuroscience*, Vol.166, No.3, (Mar 31 2010a), pp. 907-916, ISSN 1873-7544 (Electronic) 0306-4522 (Linking)

Pinto, R.; Lopes, T.; Frias, B.; Silva, A.; Silva, J.A.; Silva, C.M.; Cruz, C.; Cruz, F. & Dinis, P. (2010b). Trigonal injection of botulinum toxin A in patients with refractory bladder pain syndrome/interstitial cystitis. *Eur Urol*, Vol.58, No.3, (Sep 2010b), pp. 360-365, ISSN 1873-7560 (Electronic) 0302-2838 (Linking)

Qiao, L. & Vizzard, M.A. (2002). Up-regulation of tyrosine kinase (Trka, Trkb) receptor expression and phosphorylation in lumbosacral dorsal root ganglia after chronic spinal cord (T8-T10) injury. *J Comp Neurol*, Vol.449, No.3, (Jul 29 2002), pp. 217-230, ISSN 0021-9967 (Print) 0021-9967 (Linking)

Qiao, L.Y. & Vizzard, M.A. (2002). Cystitis-induced upregulation of tyrosine kinase (TrkA, TrkB) receptor expression and phosphorylation in rat micturition pathways. *J Comp Neurol*, Vol.454, No.2, (Dec 9 2002), pp. 200-211, ISSN 0021-9967 (Print) 0021-9967 (Linking)

Robinson, D.; Anders, K.; Cardozo, L.; Bidmead, J.; Toozs-Hobson, P. & Khullar, V. (2002). Can ultrasound replace ambulatory urodynamics when investigating women with irritative urinary symptoms? *BJOG*, Vol.109, No.2, (Feb 2002), pp. 145-148, ISSN 1470-0328 (Print) 1470-0328 (Linking)

Schaub, S.; Wilkins, J.; Weiler, T.; Sangster, K.; Rush, D. & Nickerson, P. (2004). Urine protein profiling with surface-enhanced laser-desorption/ionization time-of-flight mass spectrometry. *Kidney Int*, Vol.65, No.1, (Jan 2004), pp. 323-332, ISSN 0085-2538 (Print) 0085-2538 (Linking)

Schnegelsberg, B.; Sun, T.T.; Cain, G.; Bhattacharya, A.; Nunn, P.A.; Ford, A.P.; Vizzard, M.A. & Cockayne, D.A. (2010). Overexpression of NGF in mouse urothelium leads to neuronal hyperinnervation, pelvic sensitivity, and changes in urinary bladder function. *Am J Physiol Regul Integr Comp Physiol*, Vol.298, No.3, (Mar 2010), pp. R534-547, ISSN 1522-1490 (Electronic) 0363-6119 (Linking)

Sexton, C.C.; Coyne, K.S.; Kopp, Z.S.; Irwin, D.E.; Milsom, I.; Aiyer, L.P.; Tubaro, A.; Chapple, C.R. & Wein, A.J. (2009a). The overlap of storage, voiding and postmicturition symptoms and implications for treatment seeking in the USA, UK and Sweden: EpiLUTS. *BJU Int*, Vol.103 Suppl 3, (Apr 2009a), pp. 12-23, ISSN 1464-410X (Electronic) 1464-4096 (Linking)

Sexton, C.C.; Coyne, K.S.; Vats, V.; Kopp, Z.S.; Irwin, D.E. & Wagner, T.H. (2009b). Impact of overactive bladder on work productivity in the United States: results from EpiLUTS. *Am J Manag Care*, Vol.15, No.4 Suppl, (Mar 2009b), pp. S98-S107, ISSN 1936-2692 (Electronic) 1088-0224 (Linking)

Starkman, J.S. & Dmochowski, R.R. (2008). Urgency assessment in the evaluation of overactive bladder (OAB). *Neurourol Urodyn*, Vol.27, No.1, (2008), pp. 13-21, ISSN 0733-2467 (Print) 0733-2467 (Linking)

Steers, W.D.; Kolbeck, S.; Creedon, D. & Tuttle, J.B. (1991). Nerve growth factor in the urinary bladder of the adult regulates neuronal form and function. *J Clin Invest*, Vol.88, No.5, (Nov 1991), pp. 1709-1715, ISSN 0021-9738 (Print) 0021-9738 (Linking)

Steers, W.D.; Creedon, D.J. & Tuttle, J.B. (1996). Immunity to nerve growth factor prevents afferent plasticity following urinary bladder hypertrophy. *J Urol*, Vol.155, No.1, (Jan 1996), pp. 379-385, ISSN 0022-5347 (Print) 0022-5347 (Linking)

Steers, W.D. & Tuttle, J.B. (2006). Mechanisms of Disease: the role of nerve growth factor in the pathophysiology of bladder disorders. *Nat Clin Pract Urol*, Vol.3, No.2, (Feb 2006), pp. 101-110, ISSN 1743-4270 (Print)

Thompson, S.W.; Bennett, D.L.; Kerr, B.J.; Bradbury, E.J. & McMahon, S.B. (1999). Brain-derived neurotrophic factor is an endogenous modulator of nociceptive responses in the spinal cord. *Proc Natl Acad Sci U S A*, Vol.96, No.14, (Jul 6 1999), pp. 7714-7718, ISSN 0027-8424 (Print) 0027-8424 (Linking)

Thongboonkerd, V. (2007). Practical points in urinary proteomics. *J Proteome Res*, Vol.6, No.10, (Oct 2007), pp. 3881-3890, ISSN 1535-3893 (Print) 1535-3893 (Linking)

Tillett, W.S. & Francis, T. (1930). Serological Reactions in Pneumonia with a Non-Protein Somatic Fraction of Pneumococcus. *J Exp Med*, Vol.52, No.4, (Sep 30 1930), pp. 561-571, ISSN 0022-1007 (Print) 0022-1007 (Linking)

Tramontana, M.; Catalioto, R.M.; Lecci, A. & Maggi, C.A. (2000). Role of prostanoids in the contraction induced by a tachykinin NK2 receptor agonist in the hamster urinary bladder. *Naunyn Schmiedebergs Arch Pharmacol*, Vol.361, No.4, (Apr 2000), pp. 452-459, ISSN 0028-1298 (Print) 0028-1298 (Linking)

Tyagi, P.; Barclay, D.; Zamora, R.; Yoshimura, N.; Peters, K.; Vodovotz, Y. & Chancellor, M. (2010). Urine cytokines suggest an inflammatory response in the overactive bladder: a pilot study. *Int Urol Nephrol*, Vol.42, No.3, (Sep 2010), pp. 629-635, ISSN 1573-2584 (Electronic) 0301-1623 (Linking)

van Waalwijk van Doorn, E.S.; Ambergen, A.W. & Janknegt, R.A. (1997). Detrusor activity index: quantification of detrusor overactivity by ambulatory monitoring. *J Urol*, Vol.157, No.2, (Feb 1997), pp. 596-599, ISSN 0022-5347 (Print) 0022-5347 (Linking)

Vizzard, M.A. (2000). Changes in urinary bladder neurotrophic factor mRNA and NGF protein following urinary bladder dysfunction. *Exp Neurol*, Vol.161, No.1, (Jan 2000), pp. 273-284, ISSN 0014-4886 (Print) 0014-4886 (Linking)

Yokoyama, O.; Miwa, Y.; Oyama, N.; Aoki, Y.; Ito, H. & Akino, H. (2007). Antimuscarinic drug inhibits detrusor overactivity induced by topical application of prostaglandin E2 to the urethra with a decrease in urethral pressure. *J Urol*, Vol.178, No.5, (Nov 2007), pp. 2208-2212, ISSN 0022-5347 (Print) 0022-5347 (Linking)

Yoshimura, N.; Bennett, N.E.; Hayashi, Y.; Ogawa, T.; Nishizawa, O.; Chancellor, M.B.; de Groat, W.C. & Seki, S. (2006). Bladder overactivity and hyperexcitability of bladder afferent neurons after intrathecal delivery of nerve growth factor in rats. *J Neurosci*, Vol.26, No.42, (Oct 18 2006), pp. 10847-10855, ISSN 1529-2401 (Electronic) 0270-6474 (Linking)

Zvara, P. & Vizzard, M.A. (2007). Exogenous overexpression of nerve growth factor in the urinary bladder produces bladder overactivity and altered micturition circuitry in the lumbosacral spinal cord. *BMC Physiol*, Vol.7, (2007), pp. 9, ISSN 1472-6793 (Electronic) 1472-6793 (Linking)

Part 3

Surgical Options

Preoperative Factors as Predictors of Outcome of Midurethral Sling in Women with Mixed Urinary Incontinence

Jin Wook Kim, Mi Mi Oh and Jeong Gu Lee
Korea University
Republic of Korea

1. Introduction

Mixed urinary incontinence (MUI) presents with characteristics of both stress urinary incontinence (SUI) and urge urinary incontinence (UUI). It has been generally assumed to respond less favourably to any type of interventional therapy, whether behavioural, pharmacologic, or surgical as compared with pure stress (effort) or urge urinary incontinence. These patients represent a therapeutic challenge: two pathologies coexist, and treatment of either condition may worsen the symptoms of the other. The result is likely to be a poor response to conservative or surgical interventions. (Chaliha & Khullar, 2004)

The development of midurethral sling (MUS) surgery has become the gold standard for surgical treatment of SUI. There is great variability in data regarding cure rate of MUI following mid urethral sling (MUS) surgery of both the stress and urge components. Moreover, the postoperative course of the urge component after surgery is unpredictable as it may resolve, persist or worsen. There are no consistent predictors for persistent worsening of urge components after sling surgery. While there have been various factors described in the literature to predict who will be more likely benefit, these have not been clearly defined. Further compounding the difficulty is the lack of appropriate tools in delineating the characteristics of a mixed presentation. The poor response to treatment in MUI patients have led investigators to attempt quantifying and comparing dominance of either spectrum to dictate a priority of treatment and quantitatively assess outcome.

Despite such limitations, advance of treatment has allowed more aggressive combined approach to MUI, necessitating the delineation of patient profiles appropriate for each treatment method. Here we will review the current investigations analysing the two distinct pathophysiologies of MUI, as well as the suggested factors determining the outcome following MUS treatment.

2. Prevalence of MUI

MUI is the coexistence of stress and urgency urinary incontinence and is defined as involuntary loss of urine associated with the sensation of urgency and also associated with exertion, effort, sneezing or coughing.(Haylen et al., 2010) Mixed incontinence can also be defined urodynamically as the coexistence of urinary stress incontinence (USI) and detrusor over activity (DO). DO is characterized by involuntary detrusor contractions during the filling phase and is associated with urgency or incontinence. Urge urinary incontinence is the complaint of involuntary leakage accompanied by or immediately preceded by urgency. Investigators, however, often have grouped several different pathologies together under the category of "mixed incontinence."(Khullar et al., 2010) Further compounding the definition of MUI is an acknowledged fact that stress incontinence may also be misperceived as an urgency event. The presence of urine in the posterior urethra may actually induce urinary urgency and eventuate in a secondary episode of detrusor overactivity (stress-induced detrusor overactivity). Therefore, in some individuals, stress incontinence may actually masquerade as MUI due to the significant urgency component associated with spontaneous urinary loss. Urinary frequency is superimposed over this scenario as a behavioral response to the bothersome urinary symptoms. (Dmochowski & Staskin, 2005)

As previously noted, the difficulty in collating the results of different studies primarily lies with a confusion in definition. Epidemiologic studies also vary with reports based on symptoms to those based on urodynamic parameters. While the term "mixed incontinence" remains a clinically useful concept there is debate over the utility of its use for outcomes research. Dooley et al. investigated the discrepancy of prevalence between subjective and objective definitions of MUI. The study showed that in the population of women seeking surgical treatment for stress incontinence, the majority of women fell into the category of MUI when using subjective measures to define the condition. (Dooley et al., 2008) Prevalence rates ranged from 50% to 93% depending on the questions used and severity selected; however, when using objective measures only 8% were diagnosed as having MUI on urodynamics. These data illustrate how such wide variations in prevalence rates for MUI can occur. To date, the appropriate MUI definition has not been agreed upon for either research or clinical care.

Most clinical studies, however, generally approximate the prevalence of MUI as one-third of women with urinary incontinence. (Karram & Bhatia, 1989) Recent incidence data based on urinary symptoms were obtained through the National Overactive Bladder Evaluation (NOBLE) Program, which investigated urinary incontinence in 5,204 adults residing in the United States, 2,735 of who were women. When these survey data were applied to the 2000 US census, the total number of US women with incontinence was estimated to be 14.8 million. Urge, stress, and mixed incontinence each accounted for approximately one-third of cases. (Stewart et al., 2003) The study of medical, epidemiological, and social aspects of aging (MESA), conducted by Diokno et al. reported the prevalence of different types of urinary incontinence in senior citizens aged 60 years. (Diokno et al., 1986) Of the 1,150 randomly sampled non-institutionalized women included in the study, 716 were self-reported as continent and 434 as incontinent. The study found that 55.5% of the incontinent women had mixed stress and urge incontinence, 26.7% had stress incontinence alone, 9% had urge incontinence alone, and 8.8% had other diagnoses.

The limitations of comparing MUI in epidemiologic studies to MUI in clinical settings may also be due, in part, to the fact that they require purely symptom based assessments. Thus, one would expect that evaluations of MUI in clinical samples would be superior as they tend to employ a combination of subjective and objective evaluation. Unfortunately, the variation in prevalence rates for MUI in these settings is equally broad. Lemack and

Zimmern investigated 128 women reporting lower urinary tract symptoms and found that 26.6% had mixed incontinence, 20.3% had stress incontinence, 13.3% had urge incontinence, 14.1% had urgency and frequency symptoms, and 10.1% had vaginal prolapse. (Lemack & Zimmern, 1999) However, when symptoms were matched with urodynamic findings they correlated in less than 50% of the time.

Urodynamic studies, which provide objective evidence of the type of urinary incontinence, have shown that between 8% and 56% of women with urinary disorders have proven mixed incontinence. Digesu et al. reported rates of DO in a population of stress predominant MUI was 11%. (Digesu et al., 2008) Dooley reported that the proportion of women diagnosed with MUI ranged from a low of 8.3% using only the urodynamic-based definition. (Dooley et al., 2008) Chou et al. suggested that patients may mistake the urge component for the "fear of leaking for urge", in explaining the discrepancy between subjective and objective diagnoses. (Chou et al., 2008)

The absence of a universal definition of mixed incontinence has made it difficult to compare findings from studies. Whether it is defined urodynamically or symptomatically, incontinence associated with both stress and urge is considered mixed in nature. Ideally, a reproducible instrument that would clearly segregate stress versus urge symptoms and assess the magnitude of bother for a particular patient would best define the MUI presentation; however, this entity is yet to be defined.

Another difficulty in estimating the population of MUI is the varying degrees of severity in what constitutes the urge component. In a recent, randomized study to investigate the treatment of mixed incontinence in women, Bump et al. found that 31% of patients had mixed urinary incontinence symptoms. (Bump et al., 2003) These women had more severe baseline urinary incontinence than did those with USI in terms of frequency of incontinence and impairment of quality of life. Surprisingly, the baseline severity of incontinence was less in women with urodynamically proven mixed incontinence than in those with USI. The authors performed a comprehensive nationwide survey in Korea and found 40.8% of patients aged 30-79 years reported urinary incontinence. (Choo et al., 2007) Pure stress incontinence only consisted about half of this population (22.8% overall), while the remainder reported mixed symptoms. Of note, patients with mixed symptoms reported a higher degree of impact on daily activities, social life and mental symptoms. More patients with mixed symptoms reported an insult on the overall quality of life (43.8%) compared to pure stress symptoms (28.3%). Furthermore, these patients reported a higher likelihood to seek medical attention for their problems (19.1% vs. 25.8%).

Other than semantic aspects of this question, patients may also significantly vary in their pathophysiology. This is more evident in the diverse presentation of these components pertaining to age or race. Nygaard and Lemke reported that stress incontinence occurs in a higher degree in older women (i.e., 40%). (Nygaard & Lemke, 1996) In studies of Scandinavian women, the rates of SUI peaked at approximately 60% in patients who were in their fifth decade (40–49 years). Urge incontinence began to increase in the sixth decade of their life and peaked at approximately 20% between 80 and 89 years. Racial differences have in fact been reported in a few studies. Bump identified mixed incontinence in up to 17% of African American subjects compared with only 11% of whites. (Bump, 1993) A larger proportion of white women, however, were found to have USI (61%) compared with African American women (27%).

3. Proposed mechanism of mixed urinary incontinence

There are several theories of DO in MUI. The most commonly proposed mechanism attributes MUI primarily to triggering of an involuntary bladder contraction. (Serels et al., 2000) Detrusor overactivity is, however, often not identified in many patients undergoing analysis for OAB wet symptoms. As previously noted, the underlying source of mixed incontinence may be detrusor overactivity associated with SUI which may represent a reflex stimulated by urine entering the proximal urethra during stress events. (Dmochowski & Staskin, 2005) This supposition has been shown to correlate with certain urodynamic factors including diminished urethral functional length in patients with urethral instability. Urethral instability instigates a bladder contraction response (detrusor overactivity), which is a normal physiological event. Webster et al. reported on a series of 73 patients with cystometrically diagnosed detrusor overactivity in combination with SUI. (Webster et al., 1984) A third of these patients had a period of electromyographic silence immediately preceding an unstable detrusor contraction. They concluded that the unstable contraction may have been induced by a urethral event and, therefore, was not a primary bladder abnormality.

There is a possibility that mixed symptoms may be due to a more severe form of stress component rather than two separate mechanisms for urge and stress incontinence(Bump et al., 2003); or that DO is caused by a weak urethral sphincter mechanism, resulting in funnelling of the proximal urethra. Major et al. identified that patients with detrusor overactivity had thinner urethral longitudinal smooth muscle layers and lower MUCP. (Major et al., 2002) McLennan et al. demonstrated that the functional urethral length was significantly shorter in patients with urethral instability. (McLennan et al., 2001) This shortened functional length may allow urine to enter the urethra, as there is less of a barrier, resulting in a weak urethral sphincter mechanism, which leads to funneling of the proximal urethra. When intra-abdominal pressure is increased, urine enters the proximal urethra, producing sensory stimulation and resulting in a reflex bladder contraction. (Fulford et al., 1999) This "urethrogenic" theory has also been supported by observations that patients with detrusor overactivity have significantly lower MUCP on urethral pressure profilometry, as well as lower angle of deflection measured by Q-tip cotton swab test. (Awad & McGinnis, 1983; Kim et al., 2010) The authors compared urodynamic characteristics, as well as physical examination findings in a retrospective study of 241 patients who were diagnosed with urinary incontinence. We found that patients with mixed incontinence showed lower Q-tip angle (28.6° vs. 42.1°) and lower MUCP (44.1cmH2O vs. 54.7cmH2O), in addition to higher symptom severity and lower bladder capacity. (Kim et al., 2010)

There are several possible explanations why UUI may improve after MUS surgery. One particular explanation is that MUS prevents urine from entering into the upper posterior urethra with increases in intra-abdominal pressure thereby avoiding reflex urgency. (Koonings et al., 1988; Minassian et al., 2008) Another possible explanation is that MUS may stabilize urethral overactivity, both statically and dynamically. (Kim et al., 2010) The current MUS are generally designed to be applied in a tension free manner at the urethra, theoretically providing a kinking axis, rather than a pressure aided coaptation of the urethra. Such mechanisms underscore the beneficial effects that MUS may provide to the urgency symptom per se, rather than an incidental improvement through relief of stress symptoms.

4. Outcome of midurethral sling in resolution of mixed urinary incontinence

The presenting symptoms of patients may be a guide to the approach to MUI. In those cases where either the stress or urge symptoms predominate, the most bothersome symptom should be approached first to potentially lessen the impact of the secondary symptom. Older surgical literature implies that patients with significant stress symptoms preoperatively, even if detrusor over activity is present, have a greater likelihood of success than those patients with a significant preoperative urge. The use of history (inclusive of symptomatic appraisal) associated with physical examination demonstrating (or not) stress incontinence may be very helpful in assessing the relative contributions of stress and urgency symptoms as well as the other potential insensate urinary loss that some patients experience.(Dmochowski & Staskin, 2005) Once the patient's initial response to the primary intervention is determined, further therapies can be recommended for persistent symptoms or for secondary symptoms, should those symptoms remain problematic. For instance, patients with mixed symptoms with a strong urge component and definable but less severe stress component could undergo therapy specially defined to ameliorate the urgency symptoms including anticholinergic use followed by neuromodulation (and/or botulinum toxin) and a secondary intervention for the bladder outlet, should persistent stress symptoms remain bothersome. Similarly, patients with predominant stress symptoms could undergo intervention for SUI with secondary interventions for UUI depending upon the results of the primary intervention and persistence of bothersome urinary symptoms. Therefore, the approach to MUI should be based on symptomatic segregation, with therapy promulgated on the basis of the most bothersome symptom and secondary interventions reserved for either persistence of the primary symptom or bother arising from the less prominent initial symptom. In those individuals with relatively equal bother, or who are unable to segregate their symptoms, the initial guideline to therapy may become apparent only after beginning more intensive evaluation (such as urodynamic studies). Alternatively, conservative or minimally invasive intervention may be initiated to establish response, followed by more intensive intervention for nonresponse. Ideally, patients should be informed about which symptoms may persist or become problematic post-intervention.

The role of surgery in the treatment of mixed incontinence had been historically considered highly controversial due to a high failure rate, from symptomatic or asymptomatic DO. (Stanton et al., 1978) More recently, several studies have concluded that an effective pubovaginal sling can cure stress incontinence and may also have benefit for urge symptoms. Langer et al. reported the results of a study of 30 women with mixed incontinence who underwent Burch colposuspension. (Langer, 1988) The proportion of patients with symptoms of DO decreased significantly from 73.3% before to 33.3%after surgery. In all, 50% of patients had marked improvement in clinical symptoms of DO. Normal cystometric findings were present postoperatively in 60% of patients, and only 40% had evidence of DO on postoperative urodynamic assessments. Ulmsten et al. evaluated the effect of TVT in 80 women suffering from MUI. (Ulmsten et al., 1996) They demonstrated that at a mean of 4 years, both SUI and UUI were cured in 85% of patients, significantly improved in 4%, and unchanged or worse in 11%. They concluded that TVT could be used to treat women patients with MUI. This study excluded patients with significant detrusor overactivity; therefore, the population was somewhat selected. Anger and Rodriguez reported that surgical intervention for patients with mixed incontinence resulted in incontinence resolution rates ranging from 20 to 70%. (Anger & Rodriguez, 2004) They concluded that those patients with predominant symptoms should have the primary symptoms initially managed. They further concluded that persistent symptomatology may not require secondary therapy and intervention for symptomatic persistence should be based on patient bother. In the study by Segal et al. (Segal et al., 2004), the improvement rate of the irritative subscales in the Urinary Distress Inventory for patients with MUI was 87.8%.

On the other hand, several studies have presented that these results were only transient. Several studies report good cure rates of stress component (85–97%) and lower (30–85%) and declining cure rates of urge incontinence over time following MUS in MUI. Holmgren et al. presented initial good cure rates of TVT, with up to 60% at 4 years, for MUI which did not persist after 4 years, decreasing to 30% cure rate from 4 to 8 years. (Holmgren et al., 2005) There seems to be no significant difference in the overall subjective and UUI cure between tapes used by retropubic (TVT) or transobturator routes. Colombo et al. (Colombo et al., 1996) assessed women who underwent Burch colposuspension. These investigators retrospectively compared findings from 44 women with mixed incontinence and matched controls with USI. At the 2-year follow-up point, the cure rate for stress incontinence was significantly lower in the group with mixed incontinence than in the group with stress incontinence alone (75% vs. 95%, P 0.02). One study reported that the overall cure rate was lower in women with MUI (55%) as compared with women with SUI only (81%) at 5-year follow-up after surgery. (Ankardal et al., 2006) They found type of incontinence was the only independent variable found to influence surgical outcome. In another study, when cure rate was defined as stress and urge indices of two or less (episode of incontinence one to four times a month or less), the observed subjective cure was 60% at 7 months and 53.8% at 38 months. But on the other hand, when cure was defined as complete dryness, the subjective cure rate dropped to 35.9% at 7 months and 28.4% after 38 months. (Kulseng Hanssen et al., 2007)

Another pitfall in the interpretation of these data is the discrepancy between subjective and objective determination of treatment success. Karram and Bhatia reported results in 52 women, 27 of whom underwent surgery (i.e., modified Burch colposuspension procedures). (Karram & Bhatia, 1989) Cure, defined as complete subjective relief of incontinence plus objective evidence of the disappearance of both stress incontinence and DO on repeat urodynamic testing, was achieved in 59% of the patients who underwent the surgery. Another 22% of surgically treated patients had improvement, defined as complete subjective relief of symptoms with objective evidence of the persistence of incontinence at the time of testing, or adequate relief of symptoms, such that the patient did not desire any further therapy. Of the 25 patients treated medically, 32% achieved cure and 28% were markedly improved. In another study that assessed TVT in women with either USI or mixed incontinence, the objective cure rate (89.3%) was similar for both types of incontinence, but the subjective cure rate was 66%, a significant difference (P 0.05), for objective versus subjective evaluations. (Jeffry et al., 2001) The lower subjective value was attributed to patients with de novo urge symptoms.

Appropriate case selection is of utmost importance in order to get good results after surgery. Cure rate of MUI is better in a group of women with predominant SUI symptoms in comparison to a group with predominant UUI symptoms. (Kulseng Hanssen et al., 2007) The effect of detrusor overactivity on urodyamics associated with MUI on outcomes is not as clear as the majority of studies did not include urodynamically proven MUI. MUI implies a component of detrusor dysfunction that may be motor or sensory and is associated with superimposed urethral sphincteric underactivity. Rates of incontinence improvement in pharmacologic studies are approximately 70% although a substantive percentage of these patients are improved, not cured. Potential pharmacologic approaches to the treatment of mixed incontinence include antimuscarinic agents, estrogen replacement therapy (for postmenopausal women), and dopamine, serotonin, and norepinephrine reuptake inhibitors. (Khullar et al., 2010) Electrical stimulation is another conservative measure that could potentially be used for the treatment of MUI. (Sand, 1996) Surgery should be considered after failed medical management, proper work up, and careful counselling about the lower overall success rates of around 55%.

5. Preoperative risk factors for mixed urinary incontinence

Though various factors have been described in the literature to predict the persistence of urge components following incontinence procedures, no single predictor has presented consistent value between studies. Earlier studies, investigating Burch colposuspension, suggested precedence in patient symptom history were indicative of symptom predominance within a mixed profile of incontinence, and consequently better outcomes for patients with precedent stress symtoms. Scotti et al. investigated 82 women who underwent Burch colposuspension. (Scotti et al., 1998) They found that patients with a history of stress symptoms preceding the onset of urge symptoms showed higher cure rates compared to antecedent urge patients (78.6% vs 22.2%, $p<0.001$). Langer et al. also showed similar results, also with Burch colposuspension. However, these results have not been reproduced in recent MUS procedures. (Langer, 1988)

Urodynamic studies would appear to have predictive benefit for some patients with mixed symptoms in elucidating the gravity of urethral dysfunction (stress component) and any associated detrusor dysfunction. (Lin et al., 2004) Certain aspects of detrusor dysfunction, such as high-pressure detrusor overactivity, have been suggested to be indicative of outcome, though investigators varied in their use of its reference value. The authors retrospectively reviewed 279 patients with MUI who underwent MUS with at least 2 years of follow up. (Kim et al., 2008) Patients were divided into patient with a predominance of bother symptoms and a predominance of DO, where DO patients were further divided into patients with high pressure DO and low pressure DO with a reference level of $15cmH_2O$ of maximum detrusor pressure at which involuntary contraction occurs during filling cystometry. We found that patients with high pressure DO showed improvement of urge symptoms in 70% compared to 91.4% for patient with low pressure DO ($p=0.03$). These factors also seemed to affect resolution of stress components as patients with high pressure DO showed lower resolution rates than low pressure DO patients (90% vs. 96.6%, $p=0.04$). In a retrospective study of 51 patients, Panayi et al. found that higher opening detrusor pressure, lower volume at DO during cystometry and higher detrusor pressure were predictive of persistent DO. (Panayi et al., 2009) Schrepferman et al. evaluated 84 women undergoing a pubovaginal sling surgery for MUI. (Schrepferman et al., 2000) Of those patients, 69 had urgency symptoms. Urgency was related to defined motor urge (as established on urodynamic testing) in 41 women. Twenty-eight patients experienced sensory urgency (urge symptoms with/ without urodynamic findings). Complete resolution or improvement in urge symptoms occurred in 24 (58.5%) patients with urodynamically demonstrated motor urge incontinence, and an additional 7 (17.1%) patients were improved. In those patients with sensory urgency, only 11 (39.3%) patients were cured, and 9 (32.1%) patients were improved. Additionally, in those patients with urodynamic motor urge overactivity, 21 of 23 (91.3%) patients were cured, and 2 (8.7%) patients were improved if low pressure overactivity was present. High-pressure instability was associated with a cure in only 5 (27.8%) patients, and improvement in another 5 (27.8%) patients. The investigators used 15 cm of water as a cutoff for low-pressure versus high-pressure motor overactivity of the bladder. They suggested that patients with low-pressure motor urgency are more likely to experience resolution than those with high-pressure. Despite the fact that the International Continence Society no longer utilizes motor versus sensory urgency, the application of this trial is limited; however, these findings are interesting and provocative for potential subsequent clinical trials. Finally, on the basis of the symptoms present, Scotti et al. reported that high-pressure detrusor overactivity presented commonly with stress symptoms is a significantly poor prognostic indicator with pressures of 25cmH_2O or greater being consistent with poor surgical results. (Scotti et al., 1998)

Recently, Paick et al. evaluated factors that might predict persistency of urge incontinence in patients after undergoing tension-free vaginal tape (TVT) procedures. (Paick et al., 2007) They evaluated 274 patients of which 73 had mixed urinary symptoms. They found cure rates for stress incontinence to be different (78.1% for the mixed symptom group versus 95.5% for the pure group). Their analysis revealed that maximal urethral pressure was associated with a greater risk of persistent urge symptoms, suggesting that profound urethral dysfunction may be contributory to persistent symptoms after TVT. These findings are again intriguing and suggest the possibility that urethral dysfunction and resultant effects upon the severity of SUI may affect detrusor function. This paper gives further support to the fact that correction of the low-pressure outlet may benefit at least some individuals with detrusor overactivity although the overall benefit may be less than that experienced by patients with only SUI.

Other studies have failed to find significant predictive value for successful treatment of MUI in urodynamic studies. Houwert et al. retrospectively reviewed 437 patients who received MUS, in which the diagnosis of MUI itself was also used as a factor in analysis. (Houwert et al., 2009) Results showed that a diagnosis of MUI, a history of previous incontinence surgery and the presence of detrusor overactivity was predictive, while urodynamic parameters failed to suggest insight to outcomes in multivariate analyses. However, relative symptom components are most frequently reported as predominant and nonpredominant (assuming a rough estimate of percentage contribution). As noted previously, this method can be inaccurate and begs the need for better methods of symptom quantification. Given the confusing terminology for both patients and surgeons of what constitutes MUI, as well as the higher failure rate of surgical outcomes, treatment should be individualized based on clinical scenario along with urodynamic findings.

6. Conclusion

Recent advances in surgical treatment for stress urinary incontinence have provided effective resolution with limited morbidity. However, preoperative components of urgency complicate the treatment outcomes in a significant number of patients. Detrusor overactivity and urgency symptoms represent a separate and distinct pathophysiology, of which the possible occurrence or persistence must be addressed before management of stress incontinence symptoms. Several studies have suggested high pressure detrusor overactivity or maximal urethral pressure during preoperative urodynamic studies may implicate a higher rate of treatment failure in mixed urinary incontinence. Other studies have suggested insights into the predominance or antecedence in urgency symptoms may be indicative of treatment difficulty. Currently, no definite conclusions have been reached. Future studies require a cohesive approach in determining risks and treatment methods, while clinically, patients should be warned of risks and possibility of continued medical treatment associated with mixed symptoms.

7. References

Anger, J. T. & Rodriguez, L. V. (2004). Mixed incontinence: stressing about urge. *Current Urology Reports*, Vol. 5, No.6, pp. (427-431), ISSN 1527-2737

Ankardal, M., Heiwall, B., Lausten Thomsen, N., Carnelid, J. & Milsom, I. (2006). Short and long term results of the tension free vaginal tape procedure in the treatment of female urinary incontinence. *Acta Obstetricia et Gynecologica Scandinavica*, Vol. 85, No.8, pp. (986-992), ISSN 1600-0412

Awad, S. A. & McGinnis, R. H. (1983) Factors that influence the incidence of detrusor instability in women. *The Journal of Urology*, Vol. 130, No.1, pp. (114-115), ISSN 0022-5347

Bump, R. (1993). Racial comparisons and contrasts in urinary incontinence and pelvic organ prolapse. *Obstetrics and Gynecology*, Vol. 81, No.3, pp. (421-425), ISSN 0029-7844

Bump, R., Norton, P., Zinner, N. & Yalcin, I. (2003). Duloxetine Urinary Incontinence Study Group. Mixed urinary incontinence symptoms: urodynamic findings, incontinence severity, and treatment response. *Obstetrics and Gynecology*, Vol. 102, No.1, pp. (76-83), ISSN

Chaliha, C. & Khullar, V. (2004). Mixed incontinence. *Urology*, Vol. 63, No.3, pp. (51-57), ISSN 0090-4295

Choo, M. S., Ku, J. H., Oh, S. J, Lee, K. S., Paick, J. S., Seo, J. T., Kim, D. Y., Lee, J. J., Lee, J.G., Na, Y. G., Kwon, D. D. & Park, W. H. (2007). Prevalence of urinary incontinence in Korean women: an epidemiologic survey. *International Urogynecologic Journal of Pelvic Floor Dysfunction*, Vol. 18, No. 18, pp. (1309-1315), ISSN 0937-3462

Chou, E. C. L., Blaivas, J. G., Chou, L. W., Flisser, A. J. & Panagopoulos, G. (2008). Urodynamic characteristics of mixed urinary incontinence and idiopathic urge urinary incontinence. *Neurourology and Urodynamics*, Vol. 27, No.5, pp. (376-378), ISSN 1520-6777

Colombo, M., Zanetta, G., Vitobello, D. & Milani, R. (1996). The Burch colposuspension for women with and without detrusor overactivity. *BJOG: An International Journal of Obstetrics & Gynaecology*, Vol. 103, No.3, pp. (255-260), ISSN 1471-0528

Digesu, G. A., Salvatore, S., Fernando, R. & Khullar, V. (2008). Mixed urinary symptoms: What are the urodynamic findings? *Neurourology and Urodynamics*, Vol. 27, No.5, pp. (372-375), ISSN 1520-6777

Diokno, A., Brock, B., Brown, M. & Herzog, A. (1986). Prevalence of urinary incontinence and other urological symptoms in the noninstitutionalized elderly. *The Journal of Urology*, Vol. 136, No.5, pp. (1022-1025), ISSN 0022-5347

Dmochowski, R. & Staskin, D. (2005). Mixed incontinence: definitions, outcomes, and interventions. *Current Opinion in Urology*, Vol. 15, No.6, pp. (374-379), ISSN 0963-0643

Dooley, Y., Lowenstein, L., Kenton, K., FitzGerald, M. P. & Brubaker, L. (2008). Mixed incontinence is more bothersome than pure incontinence subtypes. *International Urogynecology Journal*, Vol. 19, No.10, pp. (1359-1362), ISSN 0937-3462

Fulford, S., Flynn, R., Barrington, J., Appanna, T. & Stephenson, T. (1999). An assessment of the surgical outcome and urodynamic effects of the pubovaginal sling for stress incontinence and the associated urge syndrome. *The Journal of Urology*, Vol. 162, No.1, pp. (135-137), ISSN 0022-5347

Haylen, B. T., De Ridder, D., Freeman, R. M., Swift, S. E., Berghmans, B., Lee, J., Monga, A., Petri, E., Rizk, D. E. & Sand, P. K. (2010). An International Urogynecological Association (IUGA)/International Continence Society (ICS) joint report on the terminology for female pelvic floor dysfunction. *International Urogynecology Journal*, Vol. 21, No.1, pp. (5-26), ISSN 0937-3462

Holmgren, C., Nilsson, S., Lanner, L. & Hellberg, D. (2005). Long-term results with tension-free vaginal tape on mixed and stress urinary incontinence. *Obstetrics and Gynecology*, Vol. 106, No.1, pp. (38-43), ISSN 0029-7844

Houwert, R. M., Venema, P. L., Aquarius, A. E., Bruinse, H. W., Kil, P. J. M. & Vervest, H. A. M. (2009). Predictive value of urodynamics on outcome after midurethral sling surgery for female stress urinary incontinence. *American Journal of Obstetrics and Gynecology*, Vol. 200, No.6, pp. (649. e641-649. e612), ISSN 0002-9378

Jeffry, L., Deval, B., Birsan, A., Soriano, D. & Dara , E. (2001). Objective and subjective cure rates after tension-free vaginal tape for treatment of urinary incontinence. *Urology*, Vol. 58, No.5, pp. (702-706), ISSN 0090-4295

Karram, M. M. & Bhatia, N. N. (1989). Management of coexistent stress and urge urinary incontinence. *Obstetrics and Gynecology*, Vol. 73, No.1, pp. (4-7), ISSN 0029-7844

Khullar, V., Cardozo, L. & Dmochowski, R. (2010). Mixed incontinence: Current evidence and future perspectives. *Neurourology and Urodynamics*, Vol. 29, No.4, pp. (618-622), ISSN 1520-6777

Kim, H. M., Oh, M. M., Lee, J. G. (2010). Does the incidence of urgency symptoms increase along with the severity of stress urinary incontinence? *Korean Journal of Urology*, Vol. 51, No. 11, pp. (772-776), ISSN 2005-6737

Kim, J. J., Bae, J. H. & Lee, J. G. (2008). Preoperative factors predicting the outcome of a midurethal sling operation for treating women with mixed incontinence. *Korean Journal of Urology*, Vol. 49, No.12, pp. (1112-1118), ISSN 0494-4747

Koonings, P., Bergman, A. & Ballard, C. (1988). Combined detrusor instability and stress urinary incontinence: where is the primary pathology? *Gynecologic and Obstetric Investigation*, Vol. 26, No.3, pp. (250-256), ISSN 0378-7346

Kulseng Hanssen, S., Husby, H. & Schiotz, H. A. (2007). The tension free vaginal tape operation for women with mixed incontinence: Do preoperative variables predict the outcome? *Neurourology and Urodynamics*, Vol. 26, No.1, pp. (115-121), ISSN 1520-6777

Langer, R. (1988). Colposuspension in patients with combined stress incontinence and detrusor instability. *European Urology*, Vol. 14, No.6, pp. (437), ISSN 0302-2838

Lemack, G. E. & Zimmern, P. E. (1999). Predictability of urodynamic findings based on the Urogenital Distress Inventory-6 questionnaire. *Urology*, Vol. 54, No.3, pp. (461-466), ISSN 0090-4295

Lin, L. Y., Yeh, N. H., Lin, C. Y., Sheu, B. C. & Lin, H. H. (2004). Comparisons of urodynamic characteristics between female patients with overactive bladder and overactive bladder plus stress urinary incontinence. *Urology*, Vol. 64, No.5, pp. (945-949), ISSN 0090-4295

Major, H., Culligan, P. & Heit, M. (2002). Urethral sphincter morphology in women with detrusor instability. *Obstetrics & Gynecology*, Vol. 99, No.1, pp. (63), ISSN 0029-7844

McLennan, M. T., Melick, C. & Bent, A. E. (2001). Urethral instability: Clinical and urodynamic characteristics*. *Neurourology and Urodynamics*, Vol. 20, No.6, pp. (653-660), ISSN 1520-6777

Minassian, V. A., Stewart, W. F. & Hirsch, A. G. (2008). Why do stress and urge incontinence co-occur much more often than expected? *International Urogynecology Journal*, Vol. 19, No.10, pp. (1429-1440), ISSN 0937-3462

Nygaard, I. E. & Lemke, J. H. (1996). Urinary incontinence in rural older women: prevalence, incidence and remission. *Journal of the American Geriatrics Society*, Vol. 44, No.9, pp. (1049-1054), ISSN 0002-8614

Paick, J. S., Cho, M. C., Oh, S. J., Kim, S. W. & Ku, J. H. (2007). Factors influencing the outcome of mid urethral sling procedures for female urinary incontinence. *The Journal of Urology*, Vol. 178, No.3, pp. (985-989), ISSN 0022-5347

Panayi, D. C., Duckett, J., Digesu, G. A., Camarata, M., Basu, M. & Khullar, V. (2009). Pre-operative opening detrusor pressure is predictive of detrusor overactivity following TVT in patients with pre-operative mixed urinary incontinence. *Neurourology and Urodynamics*, Vol. 28, No.1, pp. (82-85), ISSN 1520-6777

Sand, P. K. (1996). Pelvic floor stimulation in the treatment of mixed incontinence complicated by a low-pressure urethra. *Obstetrics and Gynecology*, Vol. 88, No.5, pp. (757-760), ISSN 0029-7844

Schrepferman, C. G., Griebling, T. L., Nygaard, I. E. & Kreder, K. J. (2000). Resolution of urge symptoms following sling cystourethropexy. *The Journal of Urology*, Vol. 164, No.5, pp. (1628-1631), ISSN 0022-5347

Scotti, R. J., Angell, G., Flora, R. & Greston, W. M. (1998). Antecedent history as a predictor of surgical cure of urgency symptoms in mixed incontinence. *Obstetrics and Gynecology*, Vol. 91, No.1, pp. (30-34), ISSN 0029-7844

Segal, J. L., Vassallo, B., Kleeman, S., Silva, W. A. & Karram, M. M. (2004). Prevalence of persistent and de novo overactive bladder symptoms after the tension-free vaginal tape. *Obstetrics & Gynecology*, Vol. 104, No.6, pp. (1263-1269), ISSN 0029-7844

Serels, S. R., Rackley, R. R. & Appell, R. A. (2000). Surgical treatment for stress urinary incontinence associated with Valsalva induced detrusor instability. *The Journal of Urology*, Vol. 163, No.3, pp. (884-887), ISSN 0022-5347

Stanton, S. L., Cardozo, L., Williams, J. E., Ritchie, D. & Allan, V. (1978). Clinical and urodynamic features of failed incontinence surgery in the female. *Obstetrics and Gynecology*, Vol. 51, No.5, pp. (515), ISSN 0029-7844

Stewart, W., Van Rooyen, J., Cundiff, G., Abrams, P., Herzog, A., Corey, R., Hunt, T. & Wein, A. (2003). Prevalence and burden of overactive bladder in the United States. *World Journal of Urology*, Vol. 20, No.6, pp. (327-336), ISSN 0724-4983

Ulmsten, U., Henriksson, L., Johnson, P. & Varhos, G. (1996). An ambulatory surgical procedure under local anesthesia for treatment of female urinary incontinence. *International Urogynecology Journal*, Vol. 7, No.2, pp. (81-86), ISSN 0937-3462

Webster, G. D., Sihelnik, S. A. & Stone, A. R. (1984). Female urinary incontinence: The incidence, identification, and characteristics of detrusor instabiiity. *Neurourology and Urodynamics*, Vol. 3, No.4, pp. (235-242), ISSN 1520-6777

13

Suburethral Slingplasty Using a Self-Fashioned Mesh for Treating Urinary Incontinence and Anterior Vaginal Wall Prolapse

Chi-Feng Su, Soo-Cheen Ng, Horng-Jyh Tsai and Gin-Den Chen
Kuang Tien General Hospital, Chung Shan Medical University/Hospital, Department of Obstetrics and Gynecology
Taiwan

1. Introduction

The pelvic floor is a highly complex structure and plays a dual role in supporting the pelvic viscera (bladder, bowel, and uterus) and maintaining the functional integrity of these organs. Pelvic organ support is maintained by complex interactions between the levator ani muscles of the pelvic floor and connective tissues along with the urethra, vaginal wall, rectum, and normal innervation (Boreham et al., 2002; Wei and DeLancey, 2004). The pelvic floor and pelvic cavity is an integral structure and can be functionally divided into three compartments. Each compartment is not discrete and is comprised of different pelvic organs. The anterior compartment contains the urethra and bladder, the middle compartment holds the vagina and uterus, and the posterior compartment consists of the anus and rectum.

Conventionally, the pathophysiology of stress urinary incontinence at the bladder neck is caused by proximal urethral hypermobility and/or intrinsic sphincter deficiency (Schick et al., 2004). The urethra and bladder lie on the supportive or suspension layers which are composed of the pubourethral ligament, endopelvic fascia, pubucoccygeal muscle, and the anterior vaginal wall. The breakdown of these layers can attenuate the urethra and/or cause asymptomatic or symptomatic anterior vaginal wall prolapse.

2. Pelvic organ prolapse and stress urinary incontinence share similar risk factors

It has been noted that better pelvic-floor muscle function is associated with less severe prolapse and urinary symptoms. Poor pelvic floor muscle function is one of the inciting or contributory factors in the development of prolapse (Borello-France et al., 2007). Consistent tension from increased intra-abdominal pressure, loss of muscular support for pelvic organs, wideness of genital hiatus, and stretched or torn connective tissue might lead to prolapse (Wei and DeLancey, 2004). Furthermore, intermittent mechanical forces imposed on the prolapsed vaginal tissues or denervation of the vaginal tissues during vaginal delivery might cause decreased content of differentiated smooth muscle in the vaginal wall of women with pelvic organ prolapse. The pathogenesis of pelvic organ prolapse is not completely understood. The development of pelvic organ prolapse may be multi-factorial. Vaginal childbirth, advancing age, and increasing body mass index are the most consistent risk factors of pelvic organ prolapse (Jelovsek et al., 2007). Other factors such as prolonged second stage of labor, constipation, chronic cough previous to pelvic surgery, and increased intra-abdominal pressure caused by heavy lifting have also been reported in association with the occurrence of stress urinary incontinence and pelvic organ prolapse (Dietz, 2008). The weakness in the supportive layer of the urethra and a lax anterior vaginal wall which results in stress urinary incontinence and/or pelvic organ prolapse seems to be caused by a "multiple-hit" mechanism.

3. Prevalence of pelvic organ prolapse associated stress urinary incontinence

The exact prevalence of pelvic organ prolapse is difficult to estimate due to patient misunderstandings and misconceptions in presenting these issues to their health care providers. Most of the estimated prevalence rates for pelvic organ prolapse are derived from the incidence of surgery for this disease or from clinic-based samples (Lawreence et al., 2008). Pelvic organ prolapse has been estimated to affect about 50% of parous women aged 50 years or over whereas stress urinary incontinence occurs in 30%. These prevalence rates increase with age (Subak et al., 2001; Abou-Elela et al., 2009; Maher et al., 2010). Pelvic organ prolapse and stress urinary incontinence coexist in 15 to 80 percent of women (Bai et al., 2002). Experts estimate that up to 50% of women with pelvic organ prolapse with the uterus in situ do not have stress urinary incontinence (Gallentine and Cespedes, 2001).

This continence mechanism in advanced pelvic organ prolapse might be caused by urethral kinking or external urethral compression, which causes obstruction that can stop the demonstration of stress urinary incontinence (Romanzi et al. 2000; Elneil, 2009). However, during surgery to reduce the prolapsed uterus or anterior vaginal wall it may be noted from the urodynamic study that 36 to 80% of the women with pelvic organ prolapse have coexisting urodynamic stress incontinence. These patients have occult stress urinary incontinence (Haessler et al., 2005; Reena et al., 2007). In addition, postoperative stress urinary incontinence (de novo stress urinary incontinence) has been noted in 10 to 30% of women following prolapse repair (Bump et al., 1996; Hung et al., 2004; Reena et al., 2007). Other reports estimate that 11 to 65% of continent patients with pelvic organ prolapse develop de novo stress urinary incontinence following pelvic reconstructive procedures performed during prophylactic anti-incontinence surgery (Borstad E and Rud T, 1989; Ellerkmann et al., 2001; Gutman et al., 2008).

4. The evolution and trends in anti-incontinence treatments

More than 100 types of anti-incontinence procedures have been invented for treating urinary incontinence in the past century. The choice of surgical method and route for treating urinary incontinence is done according to the type of incontinence, the patient's condition, the surgeon's preferences, and available materials (Wu et al., 2008). Based on the evidence of treatment outcomes, trends in anti-incontinence procedures range from the vaginal route (Kelly plication, anterior repair…), cystoscopy and needle procedures (Stamey, Pereyra,

Raz...), bladder neck suspension and/or colposuspension to the conventional pubovaginal sling. Retropubic Burch colposuspension was considered the gold standard and the most popular anti-incontinence operation by 1995 (Jarvis, 1994). In recent decades, newer tension-free, patch and prosthetic tapes with minimal invasive procedures have been used such as the tension-free vaginal tape (TVT) procedure which is based on the integral theory and was introduced by Petros and Ulmsten (1993). The treatment outcomes seem promising (Wu et al., 2008). The use of macroporous monofilament mesh has become a popular treatment in anti-incontinence surgery. However, long-term complications of these synthetic materials still need to be solved.

The goals of these procedures for achieving continence have shifted from suburethral fascia plication (Kelly procedure), lifting the urethra up to a higher retropubic position (MMK), elevating the bladder neck to enhance pressure transmission ratio (colposuspension), to stabilizing the bladder neck or proximal urethra to increase urethral closure pressure (sling operation). Now, the popular minimal invasive procedures, based on the integral theory (Petros and Ulmsten 1993), are trying to create a dynamic kinking of the mid-urethra at the level of the high pressure zone in the urethral pressure profile or in the urethral knee angle (terminology used in sonographic findings) (Wu et al., 2008; Lo et al., 2004).

5. The evolution of pelvic reconstruction surgeries

The surgical treatment for pelvic organ prolapse can be categorized into obliterative and reconstructive procedures. Reconstructive surgery for treating prolapse aims to correct the prolapsed vagina, preserve (or improve) vaginal sexual function and relieve the associated pelvic symptoms. Reconstructive surgery can be performed by either the transabdominal or vaginal route. Currently, several common approaches for correcting apex or uterovaginal prolapse include abdominal sacral colpopexy, abdominal sacral cervicopexy, McCall culdoplasty, high uterosacral ligament suspension, and vaginal sacrospinous ligament suspension. Anterior and posterior colporrhaphy in combination with central plication of the fibromuscular layer of the vaginal wall are still popular techniques for correcting anterior and posterior vaginal wall prolapse (Jelovsek et al., 2007; Gomelsky et al., 2011). Paravaginal defect repair, a side-specific repair of the vaginal wall to make a reproximation of vaginal tissue that has been torn from its lateral attachment to the arcus tendineous fascia pelvis or arcus tendineous levator ani, has also been advocated by some physicians for treating anterior vaginal wall prolapse (Mallipeddi PK et al., 2001; Young et al. 2001).

In the past two decades, the efficacy of anterior colporrhaphy, associated with central plication of the pubourethral ligament or fibromuscular layers of the vaginal wall for treating urinary incontinence or anterior vaginal wall prolapse, has been controversial. Beck et al. reported the cure rate for treating 194 patients increased from 75 to 94% when a Kelly-Kennedy technique was modified to include a vaginal retropubic urethropexy (Beck et al., 1991). Jarvis's review revealed a cure rate of around 60% using anterior colporrhaphy for stress urinary incontinence (Jarvis., 1994). It has been reported that only 30 to 46% of patients experience satisfactory or optimal anatomic results with standard anterior or ultralateral anterior colporrhaphy for the treatment of anterior vaginal wall prolapse (Weber et al., 2001). However, for this group the clinically relevant definitions of success were defined as (1) no prolapse beyond the hymen, (2) the absence of prolapse symptoms (visual analog scale $\leqq 2$), and (3) the absence of re-treatment. There was a higher success rate for treating anterior vaginal wall prolapse with anterior colporrhaphy (Chmielewski et al., 2011). In the past, the discrepancy in success rates of anterior colporrhaphy for the treatment of anterior vaginal wall prolapse can be attributed to varying definitions of success. As we know, a higher success rate is associated with a higher complication rate for the treatment of pelvic organ prolapse. Physicians should base the definition of success on patient perceptions and satisfaction according to clinically relevant definitions of success rather than on physicians' perceptions of success.

The use of mesh has also become common practice in pelvic reconstructive procedures in recent decades. An increasing number of commercial kits have been designed for site-specific defect repair or total mesh-augmented vaginal repairs to reinforce the supportive function of the vagina. Recent literature demonstrates that graft-augmented repairs seem to have a high success rate and conventional standard repairs (no mesh augmentation) have relatively high recurrence rates. However, potentially high success rates resulting from use of mesh products are accompanied by a high complication rate. Complications or side-effects associated with vaginal mesh include mesh erosion or extrusion, infection, pain, and dyspareunia (Baessler et al. 2006; Maher and Baessler 2006; Natale et al., 2006; Wu MP, 2008; Jelovsek et al. 2007; Gomelsky et al., 2011). Therefore, researchers from the Third International Consultation on Incontinence concluded that because of mesh's high potential morbidity, mesh placed transvaginally should only be used in well-designed clinical trials and not in general practice until more data is available (Brubaker et al. 2005).

6. Staged or concomitant procedures for treating pelvic organ prolapse and stress urinary incontinence

Currently, choosing either a concomitant or stepwise approach to treat concurrent pelvic organ prolapse and stress urinary incontinence is still debatable. A proper balance between the risk of incomplete treatment and exposing a patient to an unnecessary operation requires consideration when explaining the treatment outcomes to the patient. Some surgeons recommend concomitant procedures to treat co-existing stress urinary incontinence and pelvic organ prolapse in order to avoid the possibility of secondary surgery. However, they may encounter some inherent risks and unexpected adverse effects such as postoperative voiding difficulty, bladder outlet obstruction, and/or de novo detrusor overactivity. Others prefer staged procedures to correct pelvic organ prolapse first, followed by re-evaluation for the presence of stress urinary incontinence after the wound has healed and stabilized (Gordon et al., 2001; Huang et al., 2005; Winters JC, 2008; Wu et al., 2010). As mentioned before, anterior colporrhaphy might also cure stress urinary incontinence and its success rate is as high as 60% (Jarvis 1994). Intuitively, staged procedures most likely prevent two-thirds of unnecessary procedures for incontinence when contrasted with concomitant operations.

7. Rationale for suburethral slingplasty

The Cochrane Database of Systematic Reviews revealed that the use of mesh or graft inlays at the time of anterior vaginal wall repair may reduce the risk of recurrent anterior vaginal wall prolapse (Maher et al. 2010). The high failure rates of pelvic reconstructive procedures for anterior compartment prolapse might be a result of a decrease in the muscularis of the prolapsed vaginal tissues which impair vaginal tone and contractility (Boreham et al., 2002). Alterations in collagen, elastin, and proteoglycan proteins of the extracellular matrix within the pelvic-support ligaments and vaginal tissue might also contribute to or be associated with causes of pelvic organ prolapse or recurrence (Connell KA., 2011).

In order to reduce the high failure rate of anterior vaginal wall repair, we developed a tension free vaginal tape, using self-fashioned Gynemesh, for treating urodynamic stress incontinence and anterior vaginal wall prolapse, concomitantly. The rationale behind our suburethral slingplasty is using tension-free mesh for augmenting and enforcing the supporting layer of the urethra and bladder to treat stress urinary incontinence and anterior vaginal wall prolapse concomitantly. This procedure has provided a relatively high success rate in curing urinary incontinence (continence was 80%, improvement was 17%) and reduced the rate of recurrence of anterior vaginal wall prolapse (none with recurrent prolapse greater than stage II). As well, there was a more acceptable rate of mesh erosion (6%) when combined with other pelvic reconstructive procedures.

8. Surgical technique

The basis of the current procedure is to place a tension-free and customized mesh underneath the proximal urethra and bladder to act as a supporting suburethral hammock to reinforce the anterior vaginal wall while undergoing pelvic reconstructive operations. The self-fashioned mesh may augment the supporting and suspension effects against an increase in mechanical forces of daily activities and gravity. Concurrently, the mesh patch may also act as a frame for inducing fibroblasts in fibrogenesis during healing (Hung et al. 2010).

8.1 Preparation of self-fashioned mesh

The self-fashioned mesh is a polypropylene mesh from Gynemesh PS (10 cm in width and 15 cm in length; 300 USD a piece; Gynecare, Ethicon inc., Somerville, NJ, USA)(Su et al. 2009). The mesh is trimmed in the shape of a body with a pair of arms (shown in Figure 1)

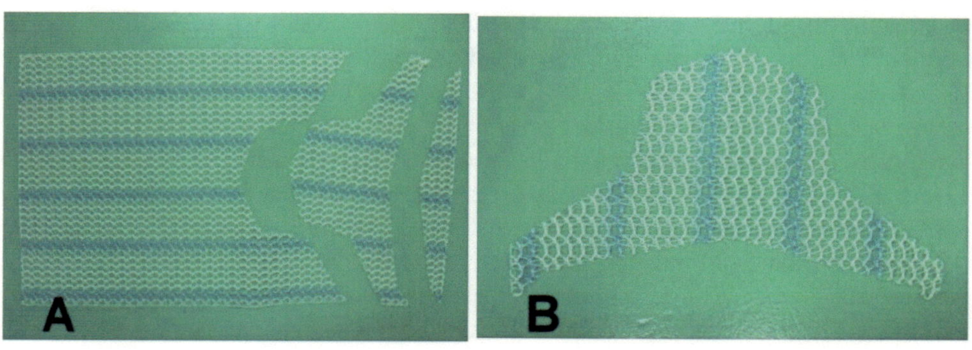

Fig. 1. The mesh is trimmed in the shape of a body with a pair of arms (B) from a Gynemesh PS (A)

and the size of the mesh is tailored to fit the patient. The length of the mesh can be adjusted according to the length of the patient's anterior vaginal wall since the end of the mesh is anchored to the vaginal apex or pubocervical fascia. The bilateral ends of the mesh are sewn using an absorbable 1-0 Vicryl suture (Ethicon inc., Somerville, NJ, USA) using a Stamey needle for the following procedures (Figure 2).

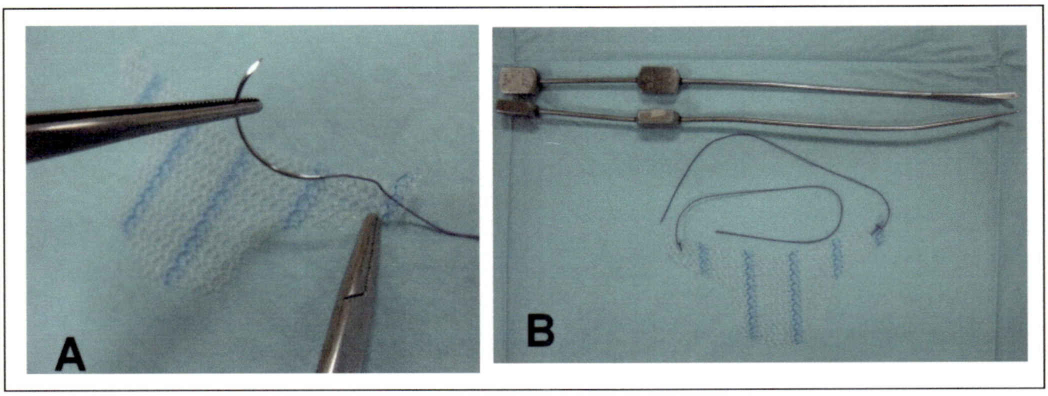

Fig. 2. The bilateral ends of the mesh are sewn using an absorbable 1-0 Vicryl suture (A). Prepared self-fashioned mesh and Stamey needles (B)

8.2 Procedures for placement of the self-fashioned mesh

The bladder neck is identified by gently pulling the Foley catheter. The anterior vaginal wall is incised in the midline from the proximal urethra to the apex of the vaginal cuff or cervix (for patients whose uterus is preserved). At the level of the proximal urethra, a tunnel underneath the pubourethral ligament is created on each side of the urethra to reach the insertion of the ligament. The vaginal mucosa layer is undermined from the fibromuscular layer of the anterior vaginal wall on each side to reach the lateral point of insertion into the paravaginal fascia. The retropubic space (Retzius space) is not entered during the dissection of the paravaginal fascia.

A Stamey needle is introduced through the suprapubic incision (less than 5 mm each side), passed blindly through the retropubic space along the posterior surface of the pubic bone (retropubis; avoiding resistance from bones and the bladder wall) (Figure 3), until the needle tip is advanced to the ventral aspect of the pubourethral ligament. The needle tip is advanced laterally along the posterior aspect of the pubis into the tip of the tunnel that was created before and passed through this fibromuscular layer (Figure 4). The 1-0 Vicryl suture is threaded through the needle hole at a certain length. The Stamey needle is withdrawn back from the suprapubic incision until the 1-0 Vicryl suture is present (Figure 5). The 1-0 Vicryl suture is pulled out through the suprapubic incision until the end of the mesh arm passes into the retropubic space (surgeon feels loss of strongest resistance while the 1-0 Vicryl suture is being pulled). The end of the mesh arm is anchored into the ventral aspect of the paravaginal fascia (paraurethral portion, near the original portion of the arcus tendineous fascia pelvis and arcus tendineous levator ani). These procedures are repeated on the other side.

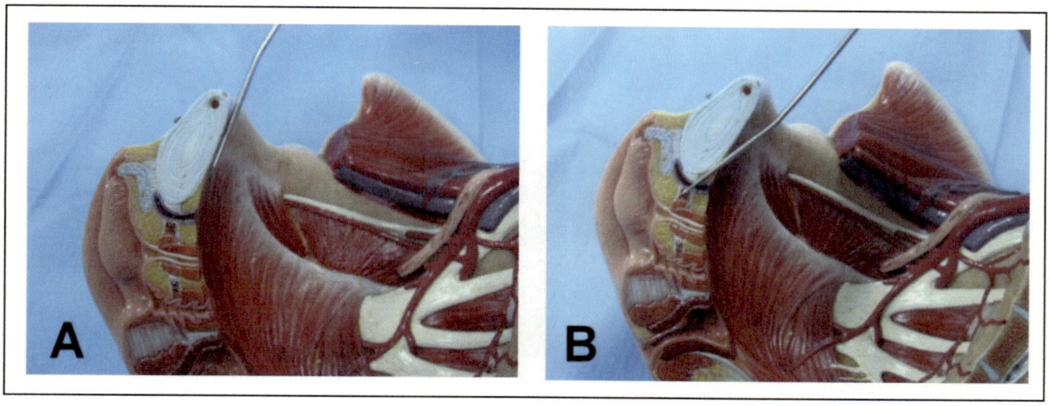

Fig. 3. Stamey needle is introduced through the suprapubic space.

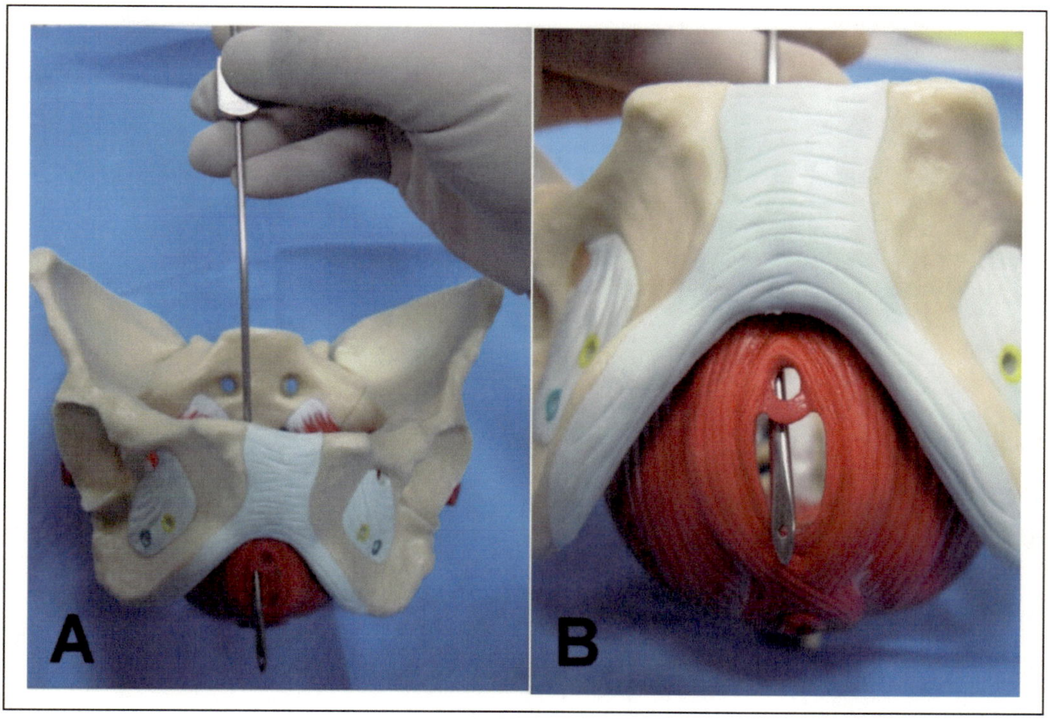

Fig. 4. The Stamey needle tip is advanced laterally into the retropubic tunnel that was created before and passed through this fibromuscular layer.

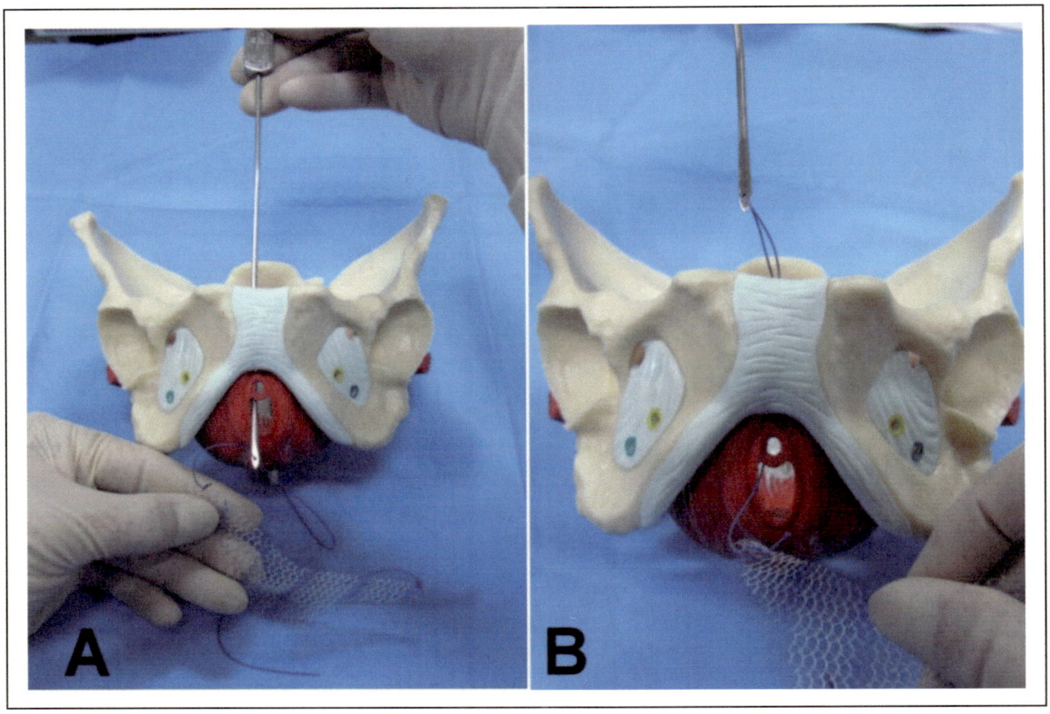

Fig. 5. The Stamey needle is withdrawn back from the suprapubic incision until the 1-0 Vicryl suture is present.

The mesh arms are adjusted by pulling the 1-0 Vicryl suture through the suprapubic incision until the mesh is placed underneath the dorsal aspect of the pubourethral ligament, proximal urethra, and bladder neck without tension and mesh unfolds. Surgeons have the option, according to their preference, of performing plication of the fibromuscular layer of the bladder before placing the mesh underneath the bladder and dorsal aspect of the paravaginal fascia. The mesh is also flattened without tension so that the bilateral edges of the mesh reach the lateral sulci of the vagina (Figure 6). The Smead-Jones suturing method is used to close the suburethral mucosa and anterior vaginal mucosa to create a mass cushion on the suburethral mucosa and anterior vaginal wall. Concomitant pelvic reconstructive procedures are performed after closing the anterior vaginal wall.

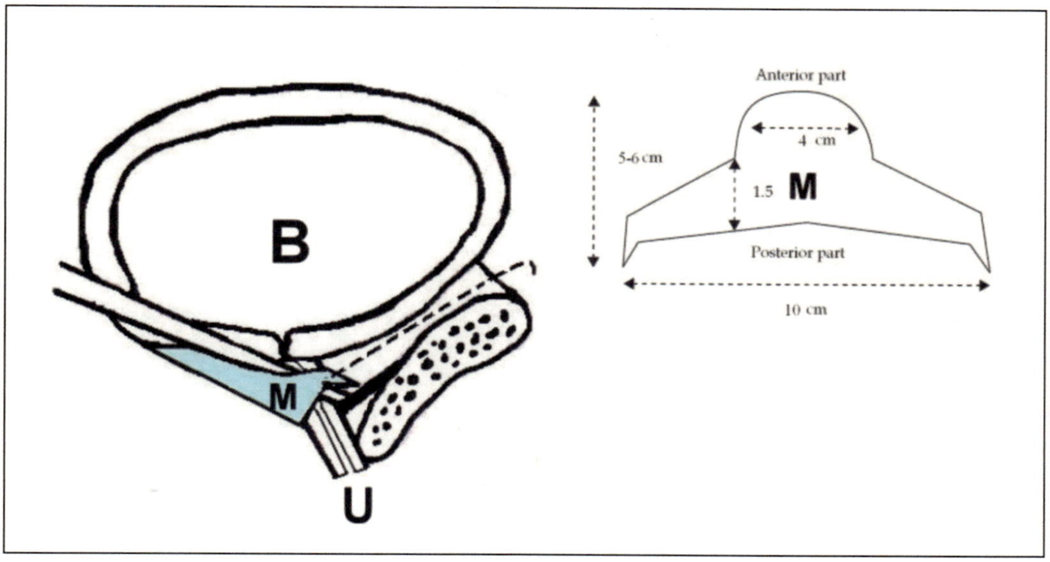

Fig. 6. The mesh is tension-free flatted under the suburethreal area. B: Bladder; U: Urethra; M: self-fashioned mesh.

9. Outcomes and complications of using self-fashioned mesh

Our results for using self-fashioned mesh for the treatment of concurrent stress urinary incontinence and pelvic organ prolapse showed a relatively high success rate in curing urinary incontinence (continence was 80%, improvement was 17%) and less recurrence of anterior vaginal wall prolapse (none with recurrent prolapse greater than stage II) in a three-year follow-up. However, mesh erosion was not completely averted. Exposed vaginal mesh was removed uneventfully. None of these patients experienced recurrent urinary incontinence and prolapse.

9.1 Comparison of relevant published articles

There are three similar articles using self-fashioned mesh for treating stress urinary incontinence and anterior vaginal wall prolapse have been found in recent five years (Mustafa and Wadie, 2006; Amrute et al., 2007; Eboue et al., 2010). Character of mesh, patient number, mean follow-up period, success rates, and complications of these articles and ours are as tabled below (Table 1). Outcomes of using self-fashioned meshes are promising. Mesh erosion rates in these case series are acceptable compared to that of commercial mesh kits (Jelovsek et al. 2007; Gomelsky et al., 2011).

The rationale for using self-fashioned mesh is: (1) to support the proximal urethra, bladder neck and anterior vaginal wall so they are simultaneously free of tension; (2) to provide a frame for augmenting the vaginal wall; (3) to fashion the size of the mesh to fit the defect in the vaginal wall; (4) to avoid complications induced by mesh arms by not using additional full-length mesh arms. A mesh patch lessens the amount of synthetic materials present in the wound bed which might diminish potential complications. Technically, it would be easier to remove the mesh patch than the full-length mesh if late complications occur (Tsui et al. 2005).

First author	Methods	Cases (n)	Mean follow up(m)	objective success (%)	Outcomes
Eboue	Trapezoidal shape with four arms, microporous multifilament polypropylene, transoburator , cystocele with/without SUI, history with/ without prior hysterectomy, no additional surgery	123	34	87.7% of SUI, 97.5% of cystocele	6.5% of erosion rate, bladder injury (1), urethral injury (2), paravesical hematoma (4), de novo SUI (9/66), de novo urgency (12/83); satisfactory outcome, maybe better with use of macroporous, monofilament mesh.
Amrute	H shaped macroporous monofilament polypropylene, retopubic route, SUI with POP, additional VH or SSLF, vaginal closure as in a Mercedes Benz or tripod fashion	76	30.7	89% of SUI, 95% of cystocele	2.1% of vaginal erosion, 2.1% of de novo SUI, 15.7% of de novo urgency; High success rate with single mesh use for SUI and cystocele and prevention of postoperative SUI
Mustafa	Placard shaped polypropylene mesh, retropubic route, SUI with/without cystocele	14	11	84.5 % of SUI, not reported of cystocele	Erosion not repoted; a simple, economic and cost-effective procedure by using placard mesh
Su	A macroporous monofilament polypropylene, SUI with/without POP, and with/without prior pelvic surgery, additional VH, SSLF or posterior repair, vaginal closure by Smead-Jones method	65	33	97% of SUI, 100% of cystocele	6% of mesh erosion, de novo urgency (1); a satisfactory outcomes, decrease the erosion rate by Smead-Jones suturing

Table 1. Clinical information self-customized mesh studies

9.2 Comparative cost of a self-fashioned mesh

The price of commercial mesh kits varies in the international market. In Taiwan, the National Health Insurance (NHI) covers some commercial kits for patients undergoing anti-incontinence surgery. The commercial mesh kits for pelvic organ prolapse are not covered by NHI. Patients choosing commercial mesh kits for treating their pelvic organ prolapse must pay 1,200-2,000 USD out of their own pockets for the additional surgical cost. In comparison, the cost of a self-fashioned mesh is relatively affordable for patients with stress urinary incontinence and pelvic organ prolapse, and the success rate is not compromised because of the lower expense of a self-fashioned mesh kit.

Stress urinary incontinence and pelvic organ prolapse are significant problems in relatively affluent countries. However, early childbearing and high fertility with early marriage, many vaginal deliveries, and frequent heavy lifting result in a high prevalence of stress urinary incontinence and pelvic organ prolapse. The situation in developing countries is far worse and cannot be overlooked (Wunasekera et al., 2007). Therefore, financial consideration for choosing a self-fashioned mesh or commercial mesh kits seems to be an important issue for treating this disease.

10. Conclusion

This procedure provides an easier placement technique, a relatively high success rate, and less recurrence. The complications of the self-fashioned mesh (monofilament and macroporous polypropylene) are acceptable compared to other commercial mesh kits. In addition, the cost of the self-fashioned mesh is cheaper than the commercial mesh kits. The self-fashioned mesh is an alternative option for treating stress urinary incontinence and anterior vaginal wall simultaneously.

11. References

Amrute, KV.; Eisenberg, ER. Rastinehad, AR. Kushner, L. & Badlani, GH. (2007). Analysis of Outcomes of Single Polypropylene Mesh in Total Pelvic Floor Reconstruction Neurourol Urodyn, Vol. 26, No.1, pp. 53-58, ISSN 0733-2467

Baessler, K. & Maher, CF. (2006). Mesh augmentation during pelvic floor reconstructive surgery: risks and benefits. *Curr Opin Obstet Gynecol,* Vol.18, No.5, (October 2006), pp. 195-201, ISSN 0147-1988

Bai, SW.; Jeon, MJ. Kim, JY. Chung, KA. Kim, SK. & Park, KH.. (2002). Relationship between stress urinary incontinence and pelvic organ prolapse. *Int Urogynecol J Pelvic Floor Dysfunct,* Vol.13, No.4, pp. 256-260, ISSN 0937-3462

Beck, RP.; McCormick, S.& Nordstrom, L.(1991). A 25-year experience with 519 anterior colporrhaphy procedures. *Obstet Gynecol,* Vol. 78, No.6, (December 1991), pp. 1011-1018, ISSN 0029-7844

Boreham, MK.; Wai, CY. Miller, RT. Schaffer, JI. & Word, RA. (2002). Morphometeric analysis of smooth muscle in the anterior vaginal wall of women with pelvic organ prolapse. *Am J Obstet Gynecol,* Vol. 187, No. 1, (July 2002), pp.56-63, ISSN 0002-9378

Borstad, E. & Rud, T. (1989). The risk of developing urinary stress incontinence after vaginal repair in continent women. A clinical and urodynamic follow-up study. *Acta Obstet Gynecol Scand Suppl,* Vol. 68, No.6, pp. 545-549, ISSN 0001-6349

Brubaker, L.; Bump, RC. Fynes, M. Jacquetin, B. Karram, K. Maher, C. Norton, B. & Cervigini, M. (2005). Surgery for pelvic organ prolapse. In: *Incontinence, 3rd International Consultation on Incontinence*, Abrams, P. Cardozo, L. Koury, S. & Wein, A., (Ed.), 1371-1402, Health Publication., ISBN 0-9546956-2-3, Paris, France

Chmielewski, L.; Walters, MD. Weber, AM. & Barber, MD. (2011). Reanalysis of a randomized trial of 3 techniques of anterior colporrhaphy using clinically relevant definitions of success. *Am J Obstet Gynecol* , [Epub ahead of print], ISSN 0002-9378

Connell, KA. (2011) Elastogenesis in the vaginal wall and pelvic-organ prolapse. *N Engl J Med*, Vol 364, No.24, (June 2011), pp. 2356-2358, ISSN 0028-4793

Eboue, C.; Marcus-Braun, N. & von Theobald P. (2010). Cystocele repair by transobturator four arms mesh: monocentric experience of first 123 patients. *Int Urogynecol J Pelvic Floor Dysfunct*, Vol.21, No.1, (January 2010), pp. 85-93, ISSN 0937-3462

Ellerkmann, RM.; Cundiff, GW. Melick, CF. Nihira, MA. Leffler, K. & Bent, AE. (2001). Correlation of symptoms with location and severity of pelvic organ prolapse. *Am J Obstet Gynecol*, Vol. 185, No. 6, (December 2001), pp. 1332-1338, ISSN 0002-9378

Gomelsky, A.; Penson, DF. & Dmochowski, RR. (2011). Pelvic organ prolapse (POP) surgery: the evidence for the repairs. *BJU Int*; Vol. 107, No. 11, (June 2011), pp. 1704-1719, ISSN 1464-4096

Gordon, D.; Gold, RS. Pauzner, D. Lessing, JB. & Groutz, A. (2001). Combined genitourinary prolapse repair and prophylactic tension-free vaginal tape in women with severe prolapse and occult stress urinary incontinence: preliminary results. *Urology*, Vol. 58, No. 4, (October 2001), pp. 547-550, ISSN 0090-4295

Gutman, RE.; Ford, DE. Quiroz, LH. Shippey, SH. & Handa, VL. (2008) Is there a pelvic organ prolapse threshold that predicts pelvic floor symptoms? *Am J Obstet Gynecol*, Vol. 199, No. 6, (December 2008), pp. 683. e1-7, ISSN 0002-9378

Haessler, AL.; Lin, LL. Ho, MH. Beston, LH. & Bhatia, NN. (2005). Reevaluating occult incontinence. *Curr Opin Obstet Gynecol*, Vol.17, No.5, (October 2005), pp. 535-540, ISSN 0147-1988

Huang, KH.; Kung, FT. Liang, HM. Chen, CW. Chang, SY. & Hwang, LL. (2006). Concomitant pelvic organ prolapse surgery with TVT procedure. *Int Urogynecol J Pelvic Floor Dysfunct*, Vol. 17, No.1, (June 2006), pp. 60-65, ISSN 0937-3462

Hung, MJ.; Liu, FS. Shen, PS. Chen, GD. Lin, LY. & Ho, ESC. (2004) Factors that affect recurrence after anterior colporrhaphy procedure reinforced with four-corner anchored polypropylene mesh. *Int Urogynecol J Pelvic Floor Dysfunct*, Vol. 15, No.6, (2004), pp. 399–406, ISSN 0937-3462

Jarvis, GJ.;(1994). Surgery for genuine stress incontinence. *Br J Obstet Gynecol*, Vol. 101, No. 5, (May 1994), pp. 371-374, ISSN 1471-0528

Jelovsek, JE.; Maher, C. & Barber, MD. (2007). Pelvic organ prolapse. *Lancet*; Vol. 369, No. 9566, (May 2007), pp.1027-1038, ISSN 0140-6736

Lo, TS.; Horng, SG. Liang, CC. Lee, SJ. & Soong, YK. (2004).Ultrasound assessment of mid-urethral tape at three-year follow-up after tension-free vaginal tape procedure. *Urology*, Vol. 63, No. 4 (April 2004), pp. 671-675, ISSN 0090-4295

Maher, C. & Baessler, K. (2006) Surgical management of anterior vaginal wall prolapse: An evidence based literature review. *Int Urogynecol J Pelvic Floor Dysfunct*, Vol.17, No.2, (February 2006), pp. 195-201, ISSN 0937-3462

Maher, C.; Baessler, K. Glazener, CMA. Adams, EJ. & Hagen, S. (2008) Surgical management of pelvic organ prolapse in women: A short version Cochrane Review. *Neurourol Urodyn,* Vol. 27, No.1, pp. 3-12, ISSN 0733-2467

Maher, C.; Feiner, B. Basessler, K. Adams, EJ. Hagen, S. & Glazener, CM. (2010). Surgical management of pelvic organ prolapse in women. *Cochrane Database syst Rev,* Vol.14, No.4, (April 2010), CD004014, ISSN 1469-493X

Mallipeddi, PK.; Steele, AC. Kohli, N. & Karram, MM.(2001).Anatomic and functional outcome of vaginal paravaginal repair in the correction of anterior vaginal wall prolapse. *Int Urogynecol J Pelvic Floor Dysfunct,* Vol.12, No.2, pp. 83-88, ISSN 0937-3462

Mustafa, M. & Wadie, BS. (2006). Placard-shaped in situ vaginal wall sling for the treatment of stress urinary incontinence. *Int J Urol,* Vol. 13, No. 2, (February 2006), pp.132-134, ISSN 0919-8172

Natale,F.; Weir, JM. & Cervigni, M.(2006). Pelvic floor reconstructive surgery: which aspects remain controversial? *Curr Opin Urol,* Vol. 16, No.6, (November 2006), pp.407-12, ISSN 0963-0643

Petros, PE. & Ulmsten, UI. (1993). An integral theory and its method for the diagnosis and management of female urinary incontinence. *Scand J Urol Nephrol,* Vol. 153, pp.1-93, ISSN 0036–5599

Reena, C.; Kekre, AN. & Kekre, N. (2007) Occult stress incontinence in women with pelvic organ prolapse. *Int J Gynaecol Obstet,* Vol. 97, No.1 (April 2007), pp.31–34, ISSN 0020-7292

Romanzi, LJ.; Chaikin, DC. & Blaivas, JG. (1999). The effect of genital prolapse on voiding. *J Urol,* Vol. 161, No. 2, (Feburary 1999), pp. 581-586, ISSN 0022-5347

Schick, E.; Jolivet-Tremblay, M. Tessier, J. Dupont, C. & Bertrand, PE. (2004). Observations on the function of the female urethra III: An overview with special reference to the relation between urethral hypermobility and urethral incompetemce. *Neurourol Urodyn,* Vol. 23, No.1, pp. 22-26, ISSN 0733-2467

Su, CF.; Ng, SC. Tsui, KP. Chen, GD. & Tsai, HJ. (2009). Suburethral slingplasty using a self-fashioned Gynemesh for treating urinary incontinence and anterior vaginal wall prolapse. *Taiwan J Obstet Gynecol,* Vol. 48, No. 1, (March 2009), pp.53-39, ISSN 1028-4559

Tsui, KP.; Ng, SC. Tee, YT. Yeh, GP. Chen, GD. (2005). Complications of synthetic graft materials used in suburethral sling procedures. *Int Urogynecol J Pelvic Floor Dysfunct,* Vol. 16, No. 2, (Mar-Apr 2005), pp. 165-167, ISSN 0937-3462

Weber, AM. Walters, MD. Piedmonte, MR. & Ballard, LA. (2001). Anterior colporrhaphy: a randomized trial of three surgical techniques. *Am J Obstet Gynecol,* Vol. 185, No. 6, (December 2001), pp. 1299-1306, ISSN 0002-9378

Wei, J.& DeLancey, JOL. (2004). Functional anatomy of the pelvic floor and lower urinary tract. *Clin Obstet Gynecol;* Vol. 47, No. 1, (March 2004), pp. 3-17, ISSN 0009-9201

Winters, JC.(2008). A critical appraisal of preventive slings and prolapse surgery—what's a urologist to do? *J Urol,* Vol. 180, No. 3, (September 2008), pp. 809-810, ISSN 0022-5347

Wu, MP. (2008). The use of prostheses in pelvic reconstructive surgery: Joy or Toy? *Taiwan J Obstet Gynecol,* Vol. 47, No. 2, (June 2008), pp.151-156, ISSN 1028-4559

Wu, MP.& Huang, KH. (2008). Tension-free midurethral sling surgeries for stress urinary incontinence. *Incont Pelvic Floor Dysfunct,* 53-60. Vol. 2, No.2, pp.53-60, ISSN 1994-568X

Wu, MP. Long, CY & Liang, CC.(2010). Staged or concomitant surgery for correcting pelvic organ prolapse and stress urinary incontinence. *Incont Pelvic Floor Dysfunct,* Vol. 4, No.4, pp.93-98, ISSN 1994-568X

Wunasekera, P.; Sazaki, J. & Walker, G. (2007). Pelvic organ prolapse: don't forget developing countries. *Lancet;* Vol. 369, No. 9575, (May 2007), pp.1789-1790, ISSN 0140-6736

Young, SB.; Daman, JJ. & Bony, LG. (2001). Vaginal paravaginal repair: one-year outcomes. *Am J Obstet Gynecol,* Vol. 185, No. 6, (December 2001), pp. 1360-1366, ISSN 0002-9378

14

Refractory Stress Urinary Incontinence

Sara M. Lenherr and Arthur P. Mourtzinos
Lahey Clinic Medical Center, Department of Urology
USA

1. Introduction

Treatment of stress urinary incontinence (SUI) caused by urethral hypermobility or intrinsic sphincter deficiency with urethral sling procedures may yield up to a 80-90% success rate depending on the definition of success. (Nilsson et al. 2001; Liapis et al. 2002; Rodriguez & Raz 2003; Nilsson et al. 2004; Ward & Hilton 2004) In a minority of patients, however, there is persistence or worse incontinence after surgical therapy. In the general population, risk factors for midurethral sling (MUS) failure are BMI >25, mixed incontinence, intrinsic sphincter deficiency, diabetes mellitus, advanced patient age >75 years old and prior continence surgery. (Cammu et al. 2009; Stav et al. 2010) Potential surgery related reasons for failure include improper adjustment of the sling or misplacement of the suburethral tape. Female patients with urethral incompetence and severe incontinence due to multiple failed surgeries, neurologic injury, or congenital anomalies represent a unique surgical challenge.

Patients with neurologic conditions have sacral arc lesions with paralysis of the skeletal musculature and an open urethra. All other patients who have failed multiple sling and anti-incontinence procedures may have severe symptoms of SUI and an open urethra with a low valsalva leak point pressure. These patients often have an incompetent, difficult to compress, urethra likely due to a combination of urethral denervation, and violation of the periurethral fascia, as well as their underlying risk factors for SUI. (Bump & Norton 1998) These patients have been shown to have low chances of cure after repeat anti-incontinence surgery and be more likely to suffer from complications including retention, osteomyelitis, and pelvic abscess. (Petrou & Frank 2001)

In the recurrent or refractory stress urinary incontinence female patient, a routine sling procedure providing only posterior support will not typically yield an appropriate response. Management options include repeat placement of a "tight" pubovaginal sling or replacement of a different type of sling, a spiral sling, periurethral bulking agents, adjustable continence therapy (ACT) device and the artificial urinary sphincter (AUS) prior to bladder neck closure with continent urinary diversion. This manuscript will review the evaluation and management options for recurrent stress urinary incontinence in this challenging population.

2. Evaluation

There are a significant number of patients in the United States that undergo successful sling placement for SUI, however a minority will present with persistent or recurrent incontinence. Recurrent stress urinary incontinence after urethral sling surgery (transvaginal tape and transobturator tape) and common complications such as urinary tract infection and de novo urge urinary incontinence need to be fully evaluated. It is also important when determining the etiology of surgical failure to identify whether the patient has refractory SUI by determining whether there was any period of cure or improvement. Recurrent stress urinary incontinence warrants at a minimum: complete history and physical examination and urinalysis. Most physicians would advocate urodynamic testing in cases of failed previous surgery for incontinence. (Houwert et al. 2010; Walsh & Moore 2010) Cystoscopic evaluation is easy to perform in the clinic and should be utilized to determine if there is evidence of sling erosion or misplacement. Ultimately, the determination must be made whether this leakage is due to bladder or outlet dysfunction.

If there is evidence of flank or pelvic pain, a retroperitoneal ultrasound with evaluation of the bladder is necessary to evaluation for obstruction and or injury to the ureteral orifices. Urodynamics with or without fluoroscopy is useful to further characterize the physiology of the bladder. While there is no published data regarding routine use, most practices use routine urodynamic evaluation of failed anti-incontinence patients prior to a repeat procedure. (Rutman et al. 2006; Rodriguez et al. 2010; Walsh & Moore 2010)

Some urologists routinely use dynamic T2-weighted MRI to look at the anatomic defects seen in pelvic floor dysfunction. A vaginal examination might demonstrate a change in the patient's pelvic floor anatomy, such as evidence of prolapse. Many researchers have used dynamic MRI to evaluate the female pelvis and delineate the possible components of pelvic floor dysfunction. This requires experience using this modality and a radiologist that can interpret the test in a useful way. In the cost-saving climate of health care today, dynamic T2 MRI can likely only be used in the setting of severe refractory incontinence or neurologic conditions.

3. Nonsurgical management

There is a paucity of literature for the nonsurgical management of recurrent SUI following prior surgical repair. Most treatments are based on primary SUI studies, namely pelvic floor muscle training, weight loss, incontinence pessary and medications. These options have been systematically reviewed elsewhere. (Shamliyan et al. 2008)

4. Periurethral bulking agents

While the majority of patients that have failed surgical repair for SUI will opt for a more aggressive intervention, periurethral bulking agents offer a potential adjunct for the insufficient sling, especially if the patient or surgeon are hesitant to be more invasive given the history of prior urethral surgery. Periurethral bulking agents include biodegradable and nonbiodegradable agents that are injected endoscopically in the perurethral tissue to presumably further coapt the urethral mucosa. While the availability of these agents has recently changed, the primary injectable bulking agents in the United States include Contigen (Bard Inc., Murry Hill, NJ) which has recently been discontinued, Durasphere (Coloplast Inc, Minneapolis, MN), Macroplastique (Uroplasty Inc, Minneapolis, MN) and Coaptite (Bioform Inc., Franksville, WI).

Investigators have reported the use of periurethral bulking agents after failed sling procedures for SUI, but no randomized studies have been reported. However, a recent report looking at intermediate follow up has reported some success. Macroplastique and Durasphere were used as periurethral bulking agents in 23 women following a failed midurethral sling procedure. (Lee et al. 2010) Macroplastique was used in 21 patients and Durasphere was used in 2 patients with a median interval between sling placement and periurethral bulking agent injection of 12 months (range 3-65). With intermediate follow up at a median of 10 months (range 6-34 months), 8 of 23 patients (35%) of all patients reported "cure" whereas 92% reported they had benefited from the procedure. Notably, 77% of the women reported satisfaction from the procedure, perhaps noting the relative simplicity and ease of placement.

5. Revision urethral sling surgery

The literature is maturing with regard to the appropriate choice for a repeat sling following midurethral sling for SUI. Stav and colleagues reviewed the cases of 1225 retrospectively identified women who underwent either a retropubic or transobturator sling. 91% of these patients completed a telephone interview questionnaire. (Stav et al. 2010) The majority of these women had a retropubic sling as opposed to a transobturator sling. Mean follow up was 50 months. Their re-operation rate for failure was 14%. Repeat retropubic sling placement was significantly more successful than utilizing a transobturator approach (71% vs 48%, p=0.04). Repeat slings were placed without removal of the previous sling. Most surgeons will opt to use a retropubic sling for recurrent incontinence and rather than a transobturator sling because of the greater urethral tension generated. Management options also include repeat placement of a "tight" pubovaginal sling with the intent of putting the patient in urinary retention. This can be done utilizing autologous fascia as well.

6. Adjustable Continence Therapy (ACT) system

The efficacy, safety & technical feasibility of the ACT was initially reported in 2009 as a novel device for the treatment of recurrent female SUI. (Aboseif et al. 2009) The device is intended to be a minimally invasive implantable device that provides support at the urethrovesical junction and enhances urethral coaptation. Its unique advantage is that it is also adjustable allowing for further optimization of the device post-operatively.

Placement of the ACT device is via bilateral small incisions between the labia majora and minora at the level of the urethral meatus with a specially designed trocar. Fluoroscopic and digital guidance is used to identify a point just distal to the urethrovesical junction where the balloons are placed. The balloons are then inflated with 1-1.5 mL of isotonic contrast solution. The subcutaneous inflation ports are then placed in a pocket in a superior ventral portion of each labia majora and the skin is closed with subcuticular absorbable suture. (Aboseif et al. 2009; Kocjancic et al. 2010)

The initial experience with the ACT system showed a complication rate of 24.4% (38 of 156 patients). Complications included port erosion, urinary retention, balloon erosion or migration and worsening incontinence. 18.3% (28 of 153) of patients underwent explantation within the first year, however 50% of explanted cases then underwent replacement. Since the development of the device, improvement in the technical related learning curve has led to reduced rates of complications.

At a mean follow-up of 72 months (range 12-84), 68% of patients (n=29) reported themselves dry. (Kocjancic et al. 2010) All of these patients had at least one prior pelvic surgery for SUI. The researchers reported 12 month urodynamic data (n=30 patients) which showed a statistically significant increase in VLPP from a mean baseline of 51.06 ± 24.38 to 86.0 ± 21.44 cm H_2O ($p<0.01$). Complications requiring device removal developed in 21.1% of patients.

Most recently, Aboseif and colleagues presented a series of 89 patients with the ACT device. (Aboseif et al. 2011) They reported that 47% of the patients were dry at 1 year and 92% overall were subjectively improved. Pads per day and incontinence episodes were significantly improved, in addition to outcomes on standardized questionnaires. Their complication rate was similar to previously published studies with an explant rate of 21.7%. Proponents of the ACT device, that are proficient in placement and adjustment, report it is effective, simple and safe.

7. Artificial urinary sphincter

The AUS in the female population differs from the suburethral sling in that it does not provide a backboard or urethral support, but rather it attempts to mimic the sphincter mechanism of the urethra with circumferential compression. (Light & Scott 1985) The initial use of the AUS in women with incontinence was described in 1985 (Light & Scott 1985) and has since been well documented in the literature. (Vayleux et al. 2011)

Costa and colleagues evaluated the efficacy of the AMS 800 AUS in women with Type III incontinence and a negative Marshall test. (Costa et al. 2001) They described a modified surgical procedure through an abdominal approach. Of the 190 patients with working devices, continence was achieved in 88.7% and 81.8% of those with non-neurogenic and neurogenic bladders, respectively at a mean follow-up of 3.9 years. 51 patients had perioperative complications and a high percentage of patients had not undergone prior surgical therapy. Thomas and associates reported 12 year follow-up in 68 patients who underwent an AUS. (Thomas et al. 2002) Despite an 81% continence rate, 46% required removal or replacement for erosion or infection. They concluded by recommending an AUS in patients with SUI after failure of one anti-stress incontinence operation and rather than as a last resort. More recent series reports demonstrate the safety, efficacy and complication rates associated with female AUS implantation. (Chung et al. 2010; Vayleux et al. 2011) Importantly, while there is a high proportion of patients that continue to use the AUS after implantation, about 50% of them have required revision or replacement, usually within the first several years of implantation. Continence rate in these two studies indicates 65-70% for no pads and 73.5-83% for 0 to 1 pad per day. Satisfaction rates were high with a majority of patients reporting they would undergo AUS placement again if necessary. Additional modifications such as insertion of an AUS laparoscopically (Roupret et al. 2010) or with a large cuff (Revaux et al. 2010) have been proposed, however long-term data is lacking at this time.

8. Spiral sling procedure

A newer technique initially described by Raz and colleagues is a transvaginal sling procedure in adult women that encircles the urethra providing circumferential coaptation. The spiral sling is a salvage procedure for a small, yet severe group of female patients with a totally incompetent urethra. The procedure was initially described in patients with congenital or neurological diseases. (Rutman et al. 2006) It has more recently been described in patients with multiple failed surgeries for SUI. (Mourtzinos et al. 2008) The procedural details of the spiral sling are not widely published and will therefore be reviewed here in detail.

Notable surgical steps different from other suburethral slings are as follows: Two parallel distal oblique incisions are made in the anterior vaginal wall. The retropubic space is entered and a complete urethrolysis is performed by detaching the urethropelvic ligaments from the arcus tendineous fascia pelvis and freeing all retropubic adhesions. The urethral dissection is started in the mid-urethral area just proximal to the pubo-urethral ligaments and carried proximally to free the rest of the urethra and the bladder neck. Then a suburethral tunnel is created in the anterior vaginal wall 1.5 cm from the urethral meatus. Polypropylene mesh measuring approximately 1 X 15 cm is passed dorsally, between the urethra and the pubis. The ends of the mesh are crossed ventrally through the previously made vaginal tunnel. This maneuver creates a complete circle of mesh around the urethra. A suprapubic puncture is made just above the symphysis and a double-pronged needle (Cook Urological, Inc., Spencer, IN) is passed under finger control through the fascia and retropubic space to the vaginal incision. The previously placed 0-polyglactin sutures from the polypropylene mesh are transferred to the suprapubic incision. This is repeated on the contralateral side and the sutures are tied without tension.

Between August 1999 and October 2004, 47 patients underwent placement of a spiral sling. (Rutman et al. 2006) This initial patient population was initially selected because of congenital or neurologic diseases, however, the technique was later expanded to include those patients with multiple failed surgeries for SUI and an incompetent lead pipe urethra. Of the 47 patients, seven were lost to follow-up. The mean age of the remaining 40 patients was 59.0 years (23-86). This represented a complex cohort of patients with 98% having failed a prior anti-incontinence surgery. The patients had undergone a mean of 2.6 previous anti-incontinence surgeries and used an average of 6 pads per day. There were two patients who had previous augmentation cystoplasty and were performing self-intermittent catheterization but had significant SUI between catheterizations. All patients were considered candidates for urethral closure and continent diversion as a salvage procedure.

In this group of 40 patients, the average follow-up was 12 months (6-37). There were no intraoperative complications. The de-novo urge incontinence rate was 7.4%. Of the 27 patients with preoperative urge incontinence (UI), 9 (33%) had resolution of their symptoms with the procedure. One of the patients had persistent refractory UI and subsequently underwent a sacral neuromodulation procedure. No patient experienced de novo retention after the spiral sling. The four patients who were performing self-intermittent catheterization pre-operatively continued to do so after the procedure. There were no urethral or vaginal erosions. The mean number of pads decreased from 6.0 preoperatively to 0.9 postoperatively ($P<0.005$). 78% of patients reported improvements of 90% or greater. Patients reported a mean improvement of symptoms of 87% after surgery. Ultimately, three patients underwent bladder neck closure and continent augmentation and were considered failures.

More recently, the spiral sling technique was described in 46 patients with multiple failed surgeries for SUI excluding patients with neurologic or congenital anomalies. (Mourtzinos, et al. 2008) The mean age of the study population was 62 years and the mean follow-up was 15 months (6 to 45 months). All patients had failed a prior anti-incontinence surgery. There were no intraoperative complications and no cases of permanent urinary retention postoperatively requiring transvaginal urethrolysis. On patient driven subjective assessment, 49% of patients reported never experiencing SUI, and 72% experienced no or rare episodes of SUI. Overall patients reported a mean improvement of 84% with a decrease in daily pads from 5.5 to 1.0. Most patients were highly satisfied with their urinary symptoms after surgery (mean QoL of 1.4). In addition, there was no statistically significant difference between pre and postoperative symptoms of incomplete bladder emptying ($P>0.05$).

A review of the literature for alternatives to bladder neck closure revealed no existing circumferential sling procedure in the adult population. Mingin and colleagues described a transabdominal technique of a urethral sling using rectus muscle wrapped around the urethra for pediatric patients with congenital urethral incompetence. (Mingin et al. 2002) Of the 37 patients reported, 92% remained dry between catheterizations. The pediatric population is unlike this population since these patients had roughly three anti-incontinence surgeries with subsequent scarring and more difficult coaptation. The mechanism of cure of the transvaginal spiral sling is not completely understood. It likely supports the midurethral segment while preventing urethral descent and improving pressure transmission to the urethra. In addition, unlike a routine sling procedure, the spiral sling also provides circumferential coaptation to the urethra at the time of increases in intrabdominal pressure.

Raz and colleagues concluded that the spiral sling is an effective salvage transvaginal procedure that may be considered for a small subset of female patients with non-functional urethras as a last resort prior to urethral closure procedures. This includes patients with urethral incompetence caused by neurologic disease, congenital anomalies or iatrogenic injury from multiple failed anti-incontinence surgeries. The most comparable surgical alternative is the AUS which requires manual dexterity to operate the device and a more extensive dissection to implant all components. The initial outcomes look promising but longer follow-up will better define its role in refractory female incontinence and demonstrate the durability of the spiral sling.

9. New technologies

Efficacy, safety & technical feasibility of intrasphincteric injections of autologous muscle derived stem cells have been shown by several groups in both animal models and humans. (Mitterberger et al. 2008; Sebe et al. 2011) In the human studies, myoblasts and fibroblasts were obtained from muscle biopsies of the patient. Cells are then grown in a culture facility to yield more myoblasts. After amplification, the cells are collected and frozen in a pellet, which is transferred to the urologist and thawed immediately prior to endourethral injection under endoscopic control. A recent review of stem cells for the treatment of urinary incontinence nicely describes the theory behind the use of stem cells for the treatment of urinary incontinence. (Staack & Rodriguez 2011) Ideally, these autologous cells provide additional mucosal coaptation in order to restore resting urethral closing pressures. These studies are in their infancy and no data has been reported on women with refractory stress urinary incontinence, however this might provide a more effective means of endoscopic bulking without the use of collagen and other synthetic materials.

10. Conclusion

Traditional first-line therapies for stress urinary incontinence are not successful in all women and management of recurrent incontinence can be quite difficult. Options for these patients include conservative management, endoscopic management with periurethral bulking, a repeat sling procedure, spiral slings, the artificial urinary sphincter and adjustable continence therapy devices or new technologies such as autologous stem cell injection. Variable success rates for all of these methods have been reported in the literature depending on the length of follow up and the definition of cure.

11. References

Aboseif, S. R., E. I. Franke, et al. (2009). The adjustable continence therapy system for recurrent female stress urinary incontinence: 1-year results of the North America Clinical Study Group. *J Urol* 181(5): 2187-91.

Aboseif, S. R., P. Sassani, et al. (2011). Treatment of moderate to severe female stress urinary incontinence with the adjustable continence therapy (ACT) device after failed surgical repair. *World J Urol* 29(2): 249-53.

Bump, R. C. and P. A. Norton (1998). Epidemiology and natural history of pelvic floor dysfunction. *Obstet Gynecol Clin North Am* 25(4): 723-46.

Cammu, H., E. Van Den Abbeele, et al. (2009). Factors predictive of outcome in tension-free vaginal tape procedure for urinary stress incontinence in a teaching hospital. *Int Urogynecol J Pelvic Floor Dysfunct* 20(7): 775-80.

Chung, E., A. Navaratnam, et al. (2010). Can artificial urinary sphincter be an effective salvage option in women following failed anti-incontinence surgery? *Int Urogynecol J* 22(3): 363-6.

Costa, P., N. Mottet, et al. (2001). The use of an artificial urinary sphincter in women with type III incontinence and a negative Marshall test. *J Urol* 165(4): 1172-6.

Houwert, R. M., J. P. Roovers, et al. (2010). When to perform urodynamics before mid-urethral sling surgery for female stress urinary incontinence? *Int Urogynecol J* 21(3): 303-9.

Kocjancic, E., S. Crivellaro, et al. (2010). Adjustable continence therapy for severe intrinsic sphincter deficiency and recurrent female stress urinary incontinence: long-term experience. *J Urol* 184(3): 1017-21.

Lee, H. N., Y. S. Lee, et al. (2010). Transurethral injection of bulking agent for treatment of failed mid-urethral sling procedures. *Int Urogynecol J* 21(12): 1479-83.

Liapis, A., P. Bakas, et al. (2002). Burch colposuspension and tension-free vaginal tape in the management of stress urinary incontinence in women. *Eur Urol* 41(4): 469-73.

Light, J. K. and F. B. Scott (1985). Management of urinary incontinence in women with the artificial urinary sphincter. *J Urol* 134(3): 476-8.

Mingin, G. C., K. Youngren, et al. (2002). The rectus myofascial wrap in the management of urethral sphincter incompetence. *BJU Int* 90(6): 550-3.

Mitterberger, M., G. M. Pinggera, et al. (2008). Adult stem cell therapy of female stress urinary incontinence. *Eur Urol* 53(1): 169-75.

Mourtzinos, A., M. G. Maher, et al. (2008). Spiral sling salvage anti-incontinence surgery for women with refractory stress urinary incontinence: surgical outcome and satisfaction determined by patient-driven questionnaires. *Urology* 72(5): 1044-8; discussion 1048-50.

Nilsson, C. G., C. Falconer, et al. (2004). Seven-year follow-up of the tension-free vaginal tape procedure for treatment of urinary incontinence. *Obstet Gynecol* 104(6): 1259-62.

Nilsson, C. G., N. Kuuva, et al. (2001). Long-term results of the tension-free vaginal tape (TVT) procedure for surgical treatment of female stress urinary incontinence. *Int Urogynecol J Pelvic Floor Dysfunct* 12 Suppl 2: S5-8.

Petrou, S. P. and I. Frank (2001). Complications and initial continence rates after a repeat pubovaginal sling procedure for recurrent stress urinary incontinence. *J Urol* 165(6 Pt 1): 1979-81.

Revaux, A., M. Roupret, et al. (2010). Is the implantation of an artificial urinary sphincter with a large cuff in women with severe urinary incontinence associated with worse perioperative complications and functional outcomes than usual? *Int Urogynecol J.*

Rodriguez, A. R., T. Hakky, et al. (2010). Salvage spiral sling techniques: alternatives to manage disabling recurrent urinary incontinence in females. *J Urol* 184(6): 2429-33.

Rodriguez, L. V. and S. Raz (2003). Prospective analysis of patients treated with a distal urethral polypropylene sling for symptoms of stress urinary incontinence: surgical outcome and satisfaction determined by patient driven questionnaires. *J Urol* 170(3): 857-63; discussion 863.

Roupret, M., V. Misrai, et al. (2010). Laparoscopic approach for artificial urinary sphincter implantation in women with intrinsic sphincter deficiency incontinence: a single-centre preliminary experience. *Eur Urol* 57(3): 499-504.

Rutman, M. P., D. Y. Deng, et al. (2006). Spiral sling salvage anti-incontinence surgery in female patients with a nonfunctional urethra: technique and initial results. *J Urol* 175(5): 1794-8; discussion 1798-9.

Sebe, P., C. Doucet, et al. (2011). Intrasphincteric injections of autologous muscular cells in women with refractory stress urinary incontinence: a prospective study. *Int Urogynecol J* 22(2): 183-9.

Shamliyan, T. A., R. L. Kane, et al. (2008). Systematic review: randomized, controlled trials of nonsurgical treatments for urinary incontinence in women. *Ann Intern Med* 148(6): 459-73.

Staack, A. and L. V. Rodriguez (2011). Stem cells for the treatment of urinary incontinence. *Curr Urol Rep* 12(1): 41-6.

Stav, K., P. L. Dwyer, et al. (2010). Repeat synthetic mid urethral sling procedure for women with recurrent stress urinary incontinence. *J Urol* 183(1): 241-6.

Stav, K., P. L. Dwyer, et al. (2010). Risk factors of treatment failure of midurethral sling procedures for women with urinary stress incontinence. *Int Urogynecol J* 21(2): 149-55.

Thomas, K., S. N. Venn, et al. (2002). Outcome of the artificial urinary sphincter in female patients. *J Urol* 167(4): 1720-2.

Uebersax, J. S., J. F. Wyman, et al. (1995). Short forms to assess life quality and symptom distress for urinary incontinence in women: the Incontinence Impact Questionnaire and the Urogenital Distress Inventory. Continence Program for Women Research Group. *Neurourol Urodyn* 14(2): 131-9.

Vayleux, B., J. Rigaud, et al. (2011). Female urinary incontinence and artificial urinary sphincter: study of efficacy and risk factors for failure and complications. *Eur Urol* 59(6): 1048-53.

Walsh, C. A. and K. H. Moore (2010). Recurrent stress urinary incontinence after synthetic midurethral sling procedure. *Obstet Gynecol* 115(6): 1296-301.

Ward, K. L. and P. Hilton (2004). A prospective multicenter randomized trial of tension-free vaginal tape and colposuspension for primary urodynamic stress incontinence: two-year follow-up. *Am J Obstet Gynecol* 190(2): 324-31.

15

Surgical Complications with Synthetic Materials

Verónica Ma. De J. Ortega-Castillo[1] and Eduardo S. Neri-Ruz[2]
[1]*Instituto Nacional de Perinatología, SSA*
[2]*Clínica de Especialidades de la Mujer, SEDENA*
México D.F.
México

1. Introduction

Many factors are involved in the pathogenesis of stress urinary incontinence (SUI) and for several decades attempts have been made to design the best device for its treatment. Experience and research have led to important breakthroughs, but there is currently no 100% effective treatment devoid of complications. As treatments have changed, the materials and access routes have given way to complications not previously reported that have sometimes been fatal. ObGyns, urologists and urogynecologists that perform surgical procedures for urinary incontinence would like to have the best kit and none of the reported complications, but in actuality, everyone has such complications. Every surgeon wonders: What was the cause of this complication? How will it be resolved? How is it classified? For future patients, how can such a complication be prevented? There have been reports of erosion and/or extrusion of material in new kits or devices for urinary incontinence in the urethra, bladder, vagina and ureter; as well as bleedings during the surgical procedure with injury to the pelvic or vaginal vessels, suburethral hematomas, intestinal perforation, voiding dysfunction, nerve lesions, bladder perforation, infections and abscesses, de novo overactive bladder, pelvic pain, necrotizing fasciitis and even death.

For decades, different types of materials have been used, such as monofilament or multifilament mesh, micropore, macropore, silicone, polyester, polypropylene and gore-tex, and none of them is free of complications.

This chapter is an overview of the complications reported according to the device or kit used, the type of mesh, with reference to the classification of complications of the International Continence Society (ICS) and the International Urogynecological Association (IUGA) and the treatments used to resolve these complications. It is necessary to adequately follow the technical procedure, check the correct position of the patient´s legs, know the anatomy and receive periodical training.

2. History

The first to use synthetic material for a female urethral sling were Williams and Te Linde in 1962, followed by Ridley in 1966 and Morgan in 1970, using a polypropylene Marlex mesh for recurrent stress urinary incontinence. Subsequently, Morgan and colleagues (1985) reported at least a 5 year follow-up of patients with a 77.4% success rate. The complications of this procedure include bladder neck obstruction and chronic cystitis. Subsequently, his patients had problems of erosion, infection and fistula formation

Vervigni and Natale (2001) described the three most important components for the use of a mesh in urological reconstructive surgery: the pore size, the type of fiber and its inflexibility. The pore size and the type of fiber may be used to classify mesh in 4 types: Mesh type 1, such as prolene, which is very soft (Ethicon, Endosurgery Inc, Summerville) and Marlex, having a long pore (>75µg) and usually made of polypropylene. This pore size allows macrophages to cross over and there is growth of fibroblasts (fibroplasias), as well as blood vessels (angiogenesis), and collagen deposits; White (1988) reported that because of these features, the mesh leads to changes to prevent infections and fibrous connective tissue grows around the tissue. Type II mesh such as Gore-tex (WL Gore & Associates Inc; Flagstaff, AZ) has a pore size under 10 µg in each one of its three dimensions (micropore). Mesh type III, such as Mersilene, is a macropore shaped naturally, but with micropore components that often include braided material and one/or multiple filaments. Mesh type IV has material with a pore size under a micron, and it is not used as a sling for urinary incontinence surgical procedures. (Table 1). Another important property is fiber composition: polypropylene mesh is made of monofilament and there are others made of multiple filaments which are commonly used. Multiple filament mesh often has a hole less than 10 µg wide, allowing small bacteria to infiltrate and proliferate. In theory, this small hole does not allow macrophages (16 to 20 µg) or white cells (9 a 15 µg) to pass through to kill bacteria, resulting in potential risk of infections. Flexibility or inflexibility of the mesh is another important feature. Prolene has a pore size twice as big as Marlex (1500 µg vs. 600 µg) and is much more flexible. Considering all of these properties, theoretically, prolene may have the lowest rate of erosion on the vagina and adjacent organs.

Type	Fiber	Pore Size
I	Monofilament	Macro(>75µm)
II	Multifilament	Micro(<75µm)
III	Multifilament	Variable
IV	Monofilament	Submicro

Table 1. Classification of Mesh Types

Ulmsten et al (1996) were the first to use a tension-free polypropylene mesh (TVT) to repair female stress urinary incontinence. They used a prolene mesh to support the mid urethra. The procedure needs to be performed with cystoscopy. This procedure was designed to avoid excessive tension and the kit is adjusted according to a cough test. The authors do not report any complication during surgery and they conclude that the procedure has a good success rate. This surgical procedure was known worldwide and surgeons started to use it, however some time later, complications were reported in publications. Primicero et al (1999) used the device in 24 patients, reporting a case of a patient with perforation of the external iliac vein and needing surgical repair. Brink (2000) reported a case of intestinal injury. Already in the year 2005 Atherton and Stanton reported that the bladder perforation rate with this kit has a 4.4% incidence in up to 71% of cases, but these were not the only complications. Delorme et al (2204) was the first to use the approach through the obturator hole. In this procedure it is not necessary to use cytoscopy. But some time later, urinary tract injuries were also documented.

Lapitan et al (2009), in their systematic Cochrane review, evaluated the different treatments for urinary incontinence: open retropubic vaginal suspension, among others, and the tension-free vaginal tape. This review included 46 articles for a total of 4738 women. The total cure rate for open retropubic vaginal suspension was 68.9% to 88%. When open retropubic vaginal suspension is compared to the tension-free tape in 12 studies, there is no difference in the success rate throughout the follow-up time. The available evidence according to Lapitan´s report is that there is no high morbidity or complication rate difference between these two surgical procedures.

Several commercial houses have started to change the mesh placement, with different access routes, either inside-out or outside-in; with suprapubic or transobturator approach.

3. Classification

Haylen et al (2011) in The Standardization and Terminology Committees of the International Urogynecological Association (IUGA) and the International Continence Society (ICS) and the joint IUGA/ICS working group on Complications Terminology seek to provide a terminology and a standardized classification for those complications arising directly from the insertion of prostheses and graft in female pelvic floor surgery. A significant increase in the use of an ever widening array of prostheses and graft has occurred in female pelvic floor surgery over the last 30 years. Terminology involved in the classification (Table 2), Classification of complications related directly to the insertion of prosthesis (Table 3) and Grades of pain (Table 4)

TERMS USED	DEFINITION
PROSTHESIS	A Fabricated substitute to assist a damaged body part or to augment or stabilize a hypoplastic structure
a. Mesh	A (prosthetic) network fabric or structure
b. Implant	A surgically inserted or embedded prosthesis
c. Tape(sling)	A flat strip of synthetic material
GRAFT	Any tissue or organ for transplantation. This term will refer to biological materials inserted.
a. Autologous Grafts	From the woman's own tissues e.g. dura mater, rectus sheath or fascia lata
b. Allografts	From post-mortem tissue banks
c. Xenografts	From other species e.g. modifies porcine dermis, porcine small intestine, bovine pericardium
COMPLICATION	A morbid process or event that occurs during the course of a surgery that is not an essential part of that surgery
CONTRACTION	Shrinkage or reduction in size
PROMINENCE	Parts that protrude beyond the surface (e.g. due to wrinkling or folding with no epithelial separation)
SEPARATION	Physically disconnected (e.g. vaginal epithelium)
EXPOSURE	A condition of displaying, revealing, exhibiting or making accessible e.g. vaginal mesh visualized through separated vaginal epithelium
EXTRUSION	Passage gradually out of a body structure or tissue
COMPROMISE	Bring into danger
PERFORATION	Abnormal opening into a hollow organ or viscus
DEHISCENCE	A bursting opening or gaping along natural or sutured line

Table 2. Terminology involved in the Classification.

		CATEGORY		
GENERAL DESCRIPTION	A ASYMPTOMATIC	B SYMPTOMATIC	C INFECTION	D ABSCESS (+)
1 VAGINAL: no epithelial separation. Includes prominence (e.g. due to wrinkling or folding), mesh fiber palpation or contraction (shrinkage	1 A : Abnormal prosthesis or graft finding on clinical examination	1 B: Symptomatic e.g. unusual discomfort/pain; dispareunia (either partner); bleeding	1C: Infection (suspected or actual)	1D: (+)
2 VAGINAL: Smaller ≤ 1cm exposure	2A : Asymptomatic	2B: Symptomatic	2C: Infection	2D: (+)
3 VAGINAL: larger >1 cm exposure, or any extrusion	3A: Asymptomatic 1-3Aa if no prosthesis or graft related pain	3B: Symptomatic 1-3B(b-e) if prosthesis or graft related pain	3C: Infection 1-3C/1-3D (b-e) if prosthesis or graft related pain	3D: (+)
4 URINARY TRACT: Compromise or perforation including prosthesis(graft) perforation, fistula and calculus	4A: Small intra-operative defect e.g. bladder perforation	4B: Other lower urinary tract complication or urinary retention	4C: Ureteric or upper urinary tract complication	
5 RECTAL OR BOWEL: Compromise or perforation including prosthesis(graft) perforation and fistula	5A: Small intra-operative defect (rectal or bowel)	5B: Rectal injury or compromise	5C: Small or large bowel injury or compromise	5D (+)
6 SKIN AND/OR MUSCULOSKELETAL Complications including discharge pain lump or sinus tract formation	6A: Asymptomatic, abnormal finding or clinical examination	6B: Symptomatic e.g. discharge, pain or lump	6C: Infection e.g. sinus tract formation	6D (+)
7 PATIENT: Compromise including hematoma or systemic compromise	7A: Bleeding complication including hematoma	7B: Major degree of resuscitation or intensive care	7C: Mortality* *additional complication *no site applicable-S0)	

TIME (CLINICALLY DIAGNOSED)			
T1: Intraoperative to 48 hours	T2: 48 hours to 2 months	T3: 2 months to 12 months	T4: Over 12 months
SITE			
S1: Vaginal area of suture line	S2: Vaginal: away from area of suture line.	S3: Trocar passage Exception: Intra-abdominal(S5)	S4: Other skin or musculoskeletal site

Table 3. A Classification of complications related directly to the insertion of prosthesis (meshes, implants, tapes) or graft in female pelvic floor surgery.

To specify the presence of pain (by the patient only, not the partner) as part or all of the abnormal findings and the grade in terms of presence and severity of symptoms	
a	Asymptomatic or no pain
b	Provoked pain only (during vaginal examination)
c	Pain during sexual intercourse
d	Pain during physical activities
e	Spontaneous pain.

Table 4. Grades of pain: Sub classification of complication category

4. Pathophysiology

Jeffry et al (2001) reported that the bladder lesion rate due to perforation, increased in patients who had a prior anti-incontinence surgical procedure, this is due to the retropubic scarring process, and they also observed that the bladder perforation site is greater on the opposite side of the surgeon's dominating hand.

Is a bladder lesion never observed during cystoscopy? Not really. Buchsbaum et al in (2004) reported that when they discarded the presence of bladder lesion after a cystoscopy, they found fluid leak through the incision or through the trocar path. Therefore, it is important to perform an appropriate bladder distension in order to separate the bladder folds and discard or confirm this complication appropriately. If necessary, methylene blue or indigo carmine can be used.

What is the anatomical relationship between vascular anatomy and placement of trocars in the insertion of a TVT? Muir et al (2003) did an anatomical dissection in cadavers and found that the TVT trocar goes through at an average distance of 4.9 cm from the external iliac artery and 3.2 cm from the obturator vessels, therefore, when the trocar goes in deviated laterally, it can cause an injury to the external iliac artery or vein. An inadequate technique when the trocar is inserted can cause severe complications.

Is the patient's position as well as position of the legs important to avoid complications? Yes. Whiteside et al (2004) reported the anatomy of the neurovascular bundle in relation to the obturator fossa when the TOT is placed; the trocar goes through at a 1.1 ± 0.4 cm average distance from the medial branch of the obturator vessels and the average distance to the obturator nerve is 2.5 ± 0.7 cm. Hubka et al (2010) reported in a study of 14 embalmed bodies with poor position of the legs (group 1), 5 fresh frozen bodies with poor leg position (group 2) and 5 fresh frozen bodies with the proper leg position (group 3). After dissection, they measured the rami of the obturator nerve; in group 1, the average distance of the anterior ramus of the obturator nerve was at 8.4 mm (left) and at 8.9 mm (right). In group 2 the average was 5 mm (left) and at 8 mm (right) and the posterior ramus of the obturator nerve was at 5 mm (left) and 8 mm (right) respectively. In group 3, the average distance of the anterior ramus of the obturator nerve was 24mm (left) and 23 mm (right). Therefore, the correct position of the patient and of the legs ensures proper placement of the TVT-O.

Several factors have been proposed for complications with these kits: broad dissection with devascularization of the vaginal tissue, estrogen deficiency, excess tension, and presence of subclinical or overt infection before surgery, poor placement of the patient's legs during surgery, poor knowledge of the surgical technique to place the kits and smoking.

Atis et al (2009) did an assessment in rats to see the reaction produced by the materials of the different slings in the bladder through histopathology (TVT, Vypro mesh, intravaginal plastic sling: IVS); they studied 30 rats with a similar control group, through laparotomy they placed a 0.5 to 1 cm mesh on the anterior bladder wall; after 12 weeks they did a hystopathological test of the bladder. They found signs of inflammation, reaction to a foreign body, subserous fibrosis, necrosis and different degrees of collagen deposits. The Kruskal-Wallis and Posthoc Dunn tests were performed, observing that the inflammatory process was greater in the IVS (p= 0.001) group than in the TVT (p= 0.006) group, and Vypro (p=0.031); this IVS group also showed greater subserous fibrosis (p=0.0001); reaction to a foreign body (p=0.0001) and more collagen deposit (p=0.0001). The bladder showed a greater inflammatory response in the IVS group than in the TVT and Vypro (p=0.041, p=0.028) groups. This can play an important role in the results or complications of the slings.

But et al (2005) reported the probability of the mesh migrating and thus presenting some of the complications mentioned above. We should recall that meshes are a foreign object in the body and there may be a response to these.

Other causes may be that the kit is placed with greater tension than necessary, the quality of the tissue may be poor for several reasons such as: estrogen deficiency or due to poor dissection that leaves tissue with significant devascularization and thus with less blood irrigation which causes a deficiency in the fibroblast migration, in angiogenesis and therefore complications may arise. Surgeons who are going to place any of these devices should be well aware of the neurovascular anatomy of the pelvis as well as of the recommendations to place the chosen device.

Letouzey et al (2011) in an experimental study in rats, used macropore and multifilament polypropylene mesh contaminated with Escherichia Coli, removing it after 30 days. They concluded that the mesh infection forms a bacterial film that acts as a lining and this may be associated to prosthetic erosion without observing changes in the polymer of the mesh. Same results have Mamy et al (2011) highlights a link between infection and shrinkage in the model used (rats).

Withagen et al (2011) reported the risk factors associated to mesh exposure after insertion of the TVT in patients with pelvic organ prolapse; 12 months later only 294 (79%) patients were studied. The risk factors identified were smoking with a RR of 3.08 (IC 95% 1.09-8.72); the surgeons lack of experience (< than 10 years) RR 0.49 (IC 95% 0.29-0.83) and placement of a total Prolift RR 2.95 (IC 95% 1.24-7.01) although this is prolapse information, the TVT mesh was used.

5. Complications

We will divide complications into: intra-operative and post-operative (immediate and late).

5.1 Intra-operative complications

5.1.1 Bladder and urethral lesions

Abouassaly et al (2004) analyzed surgical complications of the tension free tape (TVT) in six institutions; the procedures were carried out by 6 different urologists. They checked the management of each complication and the patient outcomes. Of the 241 patients, complications during surgery were bladder perforation in 48 patients (5.8%). Andonian et al (2005) compared SPARC with TVT reporting a similar percentage in both groups 24% and 23% respectively. Kristensen et al (2010) reported that out of 778 patients there was bladder perforation in 51 (6.6%). Lee et al (2010) reported 141 patients, with 9 patients (6.4%) having bladder perforation. When Novara et al (2010) in a systematic review of pubovaginal sling, retropubic tape (RT) and transobturator tape (TOT), made a comparison between procedures they reported that the TOT has less risk of bladder or vaginal perforation (OR: 2.5 IC: 1.75-3.57; $p<0.00001$); but Revicky et al (2011) reported in 342 women with TVT, that the incidence of bladder lesion was 4.7% (16/342). Pushkay et al (2011) reported in 577 patients a high incidence of bladder perforation in the TVT group vs. the TVO-O group (5.4% vs. 0.6%; $p=0.001$) George et al (2010) reported bladder perforation in 1.3% of the TVT group and none in the TOT group. Barry et al (2011) in a multicentric, randomized trial comparing TVT- Monarc at 3 months follow up, report a bladder lesion in 7/140 patients with TVT and 0/140 patients with Monarc. Rajendra et al (2011) reported 419 patients with stress urinary incontinence at 3 years follow up, 2 patients (0.5%) with bladder perforation. Latthe et al (2010) in his systematic review of 4 articles, report that bladder lesions with the TOT procedure have an OR 0.11 (IC 95% 0.05-0.25) and TVTO has an OR of 0.15 (IC 95% 0.06-0.35).

Bladder perforation during surgery due to the trocars is reported at 1.3% by George et al (2010) and up to 22% during the learning curve phase as described by Lebret et al (2001).

Up to date there have been no reports of uretheral lesion during surgery.

Alvárez-Bandrés et al (2010) reported complications with the mini-sling system (50 patients with TVT-secur and 105 with Miniarc), there were bladder perforations in 0.64% total in both groups which were resolved with conservative bladder drainage management.

6. Bleeding

Primicero et al (1999) reported one lesion of the external iliac vein in a patient with TVT which had to be repaired through laparotomy; Zilbert and Farrel (2001) reported one patient with laceration of the external iliac artery and a neurovascular bundle lesion of the obturator ramus when the TVT was applied. Kuuva and Nilssons (2002) reported in 1455 patients a lesion incidence of large vessels and nerves in 2 patients (0.1%). Flock et al (2004) reported in 7 patients with TVT, blood loss quantified at 250 to 400 ml (2.1%); Abouassaly et al (2004) reported major bleeding of 500 ml in 16 women (2.5%) (16/421) with TVT. Kristensen et al (2010) in 778 patients with TVT reported hemorrhage that needed transfusion in 5 patients (0.6%), Barry et al (2011) observed that bleeding is minor in the group of patients with Monarc, 49 ml; in the TVT group it was 64 ml ($p < 0.05$), likewise surgical time was 14.6 min with Monarc and 18.5 min with TVT ($p < 0.001$). Rajendra et al (2011) reported that of 419 patients with TVT-O, 3 patients (0.8%) had a blood loss over 200 ml. Dunn et al (2004) reported 30 cases with vascular injury including 2 fatalities.

Brink (2000) reported one case of intestinal lesion that was repaired with a good outcome for the patient. Although we have minimally invasive procedures, these also pose arterial complications as Jung et al (2010) reported in a patient with TVT-secur who presented a lesion of the internal pudendal artery. The complication was resolved with embolization of the artery guided with angiography, the treatment was successful. Jabureck et al (2011) documented that retropubic access surgery has a high lesion incidence of paraurethral, bladder and paravesical plexus vessels and even external iliac vessels.

7. Nerve lesion

Kuuva and Nilsson (2002) reported a nerve lesion 0.7/1000 with the placement of TVT.

7.1 Immediate post-surgical complications

7.1.1 Hematomas

Abouassaly et al (2004) reported a pelvic hematoma in 4 (1.9%) patients with TVT (4/421), Andonian et al (2005) reported a single case of an infected pelvic hematoma in the SPARC group and none in the TVT group. Pushky et al (2011) found that the formation of a hematoma is more frequent with TVT than with TVT-O (9.1% vs. 1.5%; p=0.001). Flock et al (2011) reported successful treatment of hematomas with retziusscopy in patients with TVT, of 685 patients, only 28 (4.1%) had a symptomatic hematoma in the Retzius space and in only 10 cases (1.5%) the volume exceeded 250 ml (range of 250-1000ml), the first case was resolved through laparotomy but the other cases were resolved successfully with a drainage through a retziusopy; this is a minimally invasive procedure. Latthe et al (2010) in a systematic review of 12 papers observed that the formation of hematomas is lower with the TOT procedure compared with the TVT with an OR of 0.06 (IC 95% 0.01-0.30). When Alvárez-Bandrés et al (2010) compared TVT -secur and Miniarc; they reported one case of hematoma of the obturator fossa (0.64%) in the Miniarc group, which resolved spontaneously.

8. Voiding disorders

Abouassaly et al (2004) reported urinary retention (>24 hours later) in 47 patients (19.7%). Of the 47 patients, retention was present in only 32 less than 48 hours later, which were managed with clean intermittent catheterization, the remaining 15 patients also had clean intermittent catheterization for several days and only one patient had catheterization for 22 days. In order to resolve retention in 7 patients, the mesh had to be released and in 3 patients the mesh had to be cut. Kristensen et al (2010) reported difficulty in voiding in 56% and 16.6% had urinary retention, 34.3% of the patients had catheterization and 8% needed continuous catheterization. They conclude that patients who had voiding dysfunction prior to surgery have an OR of 1.80 to present urinary retention post surgically. Lee et al (2010) reported that 10 patients with TVT surgery, (7.1%) had urinary retention after surgery; patients were treated with clean intermittent catheterization less than 1 week, 10 patients (7.1%) needed continuous catheterization and in 2 patients the TVT mesh had to be cut. George et al (2010) reported voiding difficulty with a follow up of 2 years; in the TVT group 9.3% it lasted less than one week and in 2.6% it lasted more than one week. In the TOT group, the voiding dysfunction was 4.1% less than 1 week and 1.4% more than 1 week. Bladder perforation has a higher incidence in the TVT group. Revicky et al (2011) reported urinary retention in 9% (31/342). Sun and Tsai (2011) reported a voiding dysfunction frequency of 6.8% with MONARC (5/73). Latthe et al (2010) in a systematic review of voiding disorder it is slightly lower in the TOT group than in the TVT-O group, but it wasn't statistically significant; for TOT the OR was 0.61 (IC 95% 0.35-1.07) and for TVT-O the OR was 0.81 (IC 95% 0.48-1.31

9. Infection

Abouassaly et al (2004) reported infection of the supra pubic wound in one patient (0.4%). Kristensen et al (2010) reported infection of the urinary tract in 3.1%.

Flam et al (2009) had a patient with necrotizing fasciitis after placement of the TVT-O; they performed extensive debridement of the affected site, a colostomy, antibiotic therapy and 8 sessions of hyperbaric oxygen. Fig. 1

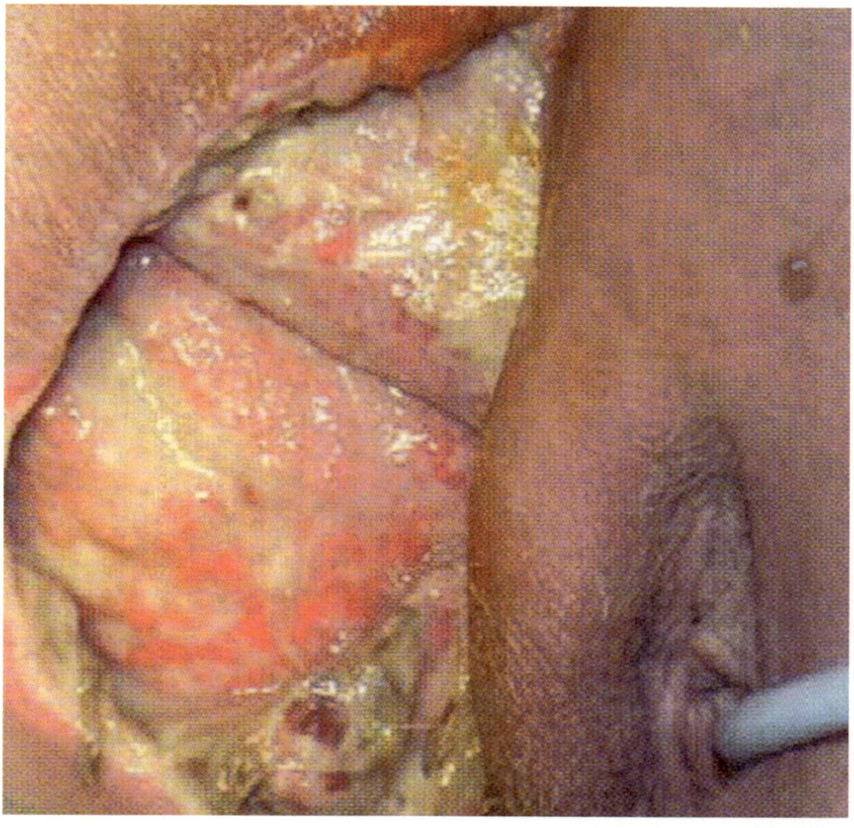

Fig. 1. 65-year-old with urinary incontinence, underwent a multifilament transobturator sling. At 14 months follow up, she experienced severe pelvic pain and vaginal discharge. Clinical examination revealed hyperthermia to 40°C, sling exposure at right vaginal sulcus and severe cellulitis in the genital-crural fold: Classification: 3C T4 S 2 and 6C T4 S3

Lee et al(2011) in four of the five patients presented with symptom of chronic vaginal discharge and these patients have a chronic infection forming a sinus tract into the vagina or other viscus, causing symptoms years after its mesh placement.

10. Late complications

10.1 De novo urgency

Abouassaly et al (2004) reported de novo urgency in 36 patients (15%), Lleberia-Juanós et al (2011) determined the incidence of de novo urgency with VT (in 243 patients) and with TVT-O (123 patients) evaluating them at 1, 6, 12 and 36 months after surgery. De novo urgency occurs in 13.4% of patients at 6 months, in 19.3 at 12 months and in 22.1% at 36 months. De novo urgency was more frequent in the TVT group than in the TVT-O group at 12 months (22.2% vs. 11.2%, P=0.025) and at 24 months (24.8% vs. 12.3%, P=0.033). Lee et al (2010) after 6 years of observation reported that de novo urgency was present in 28% (30/107) and de novo overactive bladder with incontinence was present in 27.1% (29/107) of patients. Sun and Tsai (2011) reported a frequency of de novo urgency of 2.7% with MONARC (2/73). Sabadell et al (2011) reported that 23 patients failed to TOT and a TVT was placed in a second surgery; de novo urgency occurs in 5 cases (21.7%) and it is treated with oral anticholinergics with a good clinical response.

11. Voiding disorders

Rajendra et al (2011) reported after a 3 year follow up, that 11 patients with TVT-O (2.6%) (11/419) were readmitted since 10 patients had voiding dysfunction, in 6 patients it was necessary to remove or cut the tape. Reich et al (2011) reported it in 108 patients in a follow up period of 102 months (range of 85-124). They did not find adverse effects of the mesh; 90% of these patients presented urgency incontinence and were dissatisfied with the surgical procedure. The same group studied 478 with TVT and voiding dysfunction, documenting it by measuring residual volume pre and post surgery; they reported micturition dysfunction in the first 2 weeks in 4 patients (0.8%), 7.1% had a residual volume of 50-100 ml at 3 months of surgery and 2.6% had a residual urine volume of over 100 ml. Therefore, a total of 93% of patients did not show bladder voiding disorders after a follow up of 12 to 74 months, which was documented through translabial ultrasound. Alvárez-Bandrés et al (2010) reported that the Miniarc group had urethral obstruction and thus the mesh had to be cut.

12. Pain and suprapubic discomfort

Abouassaly et al (2004) reported persisting suprapubic discomfort in 18 (7.5%) (18/241 patients). Rajendra et al (2011) after following up 419 patients for 3 years reported persistent pain in 15 patients (3.6%). Ross et al (2009) reported 199 patients, 105 of these had a TVT inserted and 94 patients had a TVT-O; they documented in the vaginal examination that the mesh was palpable in 68 (80%) in the TVT-O group and in 24 (27%) of the TVT group (RR 0.22, CI 95% 0.13-0.37, P<.001); many women are also experiencing groin pain during vaginal palpation, 13 patients (15%) in the TVT-O group and 5 patients (6%) in the TVT group.

Latthe et al (2010) did a systematic review reporting that groin and/or thigh pain with the TVT-O procedure has an OR of 8.05 (IC 95% 3.78-17.16).

When Alvárez-Bandrés et al (2010) compared TVT-secur and Miniarc; the Miniarc group reported 4 (2.5%) patients with groin pain who were treated successfully with NSAID's.

12.1 Mesh extrusion

Abouassaly et al (2004) reported one patient with mesh erosion intravaginally (0.4%) (1/241); Andonian et al (2005) reported a single case of erosion in the SPARC group (1/41) and none in the TVT group (0/43). During the first year of follow up Rajendra et al (2011) reported vaginal erosion in 2.4 % (10/419); Ortega et al (2009) reported 1 case of erosion/extrusion of the mesh toward the urethra, the mesh was resected transvaginally with a good outcome. Wijffels et al (2009) reported 3 patients with urethral erosion/extrusion, treated by resection of the mesh endoscopically; Matsumura et al (2010) reported that after 2 years of surgery a 72 year old patient had an erosion/extrusion of the mesh in the urethra and a stone in the same site; management was done endoscopically with resection of the mesh and the stone was treated with lithotripsy with a good response.

Latthe et al (2010) in a systematic review reported that the mesh erosion of TVT-O has an OR 0.77 (IC 95% 0.22-2.72), while TOT and TVT have an almost similar OR 1.11 (IC 95% 0.54-2.28) Fig. 2

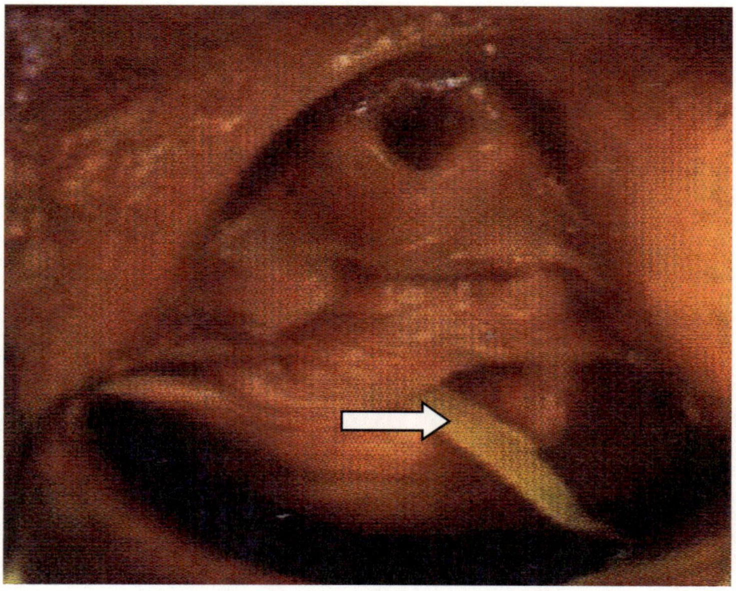

Fig. 2. A 47-years-old woman underwent a transobturator tape for USI. At 5 months follow-up, she reported vaginal discharge. Clinically she was febrile at 38ºC with a large sling extrusion as depicted. Classification: 3C T3 S1

When Alvárez-Bandrés et al (2010) compared TVT-secur and Miniarc they reported vaginal erosion in 8 patients (5%); 4 patients required removal and closure of the vaginal wall, 2 were treated with local estrogen therapy in the vagina and 2 were asymptomatic and did not require any treatment.

Lo and Nusse (2010) reported a rare case of erosion over the bladder dome with formation of a stone 11 years after insertion of the TVT. Diagnosis was made with cystoscopy after the patient referred symptoms of the lower urinary tract for 5 months. A cysto-lithotripsy was performed observing a small filament of the mesh that was removed. A control cystoscopy was made after one year showing recurrence of a stone in the same site of the previous surgery; surgery was performed in the office since the patient refused major surgery. Siegel (2006) reported one case of urethral necrosis and a urethra-vaginal fistula in a 64 year old woman, who needed 3 surgeries; initially TVT mesh fragments were removed and adjacent tissue needed debridement. A urethroplasty was performed as a second surgical procedure and in the third surgery a coaptation with an occlusive sling was made to repair the continence.

E Kobashi's (2009) reviewed the different materials and reported the rate of extrusion of these. Table 5.

Material	Fiber type	Pore Size	Extrusion Rate (%)
Silicone	Monofilament	Macro	40-71
TVT	Monofilament	Macro	2-3
Prolapse repair	Monofilament	Macro	Up to 26
Obtape	Monofilament	Micro	5.4-16.6
Sparc/Monarc	Monofilament	Macro	1.7-2.4

Table 5. Synthetic mesh types, Characteristics and Associated Vaginal Extrusion rates.

Miraliakbari and Tse (2011) reported the first case of ureteral erosion in a 78 year old woman, the erosion was located in the distal third of the ureter, and the patient was treated successfully.

Rouprêt et al (2010) reported resection of the mesh via laparoscopy in 38 women with bladder erosion, vaginal extrusion, bladder obstruction and groin pain. The resection was complete with an operating time of 110 minutes (50 to 240 minute range) all patients reported a decrease in symptoms in a follow up period of 37.9 months (2-80 months range). However, the incontinence recurrence rate is 65.7% (25 patients). Laparoscopic resection of the TVT is safe and technically possible and solves patient's symptoms.

Novara et al (2010) did a systematic review of pubovaginal sling; retropubic tape (RT) and transobturator tape (TOT) the subjective cure rate is similar among those procedures. Patients who have a TOT inserted have less risk of bladder or vaginal perforation (OR: 2.5 IC: 1.75-3.57; $p<0.00001$); less risk of hematoma (OR: 2.62; CI: 1.35-5.08; $p=0.005$) and less risk of urinary tract injury (OR: 1.35; CI: 1.05-1.72; $p=0.02$). This meta-analysis showed similar results between TVT-O and Monarc. The use of a retropubic tape had a higher objective rate than TOT, but the subjective cure is similar for both.

Mendoca et al (2011) report two cases with late urethral erosion with transobturator suburethral mesh (Obtape) the first one diagnosed 1 year after the surgery and the second one, a very late complication, occurring 4 years after the placement of the sling.

13. Intestinal lesion

With an intestinal lesion, patients refer abdominal pain, peritoneal irritation and sometimes fecal matter leak through the incisions of the kit used (TVT) as was reported by Meschia et al

(2002); Leboeuf et al (2003) and Castillo et al (2004). Leboeuf et al (2004) did a vaginal hysterectomy in a 73 year old patient due to genital prolapse followed by insertion of a TVT, during the post-op period she presented abdominal distension, and in an axial CAT scan they observed bowel distention and the bowel lesion site; they did an exploratory laparotomy where they found perforation of the mesentery without no other lesion, the perforation was repaired without complications.

Phillips et al (2009) reported a small size, thin patient with clinical signs of intestinal obstruction 3 years after the insertion of a TVT; she underwent an exploratory laparotomy where they found that the TVT mesh went through the peritoneum and was attached to the distal ileus; they did a resection and a primary anastomosis.

14. Nerve lesion

Geis and Dietl (2002) reported an ilioinguinal nerve lesion after insertion of a TVT, this due to the closeness of the nerve to the sites where the suprapubic incision was made. Rigaud et al (2010) said that pelvic or perineal pain may be a consequence of the obturator nerve or pudendal nerve lesion, a clinical sign that is underestimated.

15. Sexual function

Lau et al (2010) evaluated the impact of TVT-O insertion on sexual function in 56 women; they were evaluated through short questionnaires PISQ-12, UDI-16 and the IIQ7 before and 6 months after surgery. Their conclusion was that women perceived the surgery was successful but there was no improvement in sexual function.

16. Success and failure

Jain et al (2011) did a systematic review of TVT and TOT in the treatment of Mixed Urinary Incontinence (MUI). The subjective cure rate in 7 prospective trials was 56.4% (IC 95% 45.7-69.6%) in a follow up period of 34.9±22.9 months. The cure rate for stress urinary incontinence varied from 85% to 97% in a follow up period of 6 to 31 months. TVT and TOT have a similar cure in mixed urinary incontinence. Madhuvrata et al (2011) in a systematic review and meta-analysis of the mini-sling (SIMS) compared the retropubic procedure: TVT (9 studies were included) and TVT-O (7 studies were included). The objective short term cure rate (6-12 months) was greater in urethral sling procedures than in mini-slings (SIMS) with a RR 1.20 (IC 95% 1.01-1.43) and RR 1.18 (IC 95% 1.04-1.34); a second surgery was necessary in the SIMS group with a RR 0.15 (IC 95% 0.05-0.42). Novara et al (2010) in a systematic review and meta-analysis of 39 papers reported that patients who had a sub-urethral mesh inserted the objective cure rate had an OR: 0.38 (IC95% 0.25-0.57; p=<0.0001) compared to the patients who had a Burch colpo-suspension procedure, although they had a high bladder perforation risk with an OR of 4.94 (IC 95% 2.09-11.68; p= 0.00003). Patil (2011) in a total of 12977 surgeries performed in 68 centers in the United Kingdom, 313 patients (2.4%) failed to sub-urethral slings. Chen et al (2011) in 30 patients followed up 1 year, who had a TVT-secur inserted, the success rate decreased significantly from 83.3% one month after surgery to 60.0% one year after the procedure.

17. Risk factors for surgical failure

Abdel-Fattah et al (2010) did a randomized report of 341 patients who had an outside-in transobturator (TOT-ARIS) and an inside-out (TVT-O). The risk factors for failure in the insertion of these meshes are: prior incontinence surgery (OR 1.41; 95% CI 1.18, 1.91; P = 0.029), preoperative urgency urinary incontinence (OR 1.78; 95% CI 1.21, 3.91, P = 0.048) during the first year of follow up of these surgeries.

Revicky et al (2011) evaluated the following risk factors to predict failure of the procedure: body mass index (BMI), age, type of analgesia, concomitant prolapse repair or prior surgery and obesity. These factors were not related to bladder injury or to urinary retention. Liu et al (2011) reported that obesity was not a risk factor for surgical failure just like Revicky reported in his review.

When Pushkar et al (2011) evaluated risk factors like age, body mass index and parity; there was no correlation with the complications of TVT and TVT-O.

18. Diagnosis

All patients who have had any of the anti-incontinence kits available in the market placed through the following procedures: retropubic, transobturator, outside-in or inside-out, or any minimally invasive kit, should be followed up long term since complications have been observed up to 11 years after insertion.

For intra-operative complications it is necessary to observe the patient's vitals: heart rate, blood pressure, oxygen saturation, state of awareness, so that if a disturbance is observed in any of these parameters, any necessary additional tests can be performed; like clinical labs to diagnose a vascular complication. A cystoscopy should be performed to assess the entire bladder with proper distention (250 cc minimum of physiologic solution) and with the proper instrument like a 70^0 lens cystoscope in order to check the bladder dome and lateral bladder walls; and for the urethra a 0^0 or 30^0 lens. In the event of doubt we can use methylene blue or indigo carmine to identify any damage that may be overlooked. Hematomas are identified according to the amount or size of the hematoma, it can go from mild pain, ecchimosis or hemorrhage through the puncture sites; this can be confirmed with imaging tests (ultrasound, axial CAT scan, MRI) depending on the patient's clinical status.

For post-operative complications: signs and symptoms of a patient who refers voiding disorders, residual urine should be measured using a clean bladder catheter or with translabial or suprapubic ultrasound in order to measure urine. De novo urgency can be documented by asking the patient directly and with a multichannel Urodynamic or Video-Urodynamic test, depending on the discomfort reported by the patient. During the patient's visit to the office, the vagina and urethra must be checked to discard any extrusion complications. A cystoscopy, a urethroscopy or an additional test must be performed depending on the symptoms reported by the patient. If the patient shows any irritation symptoms in the lower urinary tract or in the bowel, hematuria, dispareunia, discomfort reported by the spouse, voiding disorders, pain, recurring infections, palpation of the mesh or recurring urinary incontinence, the integrity of the urinary tract and adjacent organs must be documented. If a patient has an intestinal injury, they will refer abdominal pain, signs of peritoneal irritation and sometimes leak of fecal matter through the incision of the kit used.

Rigaud et al (2010) said that when the patient refers perineal pain or chronic pelvic pain, immediately or shortly after insertion of a TVT or TOT Kit, this is probably associated directly or indirectly to a nerve injury (obturator nerve or pudendal nerve); diagnosis is made with the history that pain started after insertion of the kit and it can be confirmed with infiltration of local anesthesia through the mesh. This complication may be underestimated.

18.1 Treatment

Treatment of complications with these kits is still not standardized and it is something we will have to work on. When complications are severe, a multidisciplinary team is necessary to provide the best treatment and obtain favorable results for the patient.

18.2 Treatment of intra-operative complications

Complications due to punctures are caused by the passage of the kit's trocar, it can injure the urethra or the bladder, therefore, during the retropubic inside-out or outside-in procedure, a cystoscopy using a 70^0 lens should be performed in order to see the dome of the bladder and lateral walls; and a 0^0 to 30^0 lens to properly evaluate the urethra; so that under this direct view we can see whether the trocar is inside the bladder or urethra before placing the mesh. In the event the trocar punctures the bladder or urethra, it can be removed and inserted again. If there is no evidence of puncture to the urethra and/or bladder, it is now possible to place the mesh and a cystoscopy should be repeated. In the event of bladder injury, the size of the puncture should be measured and if small, a continuous drainage should be left with a Foley catheter for 48 to 72 hours. When the bladder damage is larger, a primary repair is necessary with 2 layers of absorbing suture (vicryl) and a continuous drainage using a Foley Catheter for 5 to 7 days should also be placed.

Flock et al (2011) reported 7 patients with TVT who had hemorrhage of 250ml to 400 ml that was managed with cautherization, compression or tamponade. Zorn et al (2005) recommend an exploratory laparotomy to repair the vascular damage and for proper hemostasis, or an embolization in patients who present massive bleeding after placement of the TVT; if we have this technique it provides good results.

Hubka et al (2010) recommend the patient be placed in a proper position in order to stay away from the obturator neurovascular bundle, this way, the success rate increases and the number of neurovascular damage decrease.

18.3 Treatment of post-operative complications

Abouassaly et al (2004) recommend in patients with voiding dysfunctions, the use of clean intermittent catheterization and if it has to be for a longer period of time, the mesh must be released, and in patients who continue with voiding disorders the mesh must be cut.

Abouassaly et al (2004) reported that when an infectious process arises, a culture must be performed and antibiotics should be prescribed depending on the sensitivity obtained; and as reported by Flam et al (2009) hyperbaric oxygen can be used to improve oxygenation of the tissue involved with excellent results. Abouassaly et al (2004) recommend for intravaginal mesh erosion, partial resection of the meshes and repair of the vaginal epithelium if the patient refers symptoms if not, she can just be observed as reported by

Alvárez-Bandrés et al (2010). Giri et al (2007) recommend a primary closure of the vaginal mucosa with a single line of a polyglactine 910, 2/0 suture avoiding inversion of the mucosa, when there is extrusion of the TVT mesh toward the vagina.

Rouprêt et al (2010) reported surgical resection of the mesh through laparoscopy, in 38 women with complications like: bladder erosion, vaginal extrusion, bladder obstruction and groin pain. Resection was complete in all patients through laparoscopy; with an operating time of 110 minutes (range of 50 to 240 minutes) all patients reported a decrease in symptoms in a follow up period of 37.9 months (range 2-80 months). However, the recurrence rate of incontinence was 65.7% (25 patients). Laparoscopic resection of the TVT is safe and technically possible and solves patient's symptoms if we have the necessary instruments as well as trained personnel since it is a minimally invasive treatment alternative. In patients with de novo urgency, the use of anticholinergics is necessary to improve the patient's quality of life and in patients who report pelvic or perineal pain we can prescribe NSAID's.

When there is mesh extrusion and there is no satisfactory response to primary management such as the use of antibiotics or application of local estrogen in the organ extruded; the appropriate management is to remove the mesh. Fig 3. Removal of the mesh has been performed vaginally, via the urethra or the ureter through cystoscopy or laparoscopy with a good success rate and it is a minimally invasive procedure.

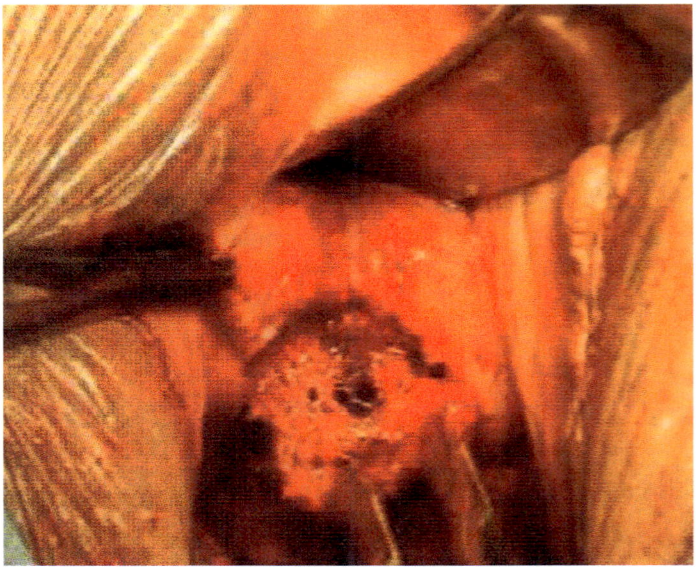

Fig. 3. The appropriated management is to remove the mesh when there is no satisfactory response to primary management.

Lo and Nusse (2010) recommend that in patients who have had a TVT or any other kit inserted to treat urinary incontinence and who show irritation symptoms of the lower urinary tract, a cystoscopy must be done to discard the presence of the mesh in the vagina, the urethra or in any other organ. If an intestinal injury is suspected, additional imaging test should be performed to document the injury and an exploratory laparotomy will be necessary to repair the injury, with an intestinal resection and/or colostomy depending on the lesion found.

Rigaud et al (2010) said that for the treatment of pelvic or perineal pain we can infiltrate local anesthesia throughout the mesh or in the nerves involved, thus achieving temporary clinical improvement. However, although there was improvement in 2 of their 3 patients, the mesh had to be removed.

Mendoca et al(2011) describe a minimally invasive trans-urethral approach for the urethral erosion under local anaesthesia. They present some "tricks of the trade" on retrieving the tape trans-urethrally while maximizing the length of tape removed.

Khong and Lam (2011) in nine patients with synthetic mesh erosion when failed to respond to conservative measures were managed surgically with Surgisis. The size erosion ranged from 1 to 4 cm in diameter. The Surgisis may prove to be a useful option in the treatment of large vaginal mesh defects.

19. Conclusion

Whenever a surgical procedure involving the use of a mesh for urinary incontinence (any sort of mesh found in the market), the patient and her family must be informed about risks and complications. It is also important to have an informed consent for the patient stating the incidence of each of the complications pertaining to the specific kit used. Surgeons should follow patients at long term, since many complications occur after a long time, and they should be prepared to act quickly and effectively to solve the complication that has arisen. The use of new technology has improved the success rate of the surgical procedures for urinary incontinence, but clinically and legally, surgeons are the ones that should determine the use of these new devices and not the representatives of the commercial houses. We suggest that all suburethral slings are not created equal and that clinical adoption of new technology should follow clinical trials demonstrating efficacy, safety and long-term outcomes.

20. References

Abdel-Fattah M, Ramsay I, Pringle S, Hardwick C, Ali H, et al(2010). Randomised prospective single-blinded study comparing 'inside-out' versus 'outside-in' transobturator tapes in the management of urodynamic stress incontinence: 1-year outcomes from the E-TOT study. *BJOG.*;117(7):870-8.

Abouassaly R, Steinberg JR, Lemieux M, Marois C, Gilchrist LI, et al. (2004) Complications of tension-free vaginal tape surgery: a multi-institutional review. *BJU Int.* 94(1):110-3.

Alvarez-Bandrés S, Hualde-Alfaro A, Jiménez-Calvo J, Cebrián-Lostal JL, Jiménez-Parra JD, et al. (2010).Complications of female urinary incontinence surgery with mini-sling system. Actas Urol Esp. 34(10):893-7.

Andonian S, Chen T, St Denis B and Corcos J. (2005). Randomized clinical trial comparing suprapubic arc (SPARC) and tension-free vaginal tape (TVT): one year results. *Eur Urol* 47(4):537-41.

Atherton MJ,Stanton SL.(2005)The tension-free vaginal tape reviewed:an evidence -based review from inception to current status.BJOG. 112 (5):534-46.

Atis G, Arisan S, Ozagari A, Caskurlu T, Dalkilinc A, et al (2009). Tissue reaction of the rat urinary bladder to synthetic mesh materials. ScientificWorldJournal. 2;9:1046-51.

Barry C, Lim YN, Muller R, Hitchins S, Corstiaans A, Foote A, Greenland H, Frazer M, Rane A (2008) . A multi-centre, randomized clinical control trial comparing the retropubic (RP) approach versus the transobturator approach (TO) for tension-free, suburethral sling treatment of urodynamic stress incontinence: The TORP study. *Int Urogynecol J Pelvic Floor Dysfunct* 19(2):171-8.

Brink DM.(2000) Bowel injury following insertion of tension-free vaginal tape. S Afr Med J. May; 90(5):450-52.

Buchsbaum GM, Moll C, Duecy EE. (2004) True occult bladder perforation during placement of tension-free vaginal tape. *Int Urogynecol J Pelvic Floor Dysfunct* 15:432.

But I, Bratus D, Faganelj M. (2005) Prolene tape in the bladder wall after TVT procedure-intramural tape placement or secondary tape migration? *Int Urogynecol J Pelvic Floor Dysfunct* 16(1): 75-76.

Castillo OA, Bodden E, Olivares RA, et al . (2004) Intestinal perforation: An infrequent complication during insertion of tension-free vaginal tape. *J Urol* 172:1364.

Chen YH, Wang YJ, Li FP, Wang Q. (2011) Efficacy and postoperative complication of tension-free vaginal tape-Secur for female stress urinary incontinence. Chin Med J 124(9):1296-9.

Delorme E, Droupy S, de Tayrac R, Delmas V.(2004) Transobturator tape (Uratape): A new minimally invasive procedure to treat female urinary incontinence. *Eur Urol* 45:203–7.

Dunn JS Jr, Bent AE, Ellerkman RM, Nihira MA, Melick CF. (2004) Voiding dysfunction after surgery for stress incontinence: literature review and survey results. *Int Urogynecol J Pelvic Floor Dysfunct* 15(1):25 -31.

Flam F, Boijsen M, Lind F.(2009) Necrotizing fasciitis following transobturator tape treated by extensive surgery and hyperbaric oxygen. *Int Urogynecol J Pelvic Floor Dys* 20(1):113-5.

Flock F, Reich A, Muche R, et al (2004) Hemorrhagic complications associated with tension-free vaginal tape procedure. Obstet Gynecol 104: 989-94.

Flock F, Kohorst F, Kreienberg R, Reich A.(2011) Retziusscopy: a minimal invasive technique for the treatment of retropubic hematomas after TVT procedure. Eur J Obstet Gynecol Reprod Biol. Sep;158(1):101-3.

Geis K, Dietl J. (2002) Illioinguinal nerve entrapment after tension-free vaginal tape (TVT) procedure. Int Urogynecol J Pelvic Floor Dysfunction 13:136.

George S, Begum R, Thomas-Philip A, Thirumalakumar L, Sorinola O.(2010) Two-year comparison of tension-free vaginal tape and transobturator tape for female urinary stress incontinence. J Obstet Gynaecol 30(3):281-4.

Giri SK, N Arsimhulu G,Flood HD, Skehan M and Drumm J (2007) Management of vaginal extrusion after tension-free vaginal tape procedure for urodynamic stress incontinence. *Urology* 69(6):1077-1080.

Haylen BT, Freeman RM, Swift SE, Cosson M, Davila GW,et al.(2011) An International Urogynecological Association (IUGA)/ International Continence Society(ICS) joint terminology and classification of the complications related directly to the insertion of prostheses(meshes, implants, tapes) & grafts in female pelvic floor surgery. *Int Urogynecol J* 22:3-15.

Hubka P, Nanka O, Martan A, Svabik K, Zvarova J, Masata J.(2010) Anatomical study of position of the TVT-O to the obturator nerve influenced by the position of the legs during the procedure: based upon findings at formalin-embalmed and fresh-frozen bodies. Arch Gynecol Obstet 284(4):901-5.

Jaburek L, Jaburkova J, Lubusky M, Prochazka M.(2011) Risk of haemorrhagic complications of retropubic surgery in females: anatomic remarks. Biomed Pap Med Fac Univ Palacky Olomouc Czech Repub.Mar;155(1):75-7.

Jain P , Jirschele K, Botros SM, Latthe P. (2011) Effectiveness of mid-urethral sling in mixed urinary incontinence: A systematic review and Meta-analysis. *Int Urogynecol J* 22 (8):923-32.

Jeffry L, Deval B, Birsan A, et al (2001). Objective and subjective cure rates after tension-free vaginal tape for treatment of urinary incontinence. *Urology* 58:702-6.

Jung YS, Lee JH, Shin TS, Han CH, Kang SH, et al.(2010) Arterial Injury Associated with Tension-Free Vaginal Tapes-SECUR Procedure Successfully Treated by Radiological Embolization. Int Neurourol J. 14(4):275-7.

Khong SY and Lam A. (2011) Use of Surgisis mesh in the management of polypropylene mesh erosion into the vagina. Int Urogynecol J. 22:41-46.

Kristensen I, Eldoma M, Williamson T, Wood S, Mainprize T, (2010). Complications of the tension-free vaginal tape procedure for stress urinary incontinence. Int Urogynecol J. 21(11):1353-7.

Kuuva N, Nilsson CG: (2002) A nationwide analysis of complications associated with tension-free vaginal tape (TVT) procedure. *Acta Obstet Gynecol Scand* 81(1):72-7.

Lapitan MC, Cody JD, Grant A. (2009) Open retropubic colposuspension for urinary incontinence in women. Cochrane Database Syst Rev. 15;(2):CD002912.

Lau HH, Su TH, Su CH, Lee MY, Sun FJ.(2010) Short-term impact of tension-free vaginal tape obturator procedure on sexual function in women with stress urinary incontinence. J Sex Med. 7(4 Pt 1):1578-84.

Latthe PM, Singh P, Foon R, Toozs-Hobson P.(2010) two routes of transobturator tape procedures in stress urinary incontinence: a meta-analysis with direct and indirect comparison of randomized trials. BJU Int. 106(1):68-76.

Lebret T, Lugagne PM, Hervé JM, Barré P, Orsoni JL, et al.(2001) Evaluation of tension-free vaginal tape procedure. Its safety and efficacy in the treatment of female stress urinary incontinence during the learning phase. Eur Urol. 40(5):543-7.

Leboeuf L, Mendez LE, Gousse AE. (2004) Small bowel obstruction associated with tension-free vaginal tape. *Urology* 63(6):1182-4.

Leboeuf L, Tellez CA, Ead D, et al. (2004) Complication of bowel perforation during insertion of tension-free vaginal tape. *J Urol* 170:1310; discussion 1310, 2003.

Lee JH, Cho MC, Oh SJ, Kim SW, Paick JS.(2010) Long-term outcome of the tension-free vaginal tape procedure in female urinary incontinence: a 6-year follow-up. Korean J Urol. 51(6):409-15.

Lee JKS, Agnew G, Dwyer. (2011) Mesh-related chronic infections in silicone-coated polyester suburethral sling. Int Urogynecol J 22:29-35.

Letouzey V, Cornille A, Mourtialon P, Garric X, Lavigne J. et al.(2011) What have we learned from basic science for mesh complication in pelvic floor reconstructive surgery? From infection to polypropylene degradation?. *Int Urogynecol J* 22 (Suppl 1): S-185-186.

Liu PE, Su CH, Lau HH, Chang RJ, Huang WC,et al(2011). Outcome of tension-free obturator tape procedures in obese and overweight women. Int Urogynecol J. 22(3):259-63.

Lleberia-Juanós J, Bataller-Sánchez E, Pubill-Soler J, Mestre-Costa M, Ribot-Luna L, et al. (2011) De novo urgency after tension-free vaginal tape versus transobturator tape procedure for stress urinary incontinence. Eur J Obstet Gynecol Reprod Biol. 155(2):229-32.

Lo TS, Nusee Z.(2010) Repeated endoscopic excision of an eroding calcified mesh sling-continued follow-up is required. J Minim Invasive Gynecol.17(3):383-5.

Madhuvrata P, Ford J, Lim CP, Fattah MA. (2011) A systematic review and meta-analysis of single-incision slings in surgical management of female stress urinary incontinence. *Int Urogynecol J*, 22(Suppl 1) S-01.

Matsumura E, Tasaki S, Ashikari A, Toyosato T, Ashimine S, et al. (2010) A case report of transurethral resection of eroding urethral mesh after a tension-free vaginal tape procedure. Hinyokika Kiyo. 56(11):655-7.

Mamy L, Letouszey V, Lavigne JP, Garric X, Gondry J, et al. Correlation between shrinkage and infection of implanted synthetic meshes using an animal model of mesh infection. Int Urogynecol J. 22:47-52.

Mendoca TM, Martinho D, Dos Reis JP.(2011) Late urethral erosion of transobturator suburethral mesh (Obtape): a minimally invasive management under local anaesthesia. Int Urogynecol J 22:37-39.

Meschia M, Busacca M, Pifarotti P, et al (2002) Bowel perforation during insertion of tension-free vaginal tape (TVT). *Int Urogynecol J Pelvic Floor Dysfunct* 13:263-5.

Miraliakbari H and Tse E.(2011) Ureteral erosion of a transvaginal tape. *Can Urol Assoc J.* 5(3): E44–E46.

Morgan JE. (1970) A sling operation using Marlex polypropylene mesh for treatment of recurrent stress incontinence. *Am J Obstet Gynecol* 106:369-377.

Morgan JE, Farrow GA, Stewart FE. (1985)The Marlex sling operation for the treatment of recurrent stress urinary incontinence: a 16-year review. Am J Obstet Gynecol. Jan 15;151(2):224-6.

Muir TW, Tulikangas PK, Fidela Paraiso M, Walters MD.(2003) The relationship of tension-free vaginal tape insertion and the vascular anatomy. *Obstet Gynecol.* 101(5 Pt 1):933-6.

Novara G, Artibani W, Barber MD, Chapple CR, Costantini E, et al(2010). Updated systematic review and meta-analysis of the comparative data on colposuspensions, pubovaginal slings, and midurethral tapes in the surgical treatment of female stress urinary incontinence. Eur Urol. 58(2):218-38.

Ortega C, Velázquez S, Kunhardt R.(2009) Urethral erosion secondary to the placing of tension-free vaginal tape. A case report. *Ginecol Obstet Mex;* 77(8):393-5.

Patil A. (2011) How do Urogynaecologists treat failed suburethral slings? Experience from the British Society of Urogynaecology database and literature review. *Int Urogynecol J*; 22 (Suppl 1) S:21

Phillips L, Flood CG, Schulz JA.(2009) Case report of tension-free vaginal tape-associated bowel obstruction and relationship to body habitus. *Int Urogynecol J Pelvic Floor* Dysfunct 20(3):367-8

Primicerio M, De Matteis G, Montanino OM, Marceca M, Alessandrini A, et al (1999) Use of the TUT (Tension-free Vaginal Tape) in the treatment of female urinary stress incontinence. Preliminary results. *Minerva Ginecol* 51(9):355-8.

Pushkar DY, Godunov BN, Gvozdev M, Kasyan GR.(2011) Complications of mid-urethral slings for treatment of stress urinary incontinence. Int J Gynaecol Obstet. Apr;113(1):54-7.

Rajendra M, Han HC, Lee LC, Tseng LA, Wong HF.(2011) Retrospective study on tension-free vaginal tape obturator (TVT-O). Int Urogynecol J. Sep 3. [Epub ahead of print]

Reich A, Kohorst F, Kreienberg R, Flock F. (2011) Long-term Results of the Tension-free Vaginal Tape Procedure in an Unselected Group: A 7-Year Follow-up Study. Urology *78(4): 774-7.*

Revicky V, Mukhopadhyay S, De Boer F, Morris EP.(2011) Obesity and the incidence of bladder injury and urinary retention following tension-free vaginal tape procedure: retrospective cohort study. Obstet Gynecol Int. ;2011:746393.

Ridley JH (1966). Appraisal of the Goebell-Frangenheim-Stoeckel sling procedure. *Am J Obstet Gynecol* 95:714-721.

Rigaud J, Delavierre D, Sibert L, Labat JJ.(2010) Management of chronic pelvic and perineal pain after suburethral tape placement for urinary incontinence. *Prog Urol* 20(12):1166-74.

Ross S, Robert M, Swaby C, Dederer L, Lier D, et al (2009). Transobturator tape compared with tension-free vaginal tape for stress incontinence: a randomized controlled trial. Obstet Gynecol. 114(6):1287-94.

Rouprêt M, Misraï V, Vaessen C, Cour F, Haertig A, (2010). Laparoscopic surgical complete sling resection for tension-free vaginal tape-related complications refractory to first-line conservative management: a single-centre experience. Eur Urol 58(2):270-4.

Siegel AL. (2006)Urethral necrosis and proximal urethro-vaginal fistula resulting from tension-free vaginal tape. Int Urogynecol J Pelvic Floor Dysfunct 17(6):661-4.

Sun MJ and Tsai HD (2011) Is transobturator suburethral sling effective for treating female urodynamic stress incontinence with low maximal urethral closure pressure? *Taiwan J Obstet Gynecol* 50(1):20-4.

Ulmsten U, Henriksson L, Johnson P, Varhos G (1996). An ambulatory surgical procedure under local anesthesia for treatment of female urinary incontinence. *Int Urogynecol* 7:81-86

Vervigni M, Natale F (2001) The use of synthetics in the treatment of pelvic organ prolapse. *Curr Opin Urol;* 11: 429-35.

Wijffels SA, Elzevier HW, Lycklama a Nijeholt AA. (2009) Transurethral mesh resection after urethral erosion of tension-free vaginal tape: report of three cases and review of literature. *Int Urogynecol J Pelvic Floor Dysfunct;* 20(2):261-3.

Withagen MI, Vierhout ME, Kluivers KB, Milani AL.(2011) Risk factors for exposure after tension-free vaginal mesh procedure. *Int Urogynecol J* 22(Suppl 1): S83-84.

Williams TJ, Telinde RW.(1962) The sling operation for urinary incontinence using mersilene ribbon. *Obstet Gynecol* 19: 241-5

Whiteside JL, Weber AM, Meyn LA, Walters MD. (2004) Risk factors for prolapse recurrence after vaginal repair. Am J Obstet Gynecol 191(5):1533-8.

Zorn KC, Daigle S, Belzile F, Tu le M, (2005) Embolization of a massive retropubic hemorrhage following a tension-free vaginal tape (TVT) procedure: case report and literature review. *Can J Urol* 12(1):2560-3.

16

Treatment of Post-Prostatic Surgery Stress Urinary Incontinence

José Anacleto Dutra de Resende Júnior, João Luiz Schiavini, Danilo Souza Lima da Costa Cruz, Renata Teles Buere, Ericka Kirsthine Valentin, Gisele Silva Ribeiro and Ronaldo Damião
Department of Urology - Pedro Ernesto University Hospital (HUPE), Rio de Janeiro State University, Rio de Janeiro, Brazil

1. Introduction

There are few long-term medical conditions and non-fatal injuries that are so inconvenient as the urinary incontinence in its various degrees. This situation effect the social life and there are consequences for the economic impact of this clinical condition in patients and health services.

The direct costs associated with urinary incontinence is related to aspects such as diagnostic tests, doctor visits, surgery, use of diapers, and others. Among the indirect costs can include the time available for patients and friends to care of incontinent patients, and the loss of productivity for the individual hours away at work. The worsening quality of life of the patient is considered an intangible cost, difficult to measure in monetary terms, but which constitutes an integral aspect of urinary incontinence.

Among the various causes of urinary incontinence, sphincter incompetence is one of the most common (Mundy, 1991). Fortunately, most patients with sphincter incompetence have simple stress incontinence, which usually responds well to one of several procedures for suspension of the bladder neck or urethra. However, surgery does not work without implants as favorably for the treatment of severe urinary sphincter, where the loss of urethral support is irrelevant (Mundy, 1991). In these circumstances, the best form of treatment is still the deployment of devices performing a specific function that compensates constrictor malfunction of the urethral sphincter (Hussain et al. 2005; Mundy, 1991; Schiavini et al. 2007; Vilar et al. , 2004).

The initial treatment of urinary incontinence with urethral devices date from 1947, when Foley described the first artificial sphincter (Foley, 1947). According to its proposal, the penile urethra was exteriorized, involved with the foreskin and, after healing, the device was placed around the urethra. This device consisted of a tube connected to a syringe, the patient carried in his pocket, and when wanted to maintain continence, insert some fluid that would exert pressure through the syringe. Foley's method fell into disuse due to the high incidence of urethral injuries.

In 1973, Scott and colleagues, based on the idea of Foley, have created a toilet model totally implantable device, the AMS 721, which was modified and optimized by Rosen, 1976 (Rosen, 1976, Scott et al., 1973). This device allowed compression of the bulbar urethra by inflating the device. Due to poor results, the device also fell into disuse.

Changes were made in the initial design and the most important was the use of a balloon to regulate the pressure valve in place.

Later models also incorporated an entirely new body of silicon, rather than a body of Dacron ®. A decrease in the number of components and connections resulted in the current AMS 800 (Fig. 01a), a device consisting of 3 parts (Hussain et al., 2005).

The AMS 800 is a body-shaped strap that is placed around the bladder neck or bulbar urethra. This body is connected to a balloon pressure regulator via a control pump, located in the scrotum of the patient. The whole system is filled with saline, hydraulic operation. The pressure in the system and therefore the strength of the occlusive balloon body is determined by the throttle, being maintained in the system except when the pump is activated voluntarily by patients who do not account for intermittent catheterization. This activation provides the rapid emptying of saline in the body, which fluid is directed to the balloon pressure regulator, momentarily removing the occlusive force of the body and allowing urination by the patient (Fig. 01b). The body is kept empty for long enough (2-3 min) so that urination is complete before returning to gain momentum due to the return of occlusive saline (Hussain et al. 2005; Mundy, 1991).

Urinary incontinence after prostate surgery represents a social problem and public health, patient and burdening the state with direct and indirect costs and affect the quality of life of patients. The AMS 800 is the best treatment for the patients with severe sphincter incontinence, but preliminary data from the Constrictor Inflatable Periurethral are encouraging (Kuznetozov et al., 2000, Montague et al. 2001; Schiavini et al., 2007).

Treatments such as collagen injections and the periurethral sling men do not appear as effective alternatives for long-term treatment of severe forms of this type of incontinence. Despite the long history of use, collagen injections are associated with success rates that generally do not exceed 40% cure rate. Due to the metabolism of collagen in the body, there is a gradual decrease in cure rates associated with the technique. This transient effectiveness usually takes the need for applying multiple injections on each patient, increasing the treatment without increasing the rates of long-term success (Carson, 2002, Cespedes et al., 1999, Kuznetsov et al., 2000).

The male sling appeared as a possible treatment for patients with sphincter incontinence after prostate surgery. However, the results were effective only in patients with mild to moderate incontinence (Castle et al., 2005). Sahaja & Terris, 2006, also pointed out that the male sling would not be as effective as a device with more physiological action, such as the artificial sphincter. For the structural similarity between the body of the AMS 800 and the Constrictor, this reasoning could be extended to the Constrictor.

Another aspect to be considered is that, despite their recognized efficacy, the greater structural complexity of the AMS 800 has a direct impact on their high cost (Mundy, 1991). This is one of the reasons that explain the low access to this device for patients with urinary sphincter in Latin America. Meanwhile, the Constrictor has provided preliminary efficacy results similar to the AMS 800, on a smaller device cost about 16 times.

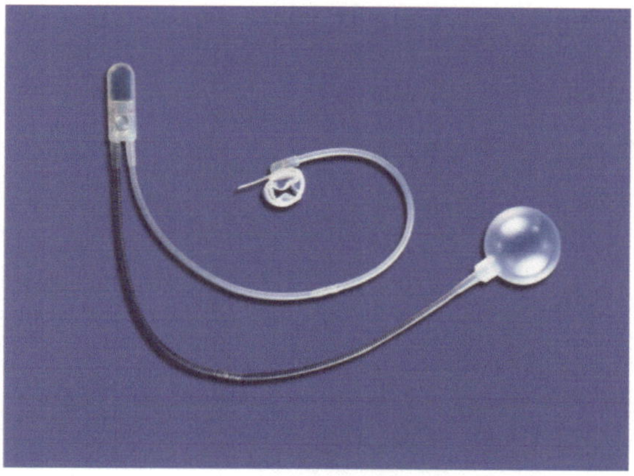

a)

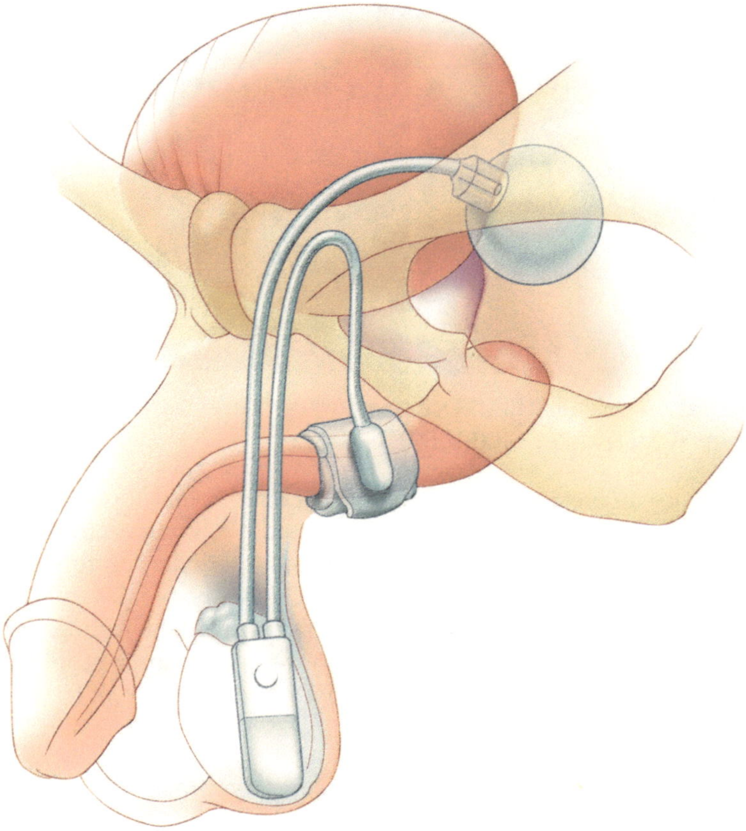

b)

Fig. 1. a) AMS 800, a device of 3 parts - body, balloon and pump. b) Operating mode of the AMS 800 (Permission by American Medical Systems®)

2. Alternatives to the AMS 800 in the treatment of urinary incontinence

Currently, the only device on the market, indicating the use and operational mode that resembles the AMS 800 in strengthening occluding the urethra is developed by Constrictor Inflatable Periurethral SILIMED (Rio de Janeiro - Brazil), a device consisting essentially of 2 parts - body and valve constriction (Fig 2).

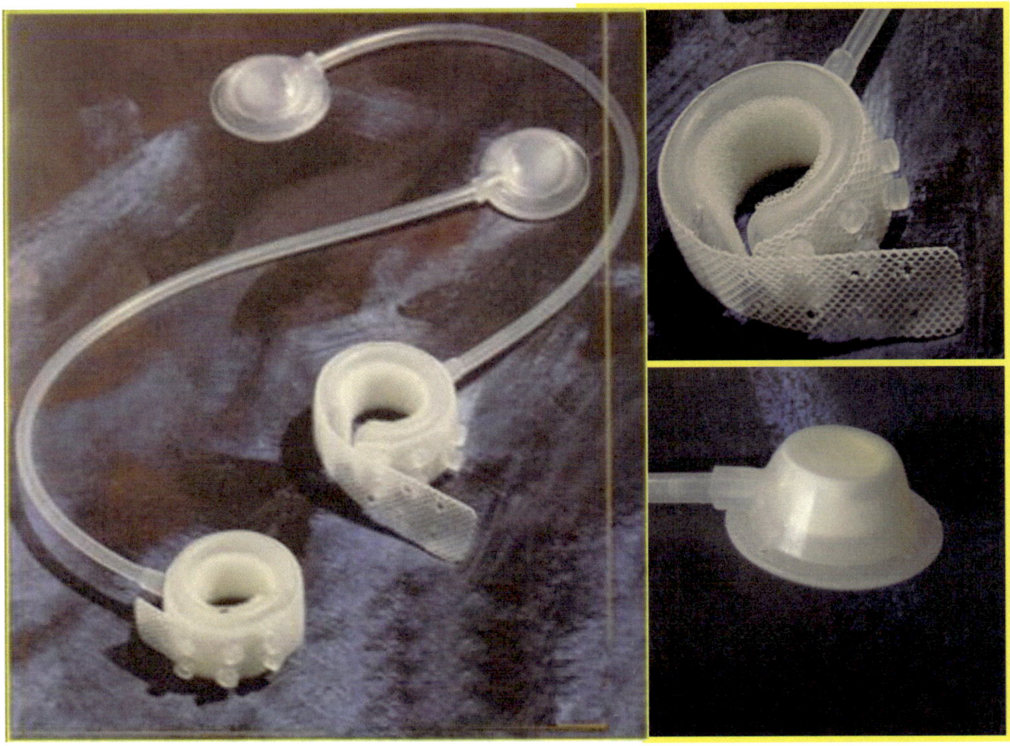

Fig. 2. Periurethral constrictor SILIMED, a two-part device (constrictor cuff and self-sealing valve with tube) (Permission by SILIMED®).

The main functional difference between the two devices is that the force of the occlusive body Constrictor Inflatable Periurethral remains constant throughout the duration of use of the device. If necessary, the patient's physician can make periodic adjustments of pressure in order to increase or decrease the force of the occlusive body, through the injection or removal of saline through the valve device in an outpatient setting. Meanwhile, the literature indicates a technical difficulty related to the change in pressure in the system of the AMS 800, possible only after revision surgery for the exchange of the balloon pressure regulator (Mundy, 1991).

The medical and scientific literature presents both AMS 800 and the Constrictor Inflatable Periurethral (preliminary data) as trusted devices and with good durability. Any problems would be reversed, in most cases, for simple or surgical outpatient review, which would ensure good continence rates, according to the criteria of effectiveness adopted by different authors (Hussain et al. 2005; Mundy, 1991; Schiavini et al. , 2007; Vilar et al. 2004; Webster & Sherman, 2005).

The relative simplicity of the Constrictor apparently does not interfere with its effectiveness. Studies of the groups of Dr. Salvador Vilar and Dr. João Schiavini Constrictor present with continence rates of around 85% during treatment, as mentioned ahead. Moreover, the Constrictor was also able to provide some patients voiding spontaneously, especially in adults with urinary incontinence after prostate surgery sphincter. Even in cases where intermittent catheterization was used, the rate of patient satisfaction were generally high (Vilar et al. 2004; Schiavini et al., 2007). The main results are described ahead.

2.1 Constrictor treatment in patients with neurogenic urinary incontinence

In 2000, Lima and colleagues from the Hospital Infantil Manoel Almeida, Federal University of Pernambuco - Recife, presented results on the use of inflatable Periurethral Constrictor for the treatment of urinary incontinence secondary to myelomeningocele. The 24 patients (14 men and 10 women) were in the age group 5 to 42 years, and were followed for an average of 4.2 years (1-84 months). Concomitant with the deployment of the device, 21 of these patients underwent cystoplasty to increase with the use of De-epithelialize colon. Twenty-one patients had a good result with the device in addition to being functional continents, giving a success rate of 87.5%. In 3 (12.5%) cases, the device was removed due to the occurrence of erosion and infection. At the end of the study, the authors stated that the use of inflatable Periurethral Constrictor would be a safe and effective in the treatment of long-term causes of neurogenic urinary incontinence (Lima et al., 2000).

In 2004, Vilar and colleagues presented a second study group related to the use of Constrictor Inflatable Periurethral the surgical treatment of urinary incontinence in 42 children (29 boys and 13 girls) with a mean age of 10.2 years (3 to 17 years). The group consisted of 29 neurogenic patients, 12 with bladder exstrophy and 1 with megalouretra. Concomitant with the deployment of the device, augmentation cystoplasty was performed in 34 patients. Patients were followed for an average of 5.2 years (4 to 104 months). In 25 patients in the neurogenic group the device was functional and provided continence, which represented a rate of continent patients during treatment of 86%. In 4 (14%) patients, the device was removed due to erosion (3) and infection (1). The patient was continent and megalouretra urinated spontaneously. In the exstrophy group, 10 patients had their devices explanted due to erosion and incontinence. Only two kept the device and performed intermittent catheterization. The authors concluded that the Constrictor Periurethral would be a long-term alternative, safe and effective for the surgical treatment of urinary incontinence cause neurogenic sphincter in children. Like previously reported for other implants, the authors emphasized that the device should be used with caution in patients with bladder exstrophy (Vilar et al., 2004).

2.2 Post-prostate surgery urinary incontinence.

In 2007, Schiavini & Resende Jr and colleagues, University Hospital Pedro Ernesto, Rio de Janeiro, showed their initial experience with the use of inflatable Periurethral Constrictor.

In this study, eighteen patients had urinary incontinence after radical retropubic prostatectomy, and five were previously submitted to procedures for the treatment of bladder neck strictures. In all patients, the body of the device was placed around the bulbar urethra, with activation of the device after 8 weeks. Patients were followed from 6 to 36 months. For the authors, successful treatment was predefined as the need to use a diaper until the day - social continence, together with patient satisfaction.

2.2.1 Preoperative evaluation

The complete urologic evaluation was performed, including urine analysis, ultrasonography, cystography and urodynamic studies before to submit the patients to the surgery, respecting the inclusion and exclusion criteria previously established, as described below.

2.2.2 Inclusion criteria

- Men;
- 18 years or more;
- Diagnosis of sphincter incontinence after prostate surgery;
- Be in good general health prior to participation in the study, no significant clinical abnormalities determined by: clinical history, physical examination, blood chemistry, blood count, urinalysis (the results of biochemical tests or hematology or urinalysis laboratory do not contain references, the patient may be included only if the researcher finds that the changes are not clinically significant);
- Informed Consent in writing and signed by the patient.

2.2.3 Exclusion criteria

- Detrusor overactivity unresponsive to clinical treatment.
- Low compliance bladder;
- Use of drugs that interfere with bladder function;
- Severe urethral stenosis,
- History of significant disease (ex. cardiovascular, pulmonary, gastrointestinal, hematological, neurological, degenerative, hormonal, autoimmune or cancer).
- History of psychological instability;
- Presence of active infection;
- Any situation that increases the possibility of infection / erosion after body contact device with the bulbar urethra (ex. sequelae of prior radiotherapy);
- History of allergenicity to foreign bodies or silicone;
- History of drug abuse in the last two years;
- Risk that prevents surgical surgery / anesthesia;
- Any condition, which in the opinion of the investigator, may interfere with the patient participation in the study (ex. difficulty of meeting the requirements of the study, attend appointments, or any other situation that may affect the response of the questionnaire on quality of life by the patient);
- Patient expected to undergo surgery during the study period, which may affect the outcome;
- Patient undergone previous surgical treatment for the treatment of sphincter incontinence.

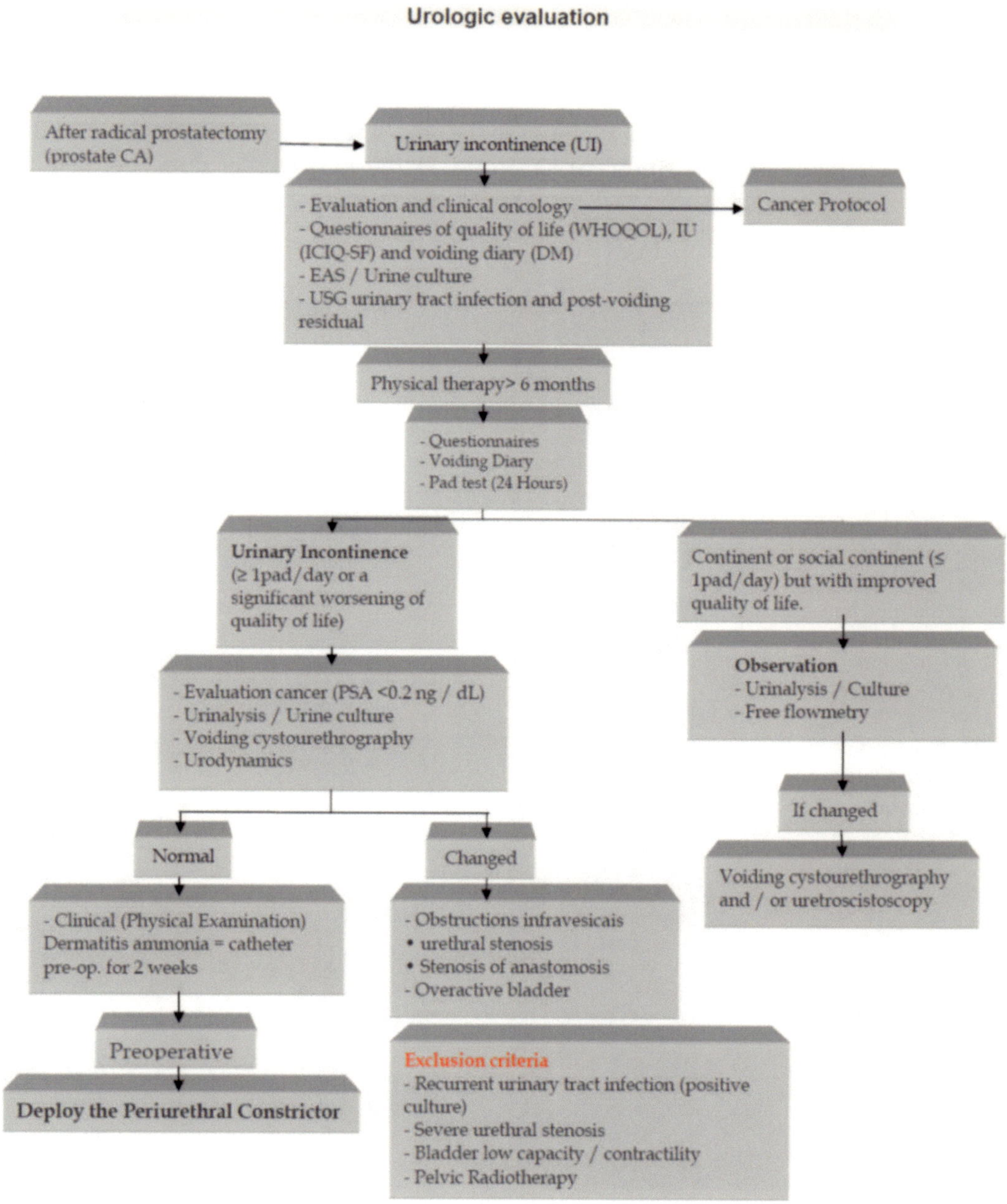

Fig. 3. Urologic Evaluation

2.3 Surgical approach and intra-operative procedures

The patient is subjected to anesthesia in the operating room after evaluation by the anesthesiologist. Prophylaxis with intravenous antibiotics (3rd generation cephalosporin) will be held 30 minutes before starting surgery. Will be held genital shaving and antisepsis genital at least 5 minutes and drapes are placed.

Ureteroscopy with internal urethrotomy was performed when it was not possible to place a bladder catheter preoperatively.

To implement the Constrictor Inflatable Periurethral around the bulbar urethra, the surgical access of up to 10cm in the perineal raphe, with the developer in the lithotomy position. The muscle fibers bulb-cavernous must be separated in the longitudinal direction, and the bulbar urethra dissected easily visible and later by creating the space for placing the constriction around her body (Fig-4).

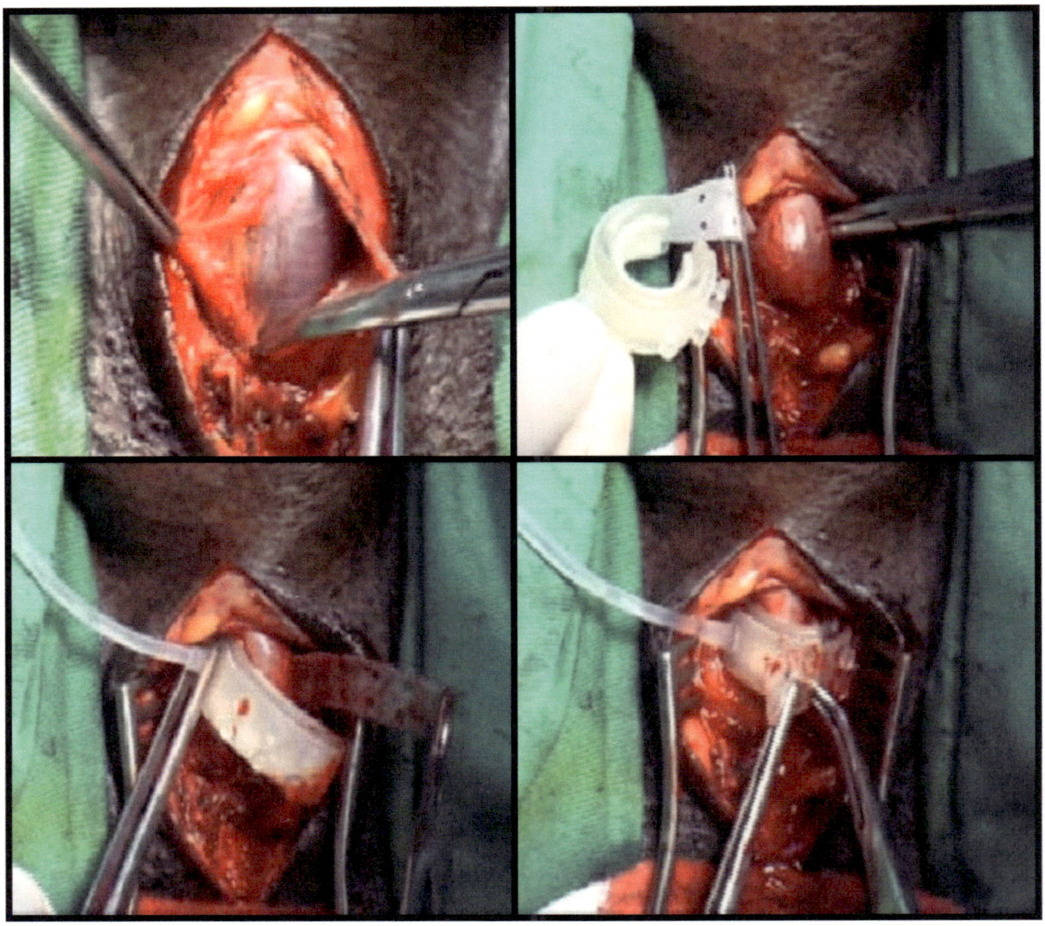

Fig. 4. Details of the constrictor cuff implantation around the bulbar urethra, after the dissection and separation of the bulbospongiosus muscle fibers.

The pipe must be routed through the subcutaneous space and the valve implanted in the suprapubic region or subdartic within the scrotum, where it can be punctured (Fig-5).

The Constrictor Inflatable Periurethral should have your air completely removed before being introduced into 2 ml of pyrogen-free saline. Meticulous haemostasis is essential to reduce risk of haematoma formation.

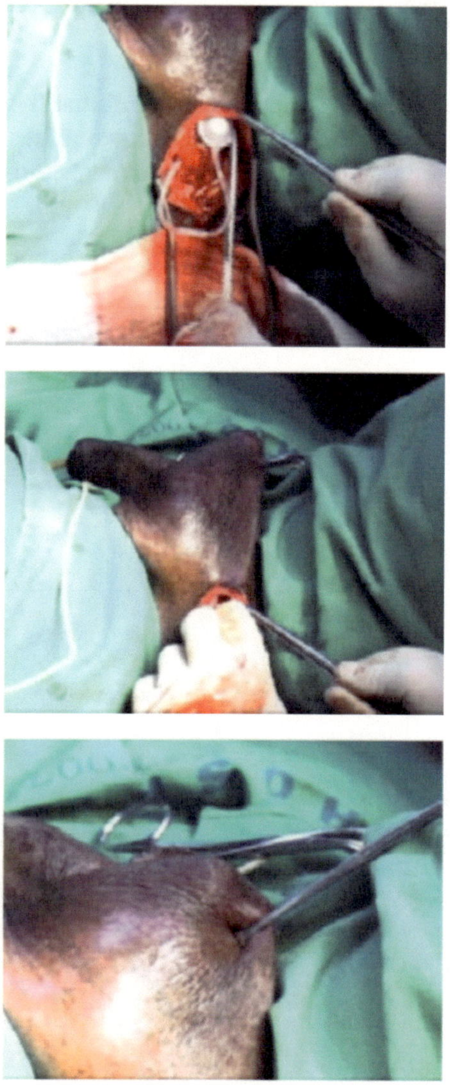

Fig. 5. Details of the valve implantation at the subdartic space of the scrotum.

2.4 Post operative care

The urethral catheter can be withdrawn on the 1st postoperative day. Activation of Inflatable Periurethral Constrictor should be held approximately 8 weeks (at least 6 and at most 12 weeks) after implantation, when a urodynamic study should be performed in conjunction with the measurement of pressure inside the device.

To enable Inflatable Periurethral Constrictor, you should use a butterfly type intravenous scalp, 25G to 27G, previously filled with sterile saline, and pyrogen, to puncture the valve. The puncture should be done in the center of the constrictor valve in 90-degree angle, avoiding the edges of this valve, where the silicon is thinner, not to damage it. Must be injected sterile saline and pyrogen in an amount sufficient to produce continence, even during sudden increase in abdominal pressure, such as episodes of coughing, but allows good urinary flow, without causing urinary retention.

During the activation step, the clinician must be careful that the needle is inserted into the valve without excessive force, which could cause bending at the end of the needle and damage to the silicone septum during their re-treatment, thus undermining the proper functioning valve device.

In addition, the use of large-caliber needles can destroy the valve.

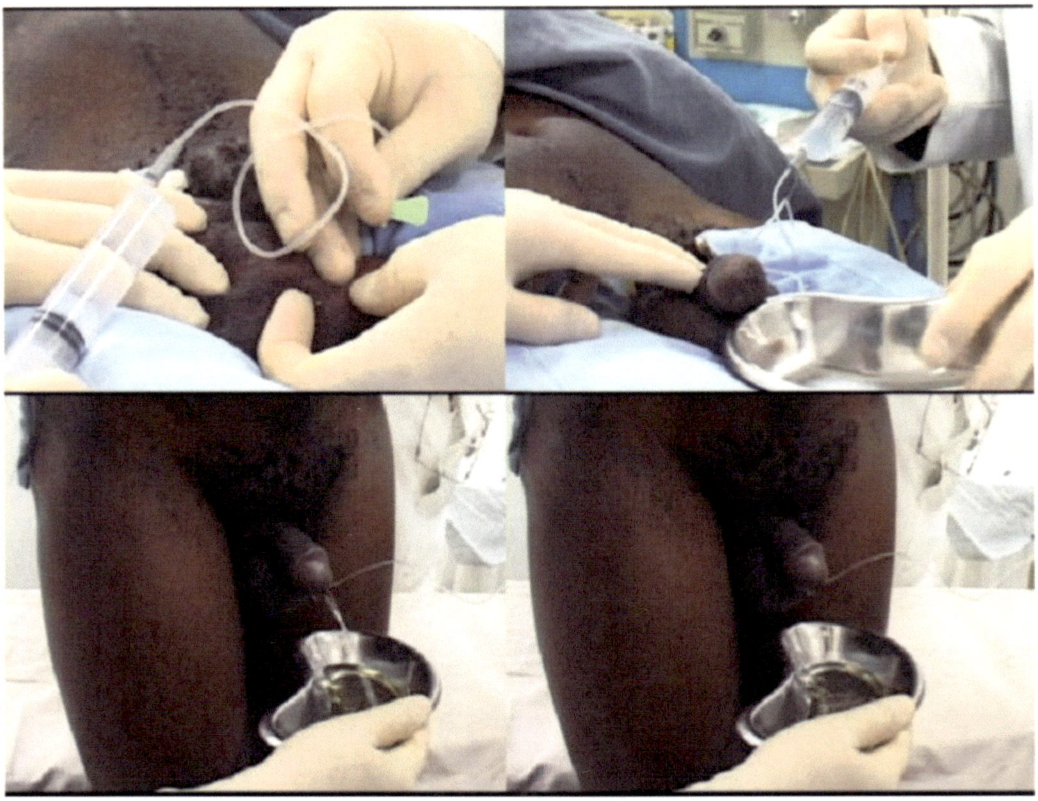

Fig. 6. Periurethral constrictor's activation by injection of saline solution through the self-sealing valve located at the scrotum. After activation, the patient had a good urine flow and achieved urinary continence.

2.5 Efficacy variables

The subjective and objective efficacy of the intervention was determined monthly in the first year and quarterly by the end of the third year (final visit) based on clinical results obtained in the patient Pad Test and questionnaires.

The questionnaires validated quality of life WHOQOL (World Health Organization - Quality of Life) and ICIQ-SF (International Consultation on Incontinence Questionnaire - Short Form) were used as an instrument of measurement.

2.6 Observations and measurements postoperative

The recommendations for postoperative monitoring are in the figure below (Fig-7).

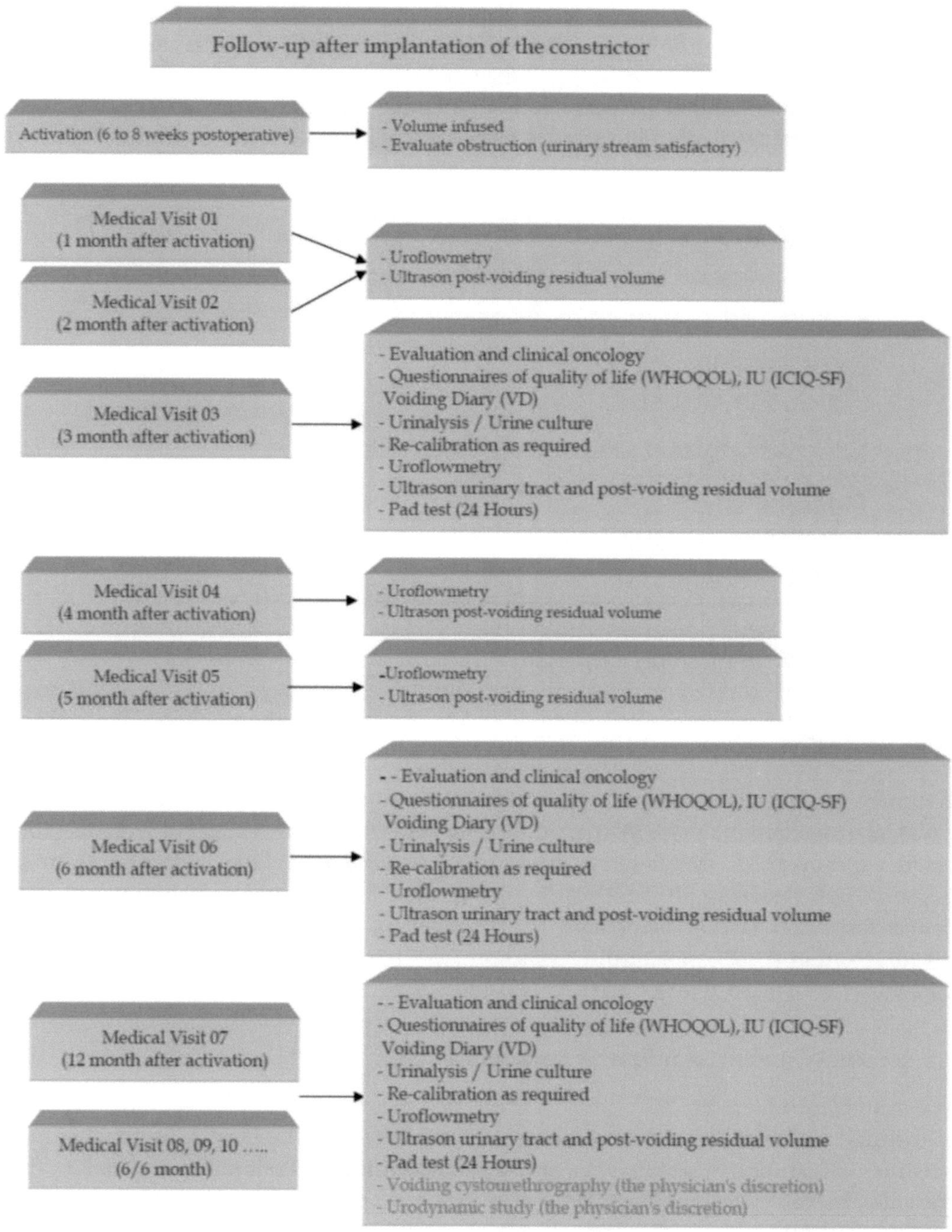

Fig. 7. Urologic Evaluation Postoperative.

2.7 Results – AMS 800®

Follow-up ranged from 27 to 132 months (mean 53.4 +- 21.4 months). There was a significant reduction in pad count from 4.0 +- 0.9 to 0.62 +- 1.07 diapers per day (*P*<0.001) leading to continence in 90%. Twenty patients (50%) were completely dry, and 16 (40%) required 1 pad per day. There was a significant reduction on the impact of incontinence decreasing from 5.0 +- 0.7 to 1.4 +- 0.93 (*P* _0.001) in a visual analogue scale (VAS). Surgical revision rate was 20%. Preoperative urodynamics was useful to identify sphincter deficiency. Except by a tendency of worse results in patients with reduced bladder compliance (RBC), other urodynamic parameters did not correlate with a worse surgical outcome. (Trigo Rocha F, et al. 2008).

Author	Number	Follow-up (yr)	Continence Rate (%)
Marks and Light	37	3.0	94.5
Light and Reynolds	126	2.3	96.7
Perez and Webster	49	3.7	85.0
Mottet *et al.*	103	1.0	86.0
Martins and Boyd	28	2.0	85.0
Fleshner and Herschorn 1996	30	3.0	87.0
Current series	40	2.5	90.0

AUS = artificial urinary sphincter; PRPUI = postradical prostatectomy urinary incontinence.

Fig. 8. Continence rates after AUS implantation in patients with PRPUI (Modified from Trigo Rocha F, et al. 2008)

The main complications related to the AMS 800 are: Revision rate of the device in 5 years (26%), malfunctioning device (8%), pain/discomfort (6,9%), slow healing of wounds (5,7%), bladder spasms (2,3%), activation difficult (2,3%), displacement of the device (3,5%), erosion tissue (2,3%), disabling difficult (1,1%), infection (2,3%), recurring incontinence (3,5%), fistula formation (1,1%), hematoma (1,1%), swelling (2,3%), hydrocele (1,1%), erosion tissue/infection (1,1%), patient dissatisfaction (1,1%), incontinence position (1,1%), wound infection (1,1%), urinary retention (1,1%) (Shellock F, et al. 1988; Litwiller SE, et al. 1996)

2.8 Results - Constrictor inflatable periurethral®

The results obtained in 2007, four patients had neurogenic functional implants. Were continents and performed intermittent catheterization. In the group of prostatectomy patients, 15 had functional implants, and 2 performed intermittent catheterization. In three patients, the valve implant some leakage of saline, after activating the device, which was easily solved by changing the valves. Only one implant fail to function properly and was removed. Other two implants were removed early due to erosion, probably caused by iatrogenic complications that occurred during dissection of the bulbar urethra. Thus, 19 patients with functional implants represented a success rate of 86%, during an mean follow up of 28 months (6 to 50 months). (Schiavini et al, 2007).

In the update made in 2010, and Schiavini & Resende Jr and colleagues, 30 patients were evaluated and followed up for a mean of 42.1 months (range, 13-72). In 22 patients (73.3%), the implanted devices were functional, 16 patients (53,3%) were completely dry, and 06 (20%) required 1 pad per day; 20 voided spontaneously, and 2 performed intermittent catheterization. Among them, 7 patients were submitted for ambulatory review—within 2 weeks of the activation of the device—to increase the occlusive static pressure of the cuff (range of volume added, 0.4-1.7 mL); and 4 were submitted for surgical exchange of the valve because of leakage of saline solution. Despite these occurrences, all of these patients claimed they were very satisfied with the results.

The main complications were urethral cuff erosion in 4 patients (13.3%) and infection in 3 patients (10%), leading in these cases to early and complete removal of the devices. An eighth patient remained incontinent after the device reactivation because of detrusor hyperreflexia. In this series, there was no occurrence of any other major complications.

3. Comment and conclusion

In the last years, the urological community has been developing new procedures to treat postprostatic surgery urinary incontinence. Despite their long history of use, collagen injections are associated with low cure rates. Moreover, collagen is gradually reabsorbed by the organism, leading to additional applications of the product, along with no significant increase in long-term cure (Cespedes.1999; Kuznetsov et al. 2000).

The male sling appeared as another alternative treatment for these patients, but seems to be effective only in mild and moderate cases of postprostate surgery urinary incontinence (Castle et al. 2005; Montague et al. 2001).

Although the artificial urinary sphincter is considered as the standard treatment for moderate and severe cases of postprostate surgery urinary incontinence, it is a high-cost device. In the present study, the authors present results of a surgical alternative for the treatment of postprostate surgery urinary incontinence. For this, we used the periurethral constrictor, a two-part device with a constrictor cuff positioned around the bulbar urethra and hydraulically activated through a self-sealing valve with a tube. Previous studies had already presented the device as a safe and effective alternative for the treatment of neurogenic urinary incontinence (Lima SVC, et al. 2000; Vilar FO, et al. 2004).

This is particularly true if we consider that the erosion and infection cases were probably caused by bulbar urethral injuries that occurred during its dissection and cuff positioning in an early phase of the study during the learning curve of the technique. Along the series, there were no new cases of erosion and infection.

Our experience indicates that the periurethral constrictor is less susceptible to mechanical problems or improper functioning, which agrees with the studies of neurogenic patients. The eventual problems were easily managed by simple surgical reviews with local anesthesia in the case of the exchange of leaking valves, or ambulatory reviews to adjust the occlusive pressure of the system—once the presence of a self-sealing valve permits suitable readjustments through simple transcutaneal injections at any time on an outpatient basis, which makes the overall procedure safer and less expensive by avoiding unnecessary surgical reviews. In the case of the valves, we verified that the leakages were inadvertedly caused by needle perforations of the edge of the valve (where the silicone is thin) during the activation of the device. As a result of this, a project alteration of the valve that greatly diminished this risk was performed, and there was no occurrence of any other improper functioning of the device afterward.

The periurethral constrictor may also be an important option in the treatment of sphincteric urinary incontinence in elderly, parkinsonian, and hemiplegic patients who have suffered cerebral vascular accident or other conditions that contribute to the decrease of manual dexterity (which would prevent the manipulation of the artificial sphincter's mechanism). Another indication would be for incontinent patients who have sustained sphincter injury with bladder atony, which can benefit from the use of the device for staying dry and voiding by intermittent catheterization.

Moreover, the low cost of the periurethral constrictor is also an important characteristic in its favor when compared with the already established AMS 800. The rates of efficacy that are apparently similar between both devices and the constrictor's lower cost may encourage its use in all cases of postprostate surgery urinary incontinence where economic aspects are an important variable to be considered, including those where the artificial sphincter may also be indicated but its high cost prevents its use.

4. References

Appell RA. Assessment and therapy for voiding dysfunction after prostatectomy. Curr Urol Rep 8: 175-8, 2007.

Carson III. Urologic prostheses : the complete practical guide to devices, their implantation, and patient follow up. *New Jersey : Humana Press,* 309p, 2002.

Castle EP, Andrews PE, Itano N, et al. The male sling for postprostate surgery incontinence: mean follow-up of 18 months. *J Urol.* 2005;173:1657-1660.

Cespedes RD et al. Collagen Injection Therapy for Posprostatectomy Incontinence. *Urology,* v. 54, p. 597-602, 1999.

Chao r & mayo ME. Incontinence after radical prostatectomy: detrusor or sphincter causes. J Urol 154: 16-8, 1995.

Foley FB. An Artificial Sphincter: a New Device and Operation for Control of Enuresis and Urinary Incontinence. *Journal of Urology,* v. 58, p. 250-4, 1947.

Hussain M et al. The Current Role of the Artificial Urinary Sphincter for the Treatment of Urinary Incontinence. *Journal of Urology,* v. 174, p. 18-24, 2005.

Klinjin AJ, Hop WCJ, Mickish G, Schroder FH, Bosch JLHR. The artificial urinary sphincter in men incontinent after radical prostatectomy: 5-year actuarial adequate function rate. Br J Urol 82: 530-3, 1998.

Kuznetsov DD, Kim HL, Steinberg GD, Bales GT. Comparison of artificial urinary sphincter and collagen for the treatment of postprostatectomy incontinence. *Urology.* 2000;56:600-603.

Lima SV et al. Periurethral Constrictor in the Treatment of Neurogenic Urinary Incontinence: the Test of Time. *Brazilian Journal of Urology*, v. 26, p. 415-7, 2000.

Lima SVC, Vilar FO, Araújo LAP. Periurethral constrictor in the treatment of neurogenic urinary incontinence: the test of time. *Braz J Urol*. 2000;26:415-417.

Litwiller SE, Kim KB, Fone PD, DeVere White RW, Stone AR.Post-Prostatectomy Incontinence and the Artificial Urinary Sphincter A Long-term Study of Patient Satisfaction and Criteria for Success. *Joumal of Urology* 1996; 156:1975-80.

Montague DK, Angermeier KW, Paolone DR. Long-term continence and patient satisfaction after artificial sphincter implantation for urinary incontinence after prostatectomy. *J Urol*. 2001;166.

Mundy A. Artificial Sphincters. *British Journal of Urology*, v. 67, p. 225-9, 1991.

Rajpurkar AD, Onur R, Singla A. Patient satisfaction and clinical efficacy of the new perineal bone-anchored male sling. Eur Urol 47: 237-42, 2005.

Rocha FT. Avaliação dos resultados do tratamento da incontinência urinária pós-prostatectomia radical por meio da implantação do esfíncter artificial AMS 800. São Paulo, 2003. *Tese apresentada à Faculdade de Medicina da Universidade de São Paulo para obtenção do Título de Professor Livre-docente junto ao Departmento de Cirurgia.*

Rosen M. A Simple Artificial Implantable Sphincter. *Bristish Journal of Urology*, v. 48, p. 675-80, 1976.

ROSNER B. Fundamentals of Biostatistics. 2nd ed. Boston: PWS Publishers.

Sajadi KP & Terris MK. Artificial Urinary Sphincter, 17p. Disponível em http://www.emedicine.com/med/topic3019.htm. Acesso eletrônico em: 21 de setembro de 2007.

Schiavini JL et al. Our Experience Using the Periurethral Constrictor, a Simplified Silicone-made Device in the Male Urinary Incontinence (Abstract). *SIU Centennial Celebration*, Paris, 2007.

Schiavini JL, Da Silva EA, Toledo JS, Damião R, Dornas MC, Resende Jr. JAD. Our experience using the Periurethral Constrictor, a simplified silicone made device in the male urinary incontinence (Abstract). Urology, 70 (Supplement 3A): 36, 2007.

Schiavini, João Luiz ; Damião, Ronaldo ; Resende Júnior, José Anacleto Dutra de; Dornas, Maria Cristina ; Cruz Lima da Costa, Danilo Souza ; Barros, Cesar Borges . Treatment of Post-prostate Surgery Urinary Incontinence With the Periurethral Constrictor: A Retrospective Analysis. Urology (Ridgewood, N.J.) JCR, v. 75, p. 1488-1492, 2010.

Schiavini, João Luiz ; Resende Júnior, José Anacleto Dutra de; Barros, Cesar Borges . Reply. Urology (Ridgewood, N.J.) JCR, v. 75, p. 1492-1493, 2010.

Schiavini JL, Dutra de Resende Júnior JA, Dornas MC, Da Silva EA, Damião R. Tratamento da incontinência urinária pós-prostatectomia radical com o constritor periuretral: análise retrospectiva de 30 casos (Abstract). Actas Urológicas Españolas (Suplemento), vol. 32 (6): 218, 2008.

Scott FB et al. Treatment of Urinary Incontinence by Implantable Prosthetic Sphincter. *Urology*, v. 1, p. 252-9, 1973.

Shellock F, *MR Imaging of Metallic Implants and Materials: A Compilation of the Literature,* AJR, outubro 1988.

Trigo Rocha F, Gomes CM, Mitre AI, Arap S, Srougi M. A prospective study evaluating the efficacy of the artificial sphincter AMS 800 for the treatment of postradical prostatectomy urinary incontinence and the correlation between preoperative urodynamic and surgical outcomes. Urology. 2008 Jan;71(1):85-9.

Venn SN, Grennwell TJ, Mundy AR. The long-term outcome of artificial urinary sphincters. J Urol 164: 702-6, 2000.

Vilar, FO et al. Periurethral Constrictor in Pediatric Urologic: Long-term Follow-up. *Journal of Urology*, v. 171, p. 2626-8, 2004.

Webster gd & sherman ND. Management of Male Incontinence Following Artificial Urinary Sphincter Failure. *Current Opinion in Urology*, v. 15, p. 386-90, 2005.

17

Continent Urinary Diversions in Non Oncologic Situations: Alternatives and Complications

Ricardo Miyaoka and Tiago Aguiar
Division of Urology, State University of Campinas, Sao Paulo, Brazil

1. Introduction

Urinary diversion is a detour of the urinary tract. It may be necessary in different scenarios and can either be continent or incontinent, catheterisable or orthotopic. Pathological situations which may demand a urinary diversion are varied and include anatomical, physiological, congenital and traumatic causes, e.g. urethral stenosis and partial or complete urethral disruption; bladder dysfunction secondary to radiotherapy or congenital pathologies (posterior urethral valve, Prune-Belly Syndrome, epispadias, bladder extrophy, cloaca); neurogenic bladder and idiopathic bladder dysfunction [1-3].

The treatment has essentially four main goals: preservation of the upper urinary tract, urinary continence, adequate reservoir emptying and avoidance of urinary tract infections [4]. With the continued development of less invasive treatments for almost all urological pathologies (including severe bladder dysfunction) surgical urinary diversion can be currently considered the end treatment for these patients [2,4,5].

Urinary diversion can be classified as either continent or incontinent. Continent urinary diversion refers to a reservoir which can be emptied through clean intermittent catheterization (CIC). Incontinent diversion refers to situations where a continuous free urinary flow through an interposed intestinal segment pours into a collecting bag [2].

Although being a realistic alternative to treat patients with a compromised bladder or urethra, one must be aware of the inherent challenges and possible complications related to urinary diversion. This encompasses not only the surgical aspects, but also the post operative care and management of complications.

We review pre and post operative aspects related to the continent urinary diversion commonly used in benign pathologies and the current literature pertaining to this.

2. Selection criteria for urinary diversion

The ultimate aim in reconstruction of the lower urinary tract in patients with adequate storage function is to attain continence. Adequate emptying can be achieved with consideration of manual dexterity, cognitive capability and patient choice. The options to create a continent or incontinent urinary system can range from long-term catheterisation, intermittent cathterisation or diversion – incontinent, or continence cutaneous.

Ultimately there is no hard and fast answer for every situation, rather an individualised decision must be made.

2.1 Pre operative evaluation

Physical examination should determine patient's cognitive capacity to perform self catheterisation. The body habitus may strongly influence the sitting position of the urinary stoma. Attention must be given on how the urine collecting bag plate will adhere to the patient's skin, whether it is going to adequately cope with the external abdominal wall when patient is sitting or standing, etc. It is a useful tip to delineate and mark the exact site where the stoma should be before patient is taken to the operating room.

Comorbidities that may impair patient's ability to properly heal such as uncontrolled diabetes or immunodeficient states must be set even beforehand.

The description by McGuire and cols. [6] that storage leak point pressures above 40 cmH_2O would jeopardize the integrity of the upper urinary tract set a reference value for urodynamic monitoring and treatment orientation. Urodynamics is also helpful in identifying or confirming detrusor overactivity and determining maximum capacity and compliance.

Upper urinary tract preservation is the corner stone of dysfunctional voiding patient management. Upper tract evaluation can be simply performed through an abdominal ultrassonography which is a non invasive procedure that provides valuable information on kidneys morphological features such as shape and size, which may preclude congenital pathologies, anatomical variances, parenchymal scars, and others [1]; and serum labs (urea, creatinine). Creatinine clearance is also recommended to assess global renal function. Evidence of renal atrophy or changes in shape that might suggest impairment of renal function, including previous history of recurrent urinary tract infection (UTI) must be confirmed with static renal scintigraphy (DMSA). This will provide precise information on the patient's baseline renal function status at the beginning of treatment and allow for future monitoring and assurance of renal preservation through comparative analysis. Renal function deterioration is an important landmark to decide upon indicating a reconstructive procedure in this specific population. As such, it seems obvious that prevention of UTIs is critical. An adequate global renal function will reduce the chance for acid/base imbalances secondary to intestinal absorption. However, regular monitoring is needed.

Whenever ureteral dilation is identified, assessment with DTPA or MAG-3 scintigraphy is recommended to rule out ureteral obstruction which may occur as a consequence of bladder wall thickening as well as urethrocistography which will identify possible associated secondary vesicoureteral reflux. In these cases ureteral reimplantation may be needed. This evaluation will not only assure ureteral patency but also determine renal split function.

Urodynamic evaluation is mandatory when bladder dysfunction is suspected. When considering a catheterizable channel, one must be certain about the bladder normal capacity and compliance. Otherwise an augmentation procedure may be necessary in association. Also, continence evaluation may indicate the need for an anti incontinence procedure such as bladder neck closure. This is recommended when urinary leak pressures are detected below 30 cm H_2O. Videourodynamics combine conventional urodynamics with contrast imaging providing both functional and morphological information at once [4,15].

Patient must present manual dexterity to firmly hold a catheter and accurately introduce it into the channel lumen. Previous abdominal surgeries and obesity may anticipate surgical difficulty to prepare and externalize the intestinal channel.

Continence must be pursued when feasible. In this sense, self catheterisation need to be adjusted in order to empty the bladder before it reaches its maximum capacity in an attempt to significantly reduce incontinence episodes in between intervals. Bladder capacity may be optimized with the rationale use of anticholinergic agents which may control unhibited detrusor contractions, maintain storage volumes and prevent the development of poor compliance [7,8].

An improvement in Quality of Life (QoL) is a consequence of the above mentioned measures. Increase in patients' self-esteem and the perception of self control and physical independence all contribute as well.

In a recent work, Lee et al. [9] reviewed QoL assessed using validated tools comparing continent x incontinent urinary diversions in cystectomized patients. Orthotopic diversions did not provide overwhelming or major QoL benefit over an incontinent cutaneous diversion at one year follow up after surgical treatment. Although cancer treated patients are not the exact same as neurogenic bladder ones, results could be extrapolated in regards to urinary habit satisfaction and adaptation.

2.2 Patient education and training

It is of utmost importance for patients to be adequately informed on the details involving intermittent self catheterization in order to avoid complications.

A review by Moore et al. [10] showed no convincing data favoring any specific catheterization technique (clean vs sterile), catheter type (coated vs uncoated), method (single vs multiple use) or person (self vs other). Different catheter types, materials and sizes can be tested depending on patient preference. Accessories may ease the procedure execution including catheter mirror, knee spreader with mirror, catheter holder. Regardless of using these, catheterization education and support is fundamental [11]. The nurse or physician should assess patient knowledge about the urinary tract; an overview of the perineum and urinary tract through pictures, figures and videos may be very helpful. Nurse should also assess the patient's ability to learn intermittent self-catheterization, awareness of problems related to it, motivation to continue long-term catheterization and the understanding of how to avoid possible complications [11].

3. Selecting the urinary diversion

As mentioned previously, urinary diversion (continent versus incontinent) must be based upon: patient's wishes; patient's manual dexterity to perform self catheterization; availability of a care provider; surgical feasibility; quality of life and life expectancy.

Whenever possible, patient's wishes regarding an incontinent conduit or an abdominal catheterizable stoma should be considered. This may result in better acceptance of the urinary diversion and therefore improve quality of life.

While a catheterizable conduit will demand a caregiver's attention every 4 to 6 hours to keep it down to the maximum storage capacity, an incontinent one may yield several hours until the urine collecting bag is full. Changing a collecting bag is incomparably easier than catheterizing a Mitroffanof channel and may significantly facilitate the caregiver's task.

Surgical feasibility of the desired urinary derivation must be assessed taking into account:

a. Previous surgical interventions:

A patient who has undergone a previous laparotomy is at risk of adhesions which can confer risk of intertinal injury and difficulty intraoperatively. If a Mitroffanof procedure is planned the presence or absence of cecal appendix will dictate whether a small bowel segment will be needed instead. In patients with previous enteric resection the residual bowel segments care must be taken not to leave the patient at high risk of a malbsorption syndrome.

With abdominal scars the resultant stoma must be fashioned without risk of ischaemia to the skin flap. Any associated abdominal wall defects will also require attention with wound closure or even access into the abdomen.

b. Obesity:

Ileal conduit externalization may be challenging in obese patients. It is important to properly anticipate the adequate intestinal loop length to assure its passage through the abdominal wall and subcutaneous tissue and also to invert the mucosal end providing an elevated "volcano-like" border. This will allow urine to flow right into the collecting bag, sparing the skin and decreasing the incidence of ammoniac dermatitis.

When externalizing a catheterizable channel, using the umbilicus may overcome the large abdominal wall width challenge.

Finally, quality of life anticipation will be most closely met when detailed preoperative planning is made in order to understand patients' expectations and the attending team is able to anticipate and clarify the patient how his routine will be with the chosen urinary diversion (frequency needed to catheterize or exchange the collecting device; changes in his physical appearance; possible related complications, etc).

The available surgical technique can be divided into continent catheterizable channels (Mitrofanoff procedure and Yang-Monti technique) and incontinent conduits (Bricker procedure and ileovesicostomy). Cutaneous ureterostomy is no longer used in current practice due to its high incidence of related complications and stomal stenosis [4].

3.1 Catheterizable channels: Mitrofanoff and Monti procedures

The principle of continent urinary diversion (Mitrofanoff principle) is similar to the one which prevents vesicoureteral reflux: to create a submucosal conduit that colapses whenever the reservoir is full preventing urinary leakage through the diversion. This is attained via a Mitrofanoff channel which is a small calibre tube that provides external access to the bladder. Clean intermittent catheterization allows for proper reservoir emptying [12,13].

This type of diversion can benefit patients with refractory urinary incontinence along with a procedure to increase the bladder outlet resistance without incontinence (bladder neck closure or tight pubovaginal sling); it may facilitate CIC execution in patients with difficulty to access their own urethra (spastic lower limbs, lack of manual dexterity) or who refuse to catheterize due to pain; and it may also offer an option for bladder emptying in patients with complex urethral stenosis [12,14].

3.2 Mitrofanoff

In 1980, Paul Mitrofanoff made the first description on the use of a continent urinary catheterizable channel utilizing the appendix which was later popularized by Duckett et al. [3,12]. The Mitrofanoff principle consists in a urinary continent derivation brought to the skin anastomosed to a low pressure reservoir utilizing an anti reflux technique through which one can perform the CIC [13]. Ideally, the stoma should be easily accessible and aesthetically pleasant [13].

The rationale behind the Mitrofanoff procedure is the maintenance of a low pressure reservoir in which filling pressures do not exceed 20 cmH_2O, while conduit pressure stands within 45-90 cmH_2O and reaches up to 80-150 cmH_2O under Valsalva maneuver [16].

3.3 The appendix

The use of the appendix by Mitrofanoff to constitute a catheterizable channel was due to several advantages: it is not a vital organ; its function is uncertain after childhood and puberty, when it has an assumed imunological role; it is easy to mobilize and has a convenient location and an adequate length; has a predictable and reliable irrigation and a steady inner lumen which permits the passage of a 10F catheter [17,18]. Mitrofanoff also described the use of the ureter as a conduit. This, however, is associated with some morbidity which are hard to overcome and limit its use: need for a transureteroureterostomy; limited mobilization; inconsistent irrigation; painful catheterization and high complication rates including stenosis and incontinence. Other options have been described such as tubularized stomach flap, cecum, colon, Meckel diverticulum, bladder, skin, prepuce, clitoris, uterine tube and vas deferens. These, however, have not reached the same acceptance as the appendix [15,17,19].

3.4 Surgical technique

Surgical approach can be accomplished through an infraumbilical median laparotomy or through a Pfannenstiel incision. The appendix is carefully dissected off of the cecum along with its mesentry. The organ is catheterized with a 12 or 14F catheter to assure adequate patency. Next, the catheterizable channel implant is performed either onto the bladder or the ileal segment when dealing with an augmented bladder. Absorbable sutures are used and care is taken to execute a 3-4 cm long anti-reflux tunnel (maintaining a length: diameter ratio of 5:1). Patency must be retested at the end of the implant [3,12,15,20].

Stomal externalization through the abdominal wall also requires attention to detail: it should be easily accessible to the patient's dominant hand and allow effortless access to the reservoir. Aesthetic appearance should also be pursued as long as it does not compromise functionality. Stoma externalization is usually made at the umbilicus or at the right lower quadrant. A stoma therapist is key for adequate positioning. There are several techniques described for the anastomosis between the conduit and the skin aiming to avoid stomal stenosis. They include V-flaps, tubular skin flaps and V-quadrilateral-Z flaps. Ideally, the conduit should be as short and straight as possible in order to avoid kinking. On the other hand, there must be no tension to the anastomosis [21-24]. Optimal drainage should be maintained post operatively. This is best accomplished with a combination of suprpubic catheterisation and a cathter through the channel.

Conduit Foley catheter is removed 3 to 6 weeks after surgery. Suprapubic cystostomy is clamped and CIC is initialized. Cystostomy may be unclamped at the end of catheterization. Once the patient is familiar with CIC technique cystostomy is definitively removed [3,12,15].

3.5 Yang-Monti

In 1993, Yang described the transversal tubularization of two previously detubularized intestinal ileal segments [25]. This technique, however, was only popularized in 1997 by Monti et al. who described its use in dogs [26].

The Monti conduit became a very important option especially in patients who are candidates for a catheterizable channel but have already undergone apendicectomy [12,15,19,26].

3.6 Surgical technique

The most important aspect for the length of the channel is the width of the abdominal wall, which should be measured in advance with the aid of a long needle [25]. The conduit short arm must be equivalent to this length. It is important to keep in mind that the diameter of the intestinal loop and not its length is the factor that is going to determine the conduit final length [27]. To obtain a longer conduit, two ileal detubularized tubes in sequence may be anastomosed [26].

In order to avoid complications secondary to malabsorption of vitamin B12 the final 15 cm of the ileum are spared [27]. A 2-2.5 cm long intestinal segment is isolated along with its vascular pedicle. This length will allow the passage of a 16F catheter. Intestine is opened longitudinally and the distance from the incision to the mesentry should be equal to the one anticipated for the conduit short arm. The segment is then tubularized transversally over a 12-14F catheter using absorbable suture [26,27,28].

Double conduits can be made of 4-5 cm of intestinal segment. Four sutures (2 at each end of the segment, one at the mesentry and the other at the anti mesenteric border) allow adequate traction and division of the intestinal loop. The two segments are incised 5 mm from the mesentry border and sutured together by the short arm with separate sutures to avoid stenosis. Tubularization is carried out in the same fashion as for single conduits. The centrifuge circulation guarantees proper perfusion and allow tailoring of the distal ends of the conduit in case it is too long [27].

The reservoir should be anchored to the deep surface of the abdominal wall immediately adjacent to the point where the channel was implanted in order to provide stability, avoid reservoir migration and conduit kinking. As mentioned for the Mitrofanoff procedure, a Foley catheter should be placed at the end of the procedure through the conduit associated with a suprapubic cystostomy [26].

On the first post operative day, irrigation of the reservoir using the suprapubic catheter is started to reduce mucus plug formation. Within 3 to 6 weeks the conduit Foley catheter is removed, cystostomy is clamped and CIC is commenced. Once the patient is familiarized with the procedure and is fully adapted suprapubic cystostomy is removed definitively [25-27,29].

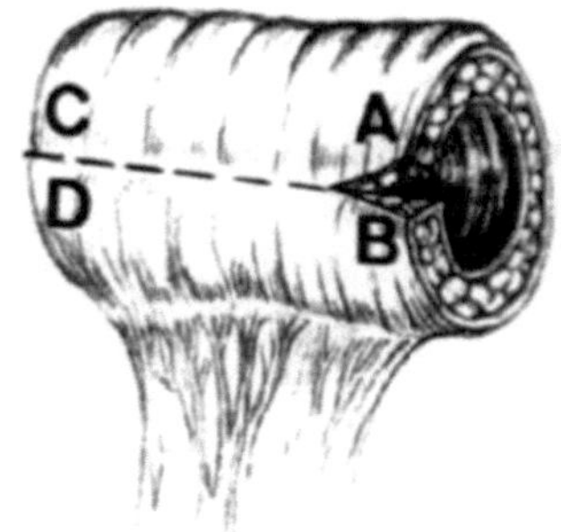

FIG. 1. Ileal segment 2 to 2.5 cm. long is excised and opened longitudinally about 1 cm. from mesentery.

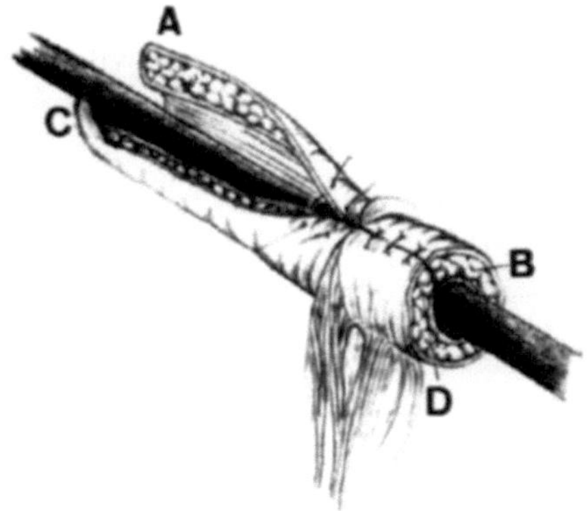

FIG. 3. Retubularization in transverse direction using interrupted sutures (4-zero chromic catgut or 5-zero polydioxanone).

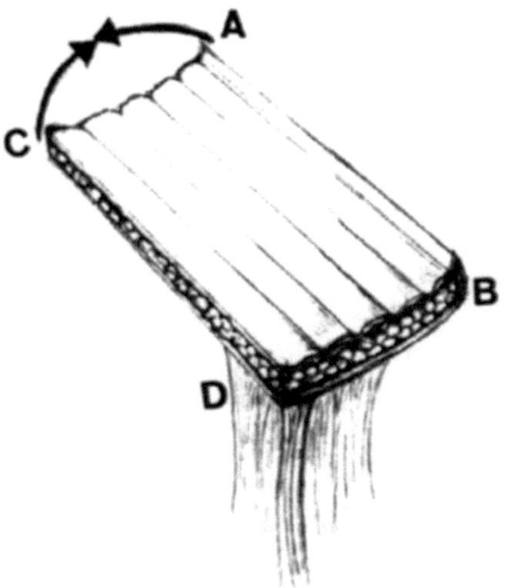

FIG. 2. Resulting pedicle rectangle (2 × 6 to 7 cm.)

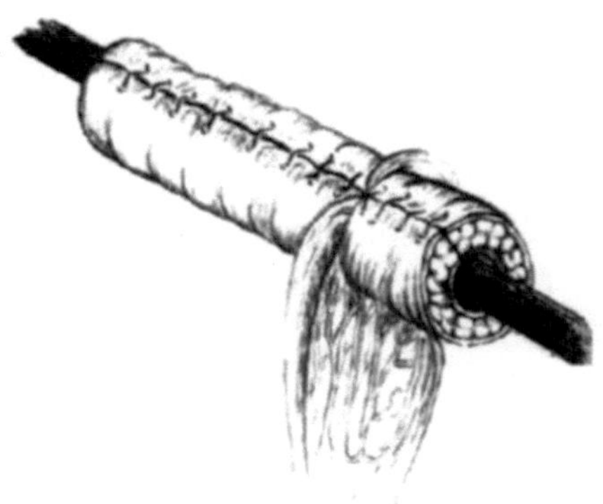

FIG. 4. Resulting small caliber tube is divided by mesentery into short and long branch.

From: Gerharz EW, Tassadaq T, Pickard RS, Shah PJ, Woodhouse CR, Ransley PG. Transverse retubularized ileum: early clinical experience with a new second line Mitrofanoff tube. J Urol 1998; 159: 525-528.

3.7 Outcomes

The risk for some early complications is common to any abdominal surgical intervention involving the urinary and gastrointestinal tracts: bleeding, infection, ileus, intestinal and urinary fistulas, intestinal obstruction, conduit ischemia, abscess, pyelonephritis and sepsis are included [1,14].

Long term follow up series show results for both Mitrofanoff and Monti interventions exceeding 90% continence rates. Sahadevan et al. reported a self-reported continence rate of 89% with a mean follow up time of 126 months [30]. Incontinence may occur through the urethra or the conduit [20,21,31,12-14,17,27-29,32-34].

Most reports comparing the two types of channel did not show differences in continence rates when comparing site of conduit implantation into the native bladder versus bowel [21,35].

Whenever there is an indication for occlusion or reinforcement of the bladder neck resistance different procedures may be considered including a "tight" sling, periurethral bulking agents injection, or bladder neck closure. In a retrospective study, De Troyer et al. [36] compared bladder neck closure with reconstructive procedures aiming to reinforce the bladder outlet resistance in a pediatric population showing a higher continence rate in the former, with no increase in morbidity (such as stone formation and stomal stenosis) or relationship with augmentation procedures. The authors highlight the need for concern when considering a bladder neck closure as access to the reservoir and to the upper urinary tract may become more difficult [36].

In Yang's original study, two main areas of elevated pressure were identified: bladder submucosal tunnel and the segment crossing the abdominal wall. Under Valsalva maneuver simultaneous pressure onto the conduit and the reservoir occurs, but not in the area through the abdominal wall [25]. As such, continence is highly dependent on the submucosal tunnel.

4. Surgical complications and treatment options

Overall complication rates are reported to be high and depend on the follow up time but may be estimated between 23 to 36% for appendicostomies [37,38].

The complications related to stoma represent the vast majority of those found in urinary diversion procedures involving a conduit. Many of these are consequences of preventable technical errors during surgery [39]. Retraction, stomal prolapse, parastomal hernia, and stenosis are the most frequent. Stenosis occurs in up to 33% of patients and is considered one of the major complications [39-43]. Stomal stenosis can result from a combination of factors, including ischemia, fascial contraction, retraction, local skin alterations, and stoma placement [37, 39]. Long term stenosis at the skin level has been shown to be preventable with the aid of a silicon device (ACE stopper, Medicina, Adlington, UK) by Lopez et al. [44]. In a retrospective study comparing VQZ technique, TSF technique and the umbilicus for stoma confection Landau et al. found VQZ plasty the most effective (patency rates 100%, 55% and 74%, $p<0.001$) hypothesizing this might be a consequence of better blood supply which would come from 3 different sources [23].

Welk et al. reported higher complication rates with Monti technique than Mitrofanoff (60% versus 19%, respectively) [18] although McAndrew et al. found more problems with appendicovesicostomy [21]. In a very recent report, Leslie et al. found no difference in complication rate comparing the two channel types [45]. CIC execution seems also to be more difficult after a Yang-Monti ileovesicostomy technique compared to the appendix. Narayanaswamy et al. reviewed patients who underwent apendicovesicostomy with those who had a Monti conduit. He found a 27% vs. 60% rate of problems to catheterize, respectively. Among Monti cases, there was a detectable stenosis in half (13 out of 25 patients). The authors observed the formation of "pouch-like dilatations" along the ileal channel and hypothesized this to be secondary to the creation of a zone of weakness resulting from the rearrangement of muscle fibers following retubularization which would facilitate "stretching-out" and false passage during catheterization [46]. Other authors reported rates of 11% [47] and 23% of problems related to catheterization of retubularized intestinal tubes [27]. Management may involve a simple Foley catheter placement for a few weeks or a surgical resection of the pouches [3].

Narayanaswamy et al. also found an incidence of conduit stenosis at the bladder implant of 6% for appendix and 8% for Monti tubes. Stomal stenosis occurred in 15% vs. 16% comparing appendix and Monti, respectively [46]. Landau et al. reported on a retrospective series comparing different techniques for stoma confection: umibilical flap, tubularized skin flap and TVZ flap. Stenosis rates were 25%, 45% and zero, respectively [23].

Problems suspected to be related to conduit patency should be evaluated using an endoscopic approach or performing a conduitogram. This will allow differentiation between stenosis, pouching or kinking. Definitive treatment may vary from calibration to conduit or stoma surgical revision [3,18,48]. D'Ancona and Miyaoka presented an innovative option for salvage treatment of stomal stenosis that fails more conservative approaches such as dilatations and corticosteroid injections and traditional surgical revisions. In patients in whose stoma was placed in the lower abdomen and had the umbilicus preserved they used an umbilical grafting to reestablish conduit superficial patency. Although follow up was short (up to 6 months) results were promising [48].

In cases where urine leakage happens the valvular mechanism may be defective, the reservoir pressure may be excessively high, or both. Urodynamic study is key to establish the diagnosis [36]. If a high pressure-reservoir is diagnosed bladder augmentation may be considered. On the other hand, if the valve mechanism is the issue a submucosal injection of a bulking agent or surgical revision making the tunnel longer may solve the problem [26]. Bulking agents have conflicting results with reported success rates up to 71% [49].

Most conduit complications will occur within 2 years from surgery, but even initially stable channels are susceptible to complications and must be reassessed throughout patients' lifetime [18].

Calculi formation and urinary tract infection have a fairly high incidence in continent reservoir patients and may vary from 26-32% and 19-63%, respectively [47,50]. They may be facilitated by mucus formation in patients who undergo bladder augmentation and by the position in which the tube is implanted into the bladder (anteriorly placed tubes drain with lower efficacy than those positioned posteriorly) [51]. Patient compliance with CIC execution may also influence these complication rates [18].

Table 1 compiles comparatively the complication rates between Mitrofanoff and Monti channels (Table 1).

	Mitrofanoff	Monti	Author
Overall	19%	60%	Welk et al. 2008
Difficulty to catheterise	27%	60%	Narayanaswamy et al. 2001
Channel stenosis at bladder implant	6%	8%	Narayanaswamy et al. 2001
Stomal stenosis	15%	16%	Narayanaswamy et al. 2001
Calculi formation	26-32%	26-32%	Clark et al. 2002; Duckett et al. 1993
Urinary Tract Infection	19-63%	19-63%	Clark et al. 2002; Duckett et al. 1993

Table 1. Surgical complications and incidence rates

5. Final considerations

Understanding the complexity involving the patients who need a urinary derivation is the cornerstone of treatment success. This includes knowing when and which urinary derivation is more suitable for each situation and assuring an appropriate preparation pre operatively. Proper patient education will facilitate patient's adherence to self catheterization and elevate chances to meet his expectations towards the treatment. It cannot be forgotten that although continent urinary conduits offer a very high rate of success, revisions are expected and may occur throughout patient's entire lifetime. Therefore, regular and thorough follow up is warranted.

6. List of abbreviations

CIC - Clean intermittent catheterization
UTI - Urinary tract infection
QoL - Quality of life

7. References

[1] Adams MC, Joseph DB. Urinary Tract Reconstruction in Children. In Campbell-Walsh Urology, 9th Ed. 2007, Chapter 124, p. 3656-3702.
[2] Metcalfe PD, Cain MP. Incontinent and Continent Urinary Diversion. Pediatric Urology 2nd Ed. 2010, Chapter 56, p. 737-747.
[3] Farrugia MK, Malone PS. Educational article: The Mitrofanoff procedure. J Ped Urol 2010; 6: 330-337.
[4] Westney OL. The Neurogenic Bladder and Incontinent Urinary Diversion Urol Clin N Am 2010; 37: 581–592.
[5] Lapides J, Diokno C, Silber SJ, et al. Clean, intermittent self- catheterization in the treatment of urinary tract disease. Trans Amer Assoc Genitourin Surg 1971; 63:92-96.
[6] McGuire EJ, Woodside JR, Borden TA, et al. Prognostic value of urodynamic testing in myelodysplastic patients. J Urol 1981; 126:205- 209.
[7] Stöhrer M, Murtz G, Kramer G, et al. Propiverine compared to oxybutynin in neurogenic detrusor: results of a randomized, double-blind, multicenter clinical study. Eur Urol 2007; 51:235-242.
[8] Goessl C, Knispel HH, Fiedler U, et al. Urodynamic effects of oral oxybutynin chloride in children with myelomeningocele and detrusor hyperreflexia. Urology 1998; 51:94-98.
[9] Lee CT. Quality of life following incontinent cutaneous and orthotopic urinary diversions. Curr Treat Options Oncol 2009; 10: 275-286.
[10] Moore KN, Fader M, Getliffe K. Long-term bladder management by intermittent catheterisation in adults and children. Cochrane Database System Review 2007, 4, CD006008.
[11] Newman DK, Willson MM. Review of intermittent catheterization and current best practices. Urol Nurs. 2011; 31:12-28.
[12] Mitrofanoff P. Cystostomie continent trans-appendiculaire dans le traitement des vessies neurologiques. Chir Pediatr 1980; 21:297- 305.

[13] Duckett JW, Snyder HM 3rd.Continent urinary diversion: variations on the Mitrofanoff principle. J Urol 1986; 136: 58–62.
[14] Liard AS, Uier-Lipszyc ES, Mathiot A, Mitrofanoff P. The Mitrofanoff Procedure: 20 Years Later. J Urol 2001; 165: 2394–2398.
[15] Kaefer M, Retik AB. The Mitrofanoff Principle in continent urinary reconstruction. Urol Clin N Am 1997; 24:795-811.
[16] Chabchoub K, Ketata H, Fakhfakh H, Bahloul A, Mhiri MN. Continent urinary diversion (Mitrofanoff principle). Physical mechanisms and urodynamic explanation of continence. Progrès en Urologie 2008; 18: 120-124.
[17] Monti PR, Lara RC, Dutra MA, de Carvalho Jr. New echniques for construction of efferent conduits based on the Mitrofanoff principle. Urology 1997; 49: 112-15.
[18] Welk BK, Afshar K, Rapoport D, MacNeily AE. Complications of the catheterizable channel following continent urinary diversion: Their nature and timing. J Urol 2008; 180: 1856-1860.
[19] McLaughlin KP, Keating MA. The appendix in reconstructive urology. Surg Ann 1995; 27: 215–231.
[20] Furness PD, Malone PSJ, Barqawi A, Koyle MA. The Mitrofanoff principle: innovative applications incontinent urinary diversion. Contemp Urol 2003; 15(1):30-45.
[21] McAndrew HF, Malone PSJ. Continent catheterizable conduits: which stoma, which conduit and which reservoir? BJU Int 2002, 89:86.
[22] Murthi GV, Kelly JH. V-Vplasty: a new technique for providing a resilient skin- lined opening for the Mitrofanoff stoma. Urology 2006; 68:661-662.
[23] Landau EH, Gofrit ON, Cipele H, Hardak B, Duvdevani M, Pode D et al. Superiority of the VQZ over the tabularized skin flap and the umbilicus for continent abdominal stoma in children. J Urol 2008; 180: 1761-1765.
[24] England RJ, Subramaniam R. Functional and cosmetic outcome of the VQ plasty for Mitrofanoff stomas. JUrol 2007; 178:2607-2610.
[25] Yang WH. Yang needle tunnelling technique in creating antireflux and continent mechanisms. J Urol 1993; 150: 830-834.
[26] Monti PR, Carvalho JR, Arap S. The Monti Procedure: Applications and Complications. Urology 2000; 55: 616–621.
[27] Castellan MA, Gosalbez R, Labbie Jr. A, Monti PR. Clinical Applications of the Monti procedure as a continent catheterizable stoma. Urology 1999; 54: 153-156.
[28] Leslie JA, Dussinger AM , Meldrum KK. Creation of continence mechanisms (Mitrofanoff) without appendix: the Monti and spiral Monti procedures. Urol Oncol 2007; 25: 148–153.
[29] Gerharz EW, Tassadaq T, Pickard RS, Shah PJ, Woodhouse CR, Ransley PG. Transverse retubularized ileum: early clinical experience with a new second line Mitrofanoff tube. J Urol 1998; 159: 525-528.
[30] Sahadevan K, Pickard RS, Neal DE, Hasan TS. Is continent diversion using the Mitrofanoff principle a viable long-term option for adults requiring bladder replacement? BJU Int 2008;102:236-240.
[31] Harris CF, Cooper CS, Hutcheson JC, Snyder HM. Appendicovesicostomy: the Mitrofanoff procedure—a 15-Year perspective. J Urol 2000; 163: 1922–1926.
[32] Keating MA, Rink RC, Adams MC. Appendicovesicostomy: a useful adjunct to continent reconstruction of the bladder. J. Urol 1993; 149: 1091-1094.
[33] Van Savage JG, Khoury AE, McLorie GA, Churchill BM. Outcome analysis of Mitrofanoff principle applications using appendix and ureter to umbilical and lower quadrant stomal sites. J Urol 1996; 158: 1794- 1797.

[34] Sylora JA, Gonzalez R, Vaughn M, Reinberg Y. Intermittent self- catheterization by quadriplegic patients via a catheterizable Mitrofanoff channel. J Urol 1997; 157: 48-50.
[35] Piaggio L, Myers S, Figueroa TE, Barthold JS, Gonzalez R. Influence of type of conduit and site of implantation on the outcome of continent catheterizable channels. J Pediatr Urol 2007; 3:230-234.
[36] De Troyer B, Van Laecke E, Groen LA, Everaert K, Hoebeke P. A comparative study between continent diversion and bladder neck closure versus continent diversion and bladder neck reconstruction in children. J Ped Urol 2011; 7: 209-212.
[37] De Ganck J, Everaert K, Van Laecke E, *et al.* A high easy-to-treat complication rate is the price for a continent stoma. BJU Int 90: 240– 243, 2002.
[38] Thomas JC, Dietrich MS, Trusler L, De Marco RT, Pope JC, Brock III JW et al. Continent catheterizable channels and the timing of their complications. JUrol 2006;176:1816-20.
[39] Farnham SB, Cookson MS. Surgical complications of urinary diversion. World J Urol 2004; 22: 157-67.
[40] Khoury AE, Van Savage JGV, McLorie GA et al. Minimizing stomal stenosis in appendicovesicostomy: using the modified umbilical stoma. J Urol 1996; 155: 2050-51.
[41] Barqawi A, Valdenebro M, Furness PD III et al. Lessons learned from stomal complications in children with cutaneous catheterizable continent stomas. BJU Int 2004; 94: 1344–1347.
[42] Blaivas JG, Weiss JP, Desai P, *et al:* Long-term follow up of augmentation enterocystoplasty and continent diversion in patients with benign disease. J Urol 2005; 173: 1631–1634.
[43] Cain MP, Casale AJ, King SJ, Rink RC. Appendicovesicostomy and newer alternatives for the Mitrofanoff procedure: results in the last 100 patients at Riley Children's Hospital. J Urol 1999; 162: 1749- 1752.
[44] Lopez PJ, Ashrafian H, Clarke SA, Johnson H, Kiely EM. Early experience with the antegrade colonic enema stopper to reduce stomal stenosis. J Pediatr Surg 2007;42:522-4.
[45] Leslie B, Lorenzo AJ, Moore K, Farhat WA, Bagli DJ, Pippi Salle JL. Long- term follow up and time to event outcome analysis of continent catheterizable channels. J Urol 2011; 185: 2298-2302.
[46] Narayanaswamy B, Wilcox DT, Cuckow PM, Duffy PG, Ransley PG. The Yang- Monti ileovesicostomy: a problematic channel? BJU Int 2001; 87: 861-865.
[47] Clark T, Pope JC, Adams MC, Wells N, Brock JW. Factors that influence outcomes of the Mitrofanoff and Malone antegrade continence enema reconstructive procedures in children. J Urol 2002;168:1537-40.
[48] D'Ancona CAL, Miyaoka R, Ikari LY, Nunes PHF. Umbilical grafting in treatment of recurrent stomal stenosis. Urology 2008; 71: 1124-1127.
[49] Prieto JC, Perez-Brayfield M, Kirsch AJ, Koyle MA. The treatment of catheterizable stomal incontinence with endoscopic implantation of dextranomer/ hyaluronic acid. J Urol 2006; 175: 709-711.
[50] Duckett JW, Lotfi AH. Appendicovesicostomy (and variations) in bladder reconstruction. J Urol 1993; 149: 567-569.
[51] Berkowitz J, North AC, Tripp R, Gearhart JP, Lakshmanan Y. Mitrofanoff continent catheterizable conduits: Top down or bottom up? J Pediatr Urol 2009; 5: 122-125.

18

Futuristic Concept in Management of Female SUI: Permanent Repair Without Permanent Material

Yasser Farahat and Ali Abdel Raheem
Tanta University Hospital
Egypt

1. Introduction

Stress urinary incontinence (SUI) is defined as the complaint of involuntary leakage of urine on exertion or on sneezing or coughing **(Abrams et al, 2002)**. Female SUI is a common distressing health problem, affecting large number of women worldwide, with prevalence rates ranging from 12.8% to 46.0% **(Botlero et al, 2008)**. SUI is considered the most common type of urinary incontinence among women and presents about 50 % of these populations, while mixed urinary incontinence presents 36 % and only 14 % are due to urge urinary incontinence **(Hannestad et al, 2000)**. SUI has a negative impact on women quality of life specially their social, physical, occupational, psychological, and sexual aspects of life.

SUI arises when the bladder pressure exceeds the urethral pressure, in the setting of sudden increases of intra-abdominal pressure (coughing, sneezing ...etc). Most researchers now identify two main etiologic mechanisms for the development of SUI: urethral hypermobility due to loss of urethral support - the hammock-like supportive layer described by DeLancey **(DeLancey, 1994)**, and intrinsic sphincter deficiency (ISD), with most patients having elements of both disorders (Table 1).

There are several options for treatment of female SUI. Conservative treatment (pelvic floor muscle exercise) is usually advocated as a 1st line therapy since it carries minimal risks and studies have shown up to 70% improvement in symptoms of SUI following appropriately performed pelvic floor exercise **(Price, Dawood and Jackson, 2010)**. Conservative management strategies include:

1. Life style changes (weight reduction, smoking cessation, ↓ fluid intake, treatment of constipation .... etc).
2. Pelvic floor muscle training ± biofeedback.
3. Vaginal cones and electrical stimulation.

Regarding pharmacotherapy, no drug till now has been approved to be used by the Food and Drug Administration (FDA) for the treatment of female SUI. Duloxetine is a serotonin-norepinephrine reuptake inhibitor (SNRI) has been investigated, it can significantly improve the quality of life of patients with SUI, but it is unclear whether or not benefits are sustainable in addition it has a common side-effects **(Mariappan et al, 2007)**.

1- Bladder neck/urethral hypermobility (due to loss of urethral support):	- Vaginal delivery. - Aging. - Estrogen deficiency. - Connective tissue disorders.
2- Intrinsic sphincter deficiency (ISD):	- Multiple anti-incontinence procedures - Radical pelvic surgery - Radiation - Menopause - Urogenital atrophy
3- Other risk factors:	- Chronic ↑ in intra-abdominal pressure. - Constipation. - Smoking. - Physical inactivity. - Genetic predisposition.

Table 1. Show various etiological factors involved in the pathophysiology of SUI.

Surgical treatment for SUI should be undertaken for women with SUI who have failed conservative treatment strategies or if the patient wants definitive treatment from the start.

Over the past years, many surgical procedures have been used for the treatment of female SUI with varying degrees of success. Recently, a number of new minimally invasive surgical techniques have been developed for treatment of female SUI that aimed to decrease the morbidity, improved safety and improvement of the surgical outcomes, while maintaining the efficacy of traditional open incontinence surgery. The Tension free vaginal tape (TVT) procedure was first described and evaluated by Ulmsten et al in Sweden in 1996 **(Ulmsten et al, 1996)**, then the Transobturator tape (TOT) procedure was developed in 2001 by DeLorme to avoid the retropubic space **(DeLorme E, 2001)**. Midurethral slings (TVT and TOT) have the following advantages:

1. The ability to be performed under local anaesthesia in patients who are unfit for major surgery.
2. Better for young aged women due to better cosmetic appearance since there is now open wound such the old traditional surgical methods.
3. Lower costs, shorter hospital stay, early recovery time and less postoperative pain.

Further improvement in surgical procedures towards less invasive sling technique has led to the innovation of a mini-sling e.g. TVT Secur system, which is a surgical device requiring only a single suburethral incision to be inserted **(Neuman and Shaare-Zedek, 2007)**. Mini-slings have the following advantages over the ordinary midurethral slings (TVT and TOT):

1. The complications associated with suprapubic and groin incisions will be eliminated.
2. Cystoscopy will not be necessary.
3. Operative time will be shorter than with other midurethral sling techniques.

2. Midurethral slings for SUI treatment

2.1 Surgical principle of midurethral slings

Petros and Ulmsten proposed the integral or midurethral theory of the female pelvic floor and urethral closure mechanism **(Petros and Ulmsten, 1993)**, which has been the basis upon which many of the newer treatments for SUI have been developed. The idea that a loss of mid-urethral support is a causative factor in female SUI led to the use of synthetic midurethral tapes which became popular because of ease of placement and excellent outcomes. After their introduction by Ulmsten and Delorme, TVT and TOT gained a great popularity and rapid widespread and become now the gold standard treatment minimally invasive treatment of female SUI. Both techniques (TVT and TOT) aimed to recreating urethral support using a polypropylene mesh placed at midurethral without tension to create an artificial collagenous neoligament, using the foreign body reaction induced by the host defense mechanism. TVT acts as a pubourethral neoligament anchored suprapubically, which tightens around the urethra in the setting of increased intra-abdominal pressure. TOT had the following advantage over TVT by avoiding the blind trocar passage in the retropubic space by passing the trocar through the obturator muscles and membrane, thus decreasing the risk of major bladder, bowel perforation and vascular injury also decreasing the need for cystoscopy use after tape placement (figure 1 and 2).

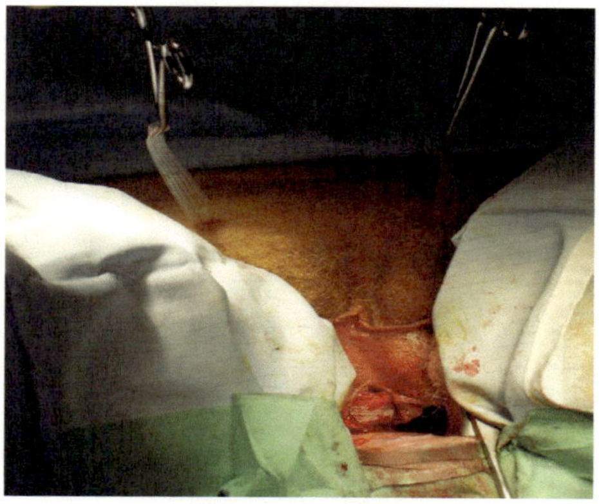

Fig. 1. TVT in position **(Morley and Nethercliffe, 2005)**.

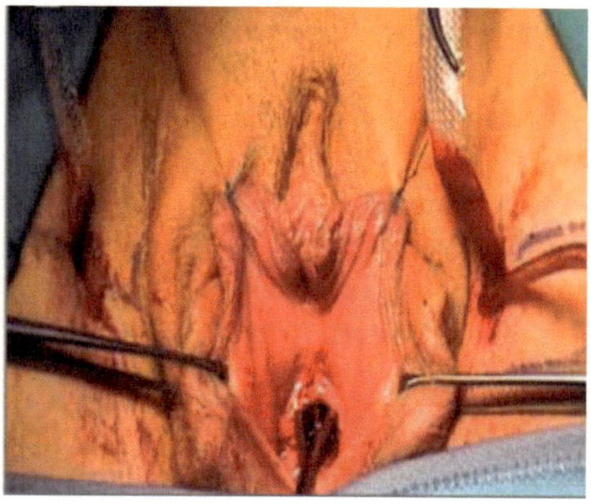

Fig. 2. TOT in position **(De Leval, 2003)**.

2.2 Clinical results of midurethral slings

2.2.1 TVT surgical outcomes

TVT has undergone the most rigorous testing all over the years, and now it is considered the gold standard treatment option for female SUI. To date it is estimated that more than 1 million cases have been performed worldwide **(Deng et al, 2007)**. There are now many prospective studies in literature with a long-term follow-up showing great success of TVT for the treatment of female SUI with cure rate > 80 % as seen in (table 2) denoting the long term durability of this procedure. In 2008, Nilsson et al reported the longest follow-up (11 years) of TVT operation and demonstrated that (90% objective cure rate) of women treated without any significant late-onset adverse effects **(Nilsson et al, 2008)**. In another study with follow-up for 10 years. TVT showed satisfactory objective (84%) and subjective (57%) cure rates with (23%) improvement **(Aigmueller et al, 2011)**.

Author	Number of patients	Patient group	Duration of follow-up (years)	Treatment outcomes (subjective/objective) % cured
Villet et al, 2002	124	SUI	32.5 months	88.7%
Rezapour et al, 2001a	34	Recurrent SUI	4	82%
Rezapour et al, 2001b	80	Mixed urinary incontinence	4	85%
Rezapour et al, 2001c	49	SUI due to (ISD)	4	74%
Deffieux et al, 2007	51	SUI	6.9	80%
Nilsson et al, 2004	90	SUI	7	81.3%

Table 2. Long term results of TVT.

TVT has replaced the old gold standard Burch colposuspension. In a randomized control trial (RCT) conducted by Ward and Hilton who compared TVT with the open colposuspension on they reported equal efficacy with subjective cure rate 81% and 80% in TVT and Burch group respectively. The duration of hospitalization, operative time and the time taken to return to normal activity seem to be shorter in the TVT group. The authors concluded that the TVT procedure is as effective as the Burch colposuspension in urodynamically proven patients with SUI at a 2-year follow-up **(Ward and Hilton, 2004)**. The same authors have published their 5-year out comes in this study where they reported subjective cure in 81% in the TVT group and 90% in the colposuspension group. They stated that the effect of both procedures on cure and improvement in quality of life has been maintained for long time **(Ward and Hilton, 2008)**.

2.2.2 TOT surgical outcomes

Short-term data regarding the efficacy of the TOT suggest that this procedure perform as well as the TVT and may perhaps cause fewer complications. TOT has shown to be of equal efficacy to TVT with cure rate > 80% (table 3), however, still long-term studies have yet to be done to evaluate the effectiveness and durability of the TOT procedure.

Author	Number of patients	Patient group	Duration of follow-up	Treatment outcomes (% cured)
Cindolo et al, 2004	80	SUI with urethral hypermobility	4 months	92
Grise et al, 2006	206	SUI	Mean (16 months)	79.1
Giberti et al, 2007	108	SUI due to urethral hypermobility	2 years	80
Roumeguere et al, 2005	120	Urodynamic SUI	1 year	80
Waltregny et al, 2008	91	SUI	3 year	88
Liapis, Bakas and Creatsas, 2010	74 (32 TVT-O and 41 TVT-O + ant. Colporrhaphy	SUI and Cystocele	4 year	82.4 and 80.5 % respectively

Table 3. Results of TOT.

2.2.3 TVT versus TOT outcomes

TVT and TOT since their introduction in the treatment of female SUI have gained a great popularity and wide spread use in a large number of studies. Both techniques showed nearly equal efficacy with more than 80% cure rate in the majority of studies as mentioned before (Table 2, table 3). Novara et al, in a large systematic review and meta-analysis showed that patients treated with TVT had slightly higher objective cure rates (OR: 0.8;CI: 0.65–0.99; p = 0.04) than those treated with TOT; however, subjective cure rates were similar in both technique **(Novara et al, 2010)**. In a long term follow-up after 5 years both TVT and TVT-O procedures were safe, with equivalent results (72.9% and 71% of patients objectively cured after TVT-O and TVT, respectively) **(Angioli et al, 2010)**.

2.3 Material used for midurethral slings

Over the past years there was a great evolution in the use of biological and synthetic materials in the treatment of different reconstructive pelvic surgery e.g. SUI and pelvic organ prolapse (POP) in an effort to improve surgical outcomes. However, the potential benefits of using grafts need to be carefully balanced against the risks of using foreign materials to the patient's body. Amid in 1997 published a classification for synthetic mesh used in abdominal hernia surgery based on the pore size (macroporous, microporous, submicro-porous) and fiber type (monofilaments or multifilament) of the synthetic mesh **(Amid, 1997)**. Synthetic grafts may be non-absorbable, absorbable, or a mixture of the two. The non-absorbable polypropylene mesh is the most common type used in reconstructive pelvic surgery. Synthetic tapes available in the market for urogynecological practice see (table 4).

The pore size and interstices distance between the fibers (figure 3) are important mesh characteristics that determine whether host inflammatory cell and fibroblasts can penetrate the mesh or not. The ideal synthetic tapes used for the treatment of SUI should have the following characters: made of polypropylene, low weight, macroporous, monofilament mesh, with an elasticity between 20 and 35%, as these tapes have a lower incidence of infection and tissue erosion **(Rosch et al, 2004; Deprest et al, 2006).**

Pore size classification	Component	Trade name	Fibre type
Type I: Totally macroporous (pore size of >75 μm)	Polypropylene Polypropylene/ Polyglactin 910 Polyglactin 910	Prolene, Gynemesh, Gynemesh PS (Ethicon) Marlex, Pelvitex a (Bard) Surgipro b SPMM (Tyco) Vypro (Ethicon) Vicryl (Ethicon)	Monofilament Monofilament Monofilament Mono- multifilament multifilament
Type II: Totally microporous (pore size of <10 μm)	Expanded PTFE	Gore-Tex (Gore)	multifilament
Type III: Micro or macro-micro	Polyethylene PTFE Braided polypropylene Braided polypropylene–open weave Perforated Expanded PTFE	Mersilene (Ethicon) Teflon (Gore) Surgipro b SPM (Tyco) Surgipro b SPMW (Tyco) Mycro-mesh (Gore)	multifilament multifilament multifilament multifilament multifilament
Type IV: Submicronic pore size (pore size of <1 μm)	Polypropylene sheet	Cellgard	Monofilament

PTFE: Polytetrafluoroethylene
a Collagen coated macroporous polypropylene materials.
b Several kinds of Surgipro (Tyco) materials are marketed under the same name and have different constructs.

Table 4. Classification and characteristics of synthetic implant materials marketed for urogynecologic indications **(Deprest et al, 2006).**

Type I macroporous mesh with (pore size >75 μm) allowing easier penetration of inflammatory cells such as leukocytes (9–15 μm), macrophages (16–20 μm), fibroblast and blood vessels into the graft to phagocytose bacteria (<1 μm) lowering the risk of infection, in addition host tissue in growth and incorporation is promoted resulting in good support. On the other hand, multifilament meshes have interstices that are <10 μm and bacteria (<1 μm) can replicate within these interstices. However, access to macrophages and ability to fight bacterial colonisation within the interstices is impaired **(Winters et al, 2006)**. Monofilament mesh does not have small interstices and the risk of mesh infection and erosion is reduced with its use.

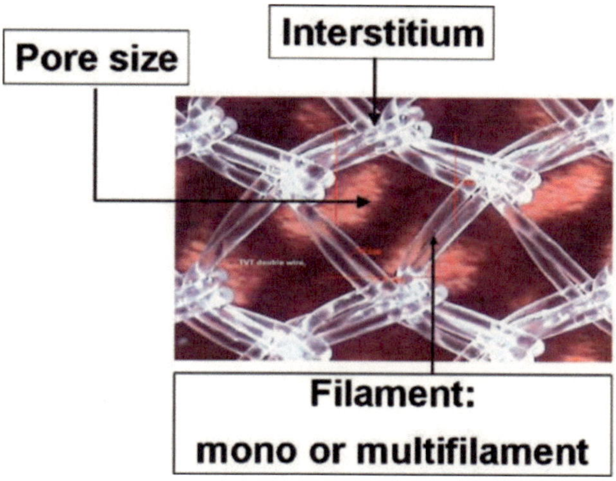

Fig. 3. Terminology used to classify synthetic implants. Magnified view of a part of a polypropylene tape as used for TVT procedure (Gynaecare, Johnson and Johnson) with identification of filament type, interstitium, and pore size **(Deprest et al, 2006).**

Biological implants have many sources; they may be an autologous graft (derived from the patient's own body tissue), allograft (derived from post-mortem tissue banks) or xenograft (derived from animals) **(Dwyer, 2006)**. Types of biologic implants available in the market that can be used in urogynecology practice (table 5):

Biological types	Component	Trade name
Autologous grafts	Rectus fascia Fascia lata Vaginal mucosa	
Allografts	Fascia lata Dura mater	Lyodura
Xenografts	Porcine non-cross-linked small intestine submucosal collagen Porcine non cross-linked dermal collagen Porcine dermal cross-linked collagen Fetal bovine skin derived collagen scaffold Bovine non-cross-linked pericardium	Surgisis (Cook) InteXen (AMS) Pelvicol, Pelvisoft, Pelvilace (Bard) Xenform (Boston Scientific) Veritas (Synovis)

Table 5. Classification of biologic implant materials marketed for urogynecologic indications **(Deprest et al, 2006).**

2.4 Complications of synthetic midurethral slings

Although midurethral slings are minimally invasive procedures with high efficacy, however they result in bothersome complications which should not be minimized. The reported complication rates for midurethral slings ranged from 4.3% to 75.1% for TVT and 10.5% to 31.3% for TOT **(Daneshgari et al, 2008).** Awareness of these complications should encourage improvements in patient counseling as well as further investigation of the underlying mechanisms. Summary of the complications of midurethral sling procedures (table 6):

a) Intraoperative complications:	- Major: Vascular lesions. Nerve injuries. Gut lesions. - Minor: Bladder injury. Urethral injury.
b) Early postoperative complications:	- Retropubic haematoma. - Blood loss > 200 ml. - Urinary tract infections. - Spondylitis.
c) Late postoperative complications:	- Transient urinary retention. - Permanent urinary retention. - Groin and thigh pain. - Genitourinary erosion. - De novo urgency. - Urethral obstruction. - Dyspareunia.

Table 6. Summary of the complications of midurethral sling procedures.

With regard to complications, most of the complications reported were intraoperative minor ones, with little or no disabling effects provided they are recognized and treated intraoperatively. A very limited number of major complications (e.g. bowel, vascular, and nerve injuries, necrotizing fasciitis, ischiorectal abscess, urethrovaginal fistulas, sepsis, and patient deaths) have been reported after placement of midurethral slings. Deng et al reported on the prevalence of major complications in the US Food and Drug Administration's Manufacturer and User Facility Device Experience database, identifying 32 cases of vascular injuries, 33 bowel injuries, and 8 patient deaths after TVT placement **(Deng et al, 2007)**.

A new terminology and classification system has been developed by the International Urogynecological Association (IUGA) and the International Continence Society (ICS) for full description of all possible physical complications related directly to the insertion of prostheses (meshes, implants, tapes) & grafts in female pelvic floor surgery (figure 4). A key advantage of a standardized classification is that all parties involved in female pelvic floor surgery including surgeons, physicians, nurses, allied health professionals and industry will be referring to the same clinical issue. It is anticipated that a category (C), time (T), and site (S) - (CTS) codified table of complications will be a necessary part of reports of surgical procedures relevant to this document. With a standardized classification in place, quicker assessment of adverse events will be achieved together with uniform reporting of prosthetic-related complications **(Haylen et al, 2011)**.

CATEGORY

	General Description	A (Asymptomatic)	B (Symptomatic)	C (Infection)	D (Abscess)
1	**Vaginal**: no epithelial separation Include prominence (e.g. due to wrinkling or folding), mesh fibre palpation or contraction (shrinkage)	**1A**: Abnormal prosthesis or graft finding on clinical examination	**1B**: Symptomatic e.g. unusual discomfort / pain; dyspareunia (either partner); bleeding	**1C**: Infection (suspected or actual)	**1D** = Abscess
2	**Vaginal**: smaller ≤ 1cm exposure	**2A**: Asymptomatic	**2B**: Symptomatic	**2C**: Infection	**2D** = Abscess
3	**Vaginal**: larger >1cm exposure, or any extrusion	**3A**: Asymptomatic 1-3A*a* if no prosthesis or graft related pain	**3B**: Symptomatic 1-3B (*b-e*) if prosthesis or graft related pain	**3C**: Infection 1-3C /1-3D (*b-e*) if prosthesis or graft related pain	**3D** = Abscess
4	**Urinary Tract**: compromise or perforation Including prosthesis (graft) perforation, fistula and calculus	**4A**: Small intraoperative defect e.g. bladder perforation	**4B**: Other lower urinary tract complication or urinary retention	**4C**: Ureteric or upper urinary tract complication	
5	**Rectal or Bowel**: compromise or perforation including prosthesis (graft) perforation and fistula	**5A**: Small intraoperative defect (rectal or bowel)	**5B**: Rectal injury or compromise	**5C**: Small or Large bowel injury or compromise	**5D** = Abscess
6	**Skin and / or musculoskeletal**: complications including discharge pain lump or sinus tract formation	**6A**: Asymptomatic, abnormal finding on clinical examination	**6B**: Symptomatic e.g. discharge, pain or lump	**6C**: Infection e.g. sinus tract formation	**6D** = Abscess
7	**Patient**: compromise including hematoma or systemic compromise	**7A**: Bleeding complication including haematoma	**7B**: Major degree of resuscitation or intensive care*	**7C**: Mortality * *(additional complication - no site applicable - **S 0**)	

TIME (clinically diagnosed)

T1: Intraoperative to 48 hours	**T2**: 48 hours to 2 months	**T3**: 2 months to 12 months	**T4:** over 12 months

SITE

S1: Vaginal: area of suture line	**S2**: Vaginal: away from from area of suture line	**S3**: Trocar passage Exception: Intra-abdominal (**S5**)	**S4**: other skin or musculoskeletal site	**S5**: Intra-abdominal

N.B.
1. **Multiple complications may occur in the same patient. There may be early and late complications in the same patient. i.e. All complications to be listed. Tables of complications may often be procedure specific.**
2. **The highest final category for any single complication should be used if there is a change over time. (patient 888)**
3. **Urinary tract infections and functional issues (apart from 4B) have not been included.**

CODE ☐☐☐- T ☐- S ☐

Fig. 4. A classification by category (C), time (T), and site (S) of complications directly related to the insertion of prostheses (meshes, implants, tapes) or grafts in female pelvic floor surgery **(Haylen et al, 2011).**

2.4.1 Intraoperative and early postoperative complications

Bladder perforation: occur during trocar passage in the retropubic space, it is a common intraoperative complication with reported rates of 0.7% to 24%. **(Laurikainen et al, 2007; Andonian et al, 2005).** Incidence of perforation increases with poor surgeon experience with the procedure or in recurrent cases. Bladder perforation is suspected intraoperatively by observation of hematuria after trocar passage and diagnosed by cystoscopy. Perforation is easily treated by correct reinsertion of the trocar and catheter drainage for 2-4 days. TOT avoids the needle passage in the retropubic space, and hence bladder perforation is much lower than that of TVT.

Bleeding and retro-pubic hematoma: ranges from 0.7% to 8% **(Laurikainen et al, 2007; Rezapour et al, 2001c)** and in majority of cases minor bleeding occur during vaginal dissection and easily controlled. Sometimes excessive bleeding may lead to retropubic hematoma formation usually arises from pelvic floor veins, epigastric, external iliac or obturator vessels injury due to inadvertent trocar passage if laterally directed or externally rotated during the course of insertion. Hematomas size < 100 ml usually asymptomatic, between 100 - 200 ml cause moderate pain, while those >300 ml associated with severe pain and require surgical evacuation of Retzius space **(Flock et al, 2004).** As perforation, bleeding is not a common complication in TOT procedures, with reported rate 0% to 2% **(Barber et al, 2006; Costa et al, 2004).**

Bowel perforation: a very rare (< 0.007%) **(Costantini et al, 2007)** but serious complication and may be fatal. A recent review revealed 7 deaths that occurred after TVT placement of which 6 were associated with bowel injury **(Nygaard and Heit, 2004).** Bowel perforation is not reported with TOT procedures. Risk factors for bowel injury include previous pelvic and abdominal surgery due to presence of adhesions in the retropubic space.

2.4.2 Late postoperative complications

De novo urgency: The rate of de novo urgency after midurethral slings placement as reported in literature ranges from 7.2% to 25% **(Costantini et al, 2007).** The mechanisms of de novo urgency after midurethral slings procedures are poorly understood. Combined outlet obstruction and urethral irritation by the sling has commonly been used as an explanation. TOT procedure is usually associated with a lower rate of de novo urgency than TVT **(Juanos et al, 2011).** Meanwhile, such complication usually does not improve by time. Holmgren et al reported 14.5% of de novo urgency after long term follow-up of 5.2 years after TVT **(Holmgren et al, 2007).**

Groin and thigh pain: On the other hand, TOT procedure has a significant risk of post-operative groin and thigh pain. This pain was observed with range of 5% to 26%. **(Meschia et al, 2007; Dobson et al, 2007).** However, the pain is usually transient and resolves spontaneously within a few months in most of cases. The exact etiology of this pain remains unknown but it may be related to the tape's presence in the adductor muscles or the foreign body reaction to the tape lying in proximity to peripheral obturator nerve branches or secondary to the trauma to the obturator membrane and muscles during the procedure.

Bladder Outlet Obstruction: Postoperative obstruction is another challenging complication after a mid urethral sling procedure which varies from urinary retention (temporary or permanent), difficulty emptying or a weak urinary stream. Obstruction usually arises from excessive tension placed over the midurethra by the tape. The reported rates of postoperative obstruction after TVT range from 1.9% to 19.7% **(Abouassaly et al, 2004; Barber et al, 2006)**, and after TOT the rates actually vary from 0% to 15.6% **(Fischer et al, 2005; Delorme et al, 2004)**. Although urine retention and voiding dysfunction are thought to be less common after TOT approach, a recent multicenter randomized trial did not reveal significant differences in postoperative urinary retention between the TVT and TOT (6% and 3%, respectively) **(Barber et al, 2008).** Early postoperative transient urinary retention could be treated with intermittent sterile self-catheterisation or indwelling catheter and usually resolve spontaneously within 12 wk with restoration of complete bladder emptying in the majority of cases. If no improvement occur, early simple sling lysis should be considered or suburethral tape transaction.

Genitourinary erosion: it is the most frequent and distressing complication after synthetic midurethral sling operations. Costantini and colleagues reported erosion rates after midurethral sling operations based on ranges as reported in the literatures a range from 0.7% - 33%, 2.7% - 33% and 0.5% - 0.6% for vaginal, urethra and urinary bladder erosion respectively **(Costantini et al, 2007)**.

The etiology of the erosion is multifactorial and includes inadequate closure of vaginal wall incision, extensive or incorrect plane of dissection, wound infection, mesh rejection, early sexual activity, tape rolling and abnormal vaginal epithelium i.e. atrophic, scarred or otherwise compromised vaginal mucosa as in post-menopausal women or after previous vaginal surgery and unrecognized vaginal laceration injury during trocar passage. The sling material also plays an important role in this complication.

Patients with genitourinary erosion may be asymptomatic discovered on routine follow-up or presented with a group of symptoms which raise the suspicion of its diagnosis such as pain, dyspareunia, dysuria, discharge and/or bleeding from the urethra or vagina or tape palpable to the patient or partner. Hammad et al, reported that 35% of vaginal erosions were asymptomatic and erosion was discovered on routine follow-up **(Hammad et al, 2005)**. Kobashi et al seemed to confirm these data. In > 90 women who received a polypropylene mesh for the treatment of SUI, 3 developed vaginal erosion, but only 1 had symptoms such as pain, discomfort during sexual activity, and vaginal discharge and erosion was discovered during a routine check-up **(Kobashi et al, 2003)**. Most cases occur in the first few months after surgery but they can also happen much later.

Mesh erosion may be treated with conservative measures or surgically treated depends on the erosion site and size, mesh material, and local tissue condition. Surgical approach ranges from partial simple excision of the exposed mesh to surgical exploration for total graft removal and tissue reconstruction with a Martius flap.

Conservative management with observation might be a viable option if erosion is limited to the vagina and the sling were made of autologous, allograft and new, loosely woven polypropylene material because the latter provides large interstices, which favour tissue ingrowth and healing **(Duckett and Constantine, 2000)**. While some authors stated that polypropylene tape erosion should be treated with complete mesh removal, without regard to erosion site, size, or local tissue condition **(Sweat et al, 2002)**. Vaginal erosion of synthetic materials, such as polyester and silicone slings, should also be treated with mesh removal because epithelialisation over these materials is unlikely **(Duckett and Constantine, 2000; Stanton, Brindley and Holmes, 1985).**

If the vaginal erosion is small (<1 cm) and local tissue does not appear infected, spontaneous healing by epithelialisation may occur in 6 to 12 weeks with pelvic rest alone **(Kobashi and Govier, 2003)**. If conservative management is unsuccessful or the erosion is (>1 cm), the exposed mesh may be excised with the patient under local anesthesia with vaginal closure after the edges have been freshened. Erosions with copious vaginal discharge or if local tissue appears to be infected may require more extensive resection of the mesh. Surgery is recommended when erosion involves the lower urinary tract (bladder or urethra), independently of sling materials **(Clemens et al, 2000; Duckett and Constantine, 2000)**. A recent meta-analysis of polypropylene midurethral slings revealed a possible trend toward increased erosion rates after TOT approach (OR 1.5, 95% CI 0.51–4.4) **(Latthe et al, 2007)**.

Although rare, erosion of mesh into the urethra can occur. A recent large retrospective series of TVT revealed urethral erosion in 0.3% of cases **(Karram et al, 2003)**.

With the new classification system of IUGA and ICS the description of the complications related to midurethral slings especially genitourinary erosion now become standardized and easy as shown in some the following reported cases of complication related to the use of midurethral tapes (figures 5, 6, 7)

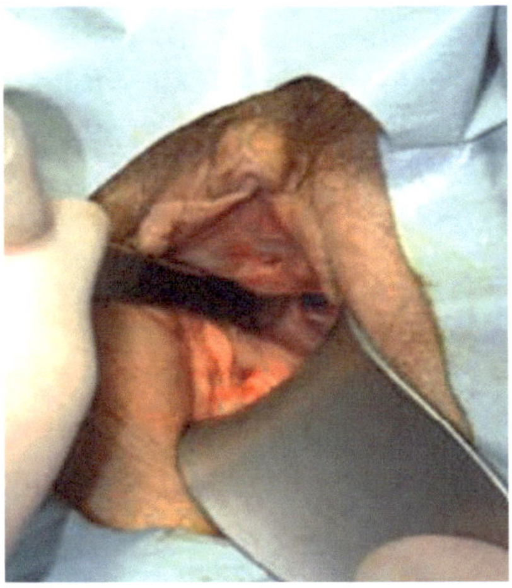

Fig. 5. 52 year old female underwent a transobturator tape. At 6 weeks, she was cured of her USI and reported no vaginal discharge. Vaginal examination revealed a smaller mesh exposure away from vaginal suture line. Classification: 2A T2 S2 **(Haylen et al, 2011)**

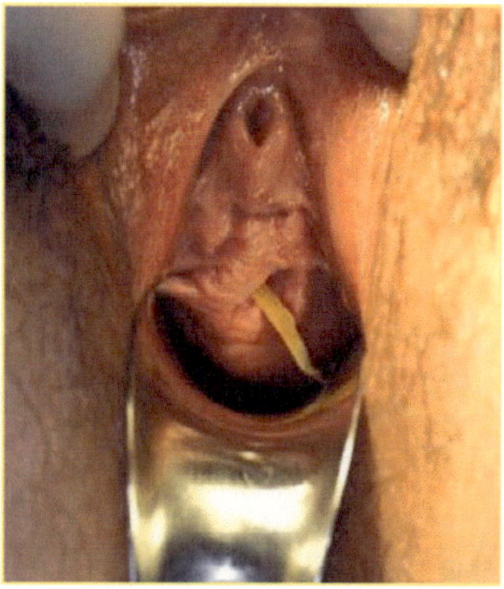

Fig. 6. A 47-year-old woman underwent a transoburator tape for USI. At 5 months follow-up, she reported vaginal discharge. Clinically she was febrile at 38°C with a large sling extrusion as depicted. Classification: 3C T3 S1 **(Haylen et al, 2011)**

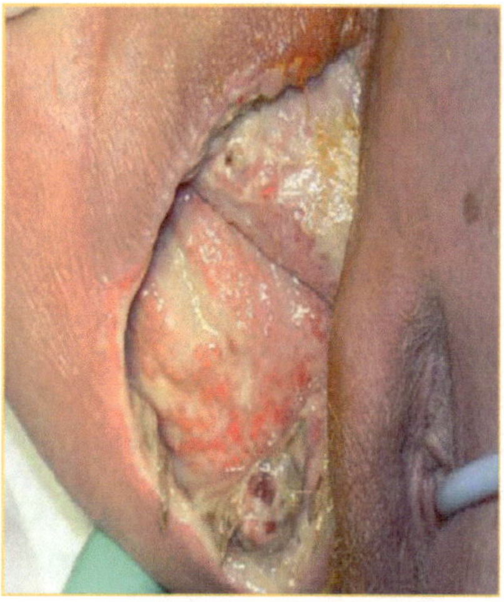

Fig. 7. 65-year-old with urinary incontinence underwent a multifilament transobturator sling. At 14 months follow up, she experienced severe pelvic pain and vaginal discharge. Clinical examination revealed hyperthermia to 40°C, (i) sling exposure at right vaginal sulcus and (ii) severe cellulitis in the genito-crural fold. Classification: 3C T4 S2; (ii) 6C T4 S3 **(Haylen et al, 2011)**

3. Use of biodegradable materials

3.1 Introduction

The perfect implant material currently is not available yet, but in general surgery there is now a consensus, that low weight, large pore (macroporus), monofilament synthetic materials are preferable. However, still serious local complications (e.g. erosion and infection) may occur and related to an increased foreign body reaction. Subsequently, biologic implants were introduced in an effort to reduce the local complications associated with synthetic materials without compromising the surgical results.

Biological xenograft is a mammalian extracellular matrix (ECM) composed of laminin, fibrinectin, elastin, and collagen. Tissue sources from which xenografts are chosen include: porcine (small intestine, dermis), bovine (pericardium, fetal, dermis) and equine. Collagen based implants can either be cross-linked or not. Cross-linking protects the implant against degradation by collagenases, so that they remain intact very long, if not ever. At present, most xenogenic materials are from porcine source and it is the most commonly used, as bovine material became less acceptable. Production is strictly controlled by Food and Drug Administration (FDA) guidelines, which include knowledge of the animal herd, vaccination status, feed source, abattoir approval and bovine spongiform encephalopathy clearance **(Deprest et al, 2006).**

We will discuss below the role of Small intestinal submucosal (SIS) graft as a futuristic biodegradable implant to substitute synthetic slings in the treatment of female SUI.

3.2 Small intestinal submucosal (SIS) graft

SIS xenograft is an acellular, nonimmunogenic, biodegradable, biocompatible, collagen matrix manufactured from porcine small intestinal submucosa, which could induce native tissue regeneration in various organs.

3.2.1 Clinical applications of SIS

SIS graft has gained popularity in the field of urogynecology and reconstructive surgery. Promising results have been reported with the use of SIS as a bladder and urethral substitute material in animals **(Kropp, 1998a; Kropp et al, 1998b; Chen, Yoo and Atala, 1999).** Also, SIS has been used in humans undergoing urogenital procedures such as cystoplasties, ureteral reconstructions, penile chordee, and even urethral reconstruction for hypospadias and strictures **(Dedecker et al, 2005; Atala et al, 1999; Le Roux, 2005; Kassaby et al, 2003; Sharma and Secrest, 2003; Liatsikos et al, 2001).** In the field of urinary incontinence, SIS has been used with encouraging results in treatment of postprostatectomy incontinence **(Jones et al, 2005a),** neuropathic incontinence **(Misseri et al, 2005),** and SUI **(Wiedemann and Otto, 2004; Rutner et al, 2003; Jones et al, 2005b; Farahat et al, 2009).** Practical concerns regarding the use of the SIS implant in clinical practice: The first practical concern is related to the graft biocompatibility and how the tissue would react to the implant. The second practical concern is related to the biomechanical properties of the SIS sling and its suitability for curing SUI **(Farahat et al, 2009).**

3.2.2 Graft biocompatibility

SIS is made by a way that all cells responsible for an eventual immune response are removed, but the ECM and natural growth factors are left intact. It contains collagen, growth factors TGF-beta and FGF-2 **(Wiedemann and Otto, 2004).** Many clinical trials and histopathological studies support the fact that the SIS graft has excellent biocompatibility as evidenced by lack of significant immunological reaction, foreign body reaction, and chronic inflammatory reaction (figure 8). In addition, the SIS sling is well known for its strength, durability, and resistance to infection **(Badylak, 2004; Jankowski, et al, 2004; Wiedemann and Otto, 2004; Rutner et al, 2003).**

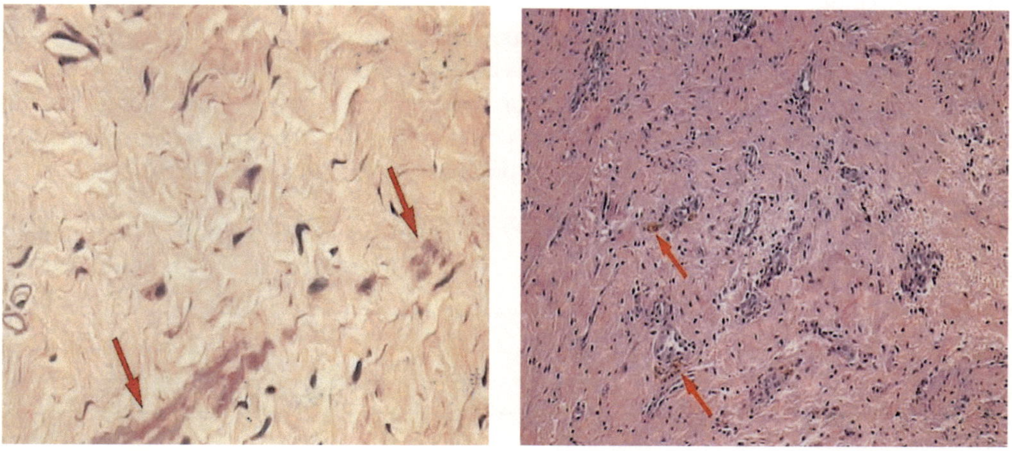

Fig. 8. First histopathological results for SIS pubovaginal slings show: submucosal biopsy with A) minimal SIS residues (red arrows) - B) minimal chronic inflammatory infiltration **(Wiedemann and Otto, 2004)**.

3.2.3 Biomechanical properties

SIS is degraded in 4 to 12 weeks by a "constructive" remodeling process that replaces the graft gradually by host connective tissue **(Clarke et al, 1996; Prevel et al, 1995).** Tensiometric strength initially decreases down to 45% 10 days after implantation, but by 1 month it is identical to that of the native tissue **(Badylak et al, 2001).** The task of the SIS sling is mainly to act as a scaffold that allows in-growth and structural organization of the native host tissue. The implant actively supports connective and epithelial tissue ingrowth and differentiation, as well as deposition, organization, and maturation of ECM components that characterize site-specific tissue remodeling. This phenomenon has been called *smart tissue remodeling* **(Badylak, 1993)** and it is important to note that the balance between implant degradation and host incorporation results in a dynamic implant strength response. The strength of the SIS sling is expected to be the net result between SIS degradation and tissue regeneration. Degradation rates that are too rapid or reconstruction rates that are too slow can result in transient minimum strengths that are below the critical threshold. Supposedly, this carries increased risk of recurrence of incontinence symptoms after an initial successful anti-incontinence surgery **(Jankowski et al, 2004).**

3.2.4 Outcome of the SIS Sling

The suitability of the SIS sling is better reflected by the clinical outcome. In terms of clinical efficacy in correction of SUI, the results of different studies showed that SIS was able to provide a strong suburethral support and durable clinical results (table 7).

Rutner et al, reported in their work utilizing SIS as a pubovaginal slings in the treatment of female SUI that all patients had minimal local reactions and pelvic pain; no cases of erosion or extrusion were noted. The authors also performed a biopsy for cases which required reoperation for correction of incontinence. They observed absence of the implanted graft on gross examination. Microscopically, only a few remnants of the SIS (< 0.4 mm) could be found **(Rutner et al, 2003)**. Farahat et al, reported also using SIS as TVT (figure 9) in the treatment of female SUI that the SIS sling was accepted nicely by the tissue after 12 months. No erosion, extrusion, or severe inflammatory reactions were noted. Most reactions were mild and usually observed as early as 10 days or as late as 45 days after the procedure. Most reactions were well tolerated and resolved spontaneously **(Farahat et al, 2009).**

Author	Number of patients	Patient group	Technique of SIS graft placement	Treatment outcomes (% cured)
Rutner et al, 2003	152	SUI	Pubovaginal slings + bone anchoring	93.4%
Jones et al, 2005b	34	SUI	TVT	80%
Farahat et al, 2009	17	SUI	TVT	82.3 %

Table 7. Treatment outcome of SIS graft.

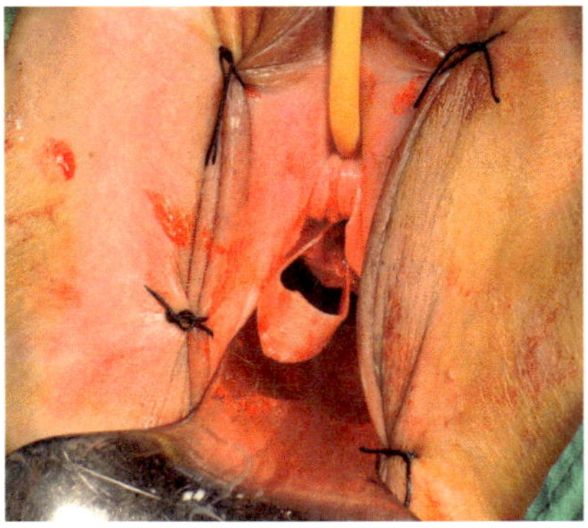

Fig. 9. SIS as TVT sling **(Farahat et al, 2009).**

3.2.5 SIS graft complications

However, unlike most reports confirming the safe use of the SIS graft in the treatment of SUI, Ho et al **(Ho et al, 2004)** reported inflammatory reactions (figure 10) at the abdominal incision (but none at the vaginal incision) in 6 out of 10 patients treated with the 8-ply SIS sling. Most cases resolved with minimal or no intervention. Abscess formation was observed in 2 patients.

John et al **(John et al, 2008)** used both the Cook 4-ply and the 8-ply Stratasis- TF in 16 women with SUI. They reported intense inflammatory complications in 5 patients (nearly one third). Most of the inflammatory reactions were related to the suprapubic region rather than near the vagina or urethra. Four of the 5 patients with complications had the new 8-ply Stratasis-TF. The remaining patient had the 4-ply SIS; however, this patient had a concomitant extensive pelvic floor reconstruction by a gynecologist prior to placement of the SIS sling. Apparently adding more layers to the SIS graft material may have a contributing role in inflammatory reactions, because these high complication rates were not observed with the older 1-ply and 4-ply formulations **(John et al, 2008; Santucci and Barber, 2005)**. No study till now compared the 1-ply, 4-ply, and 8-ply SIS grafts in humans.

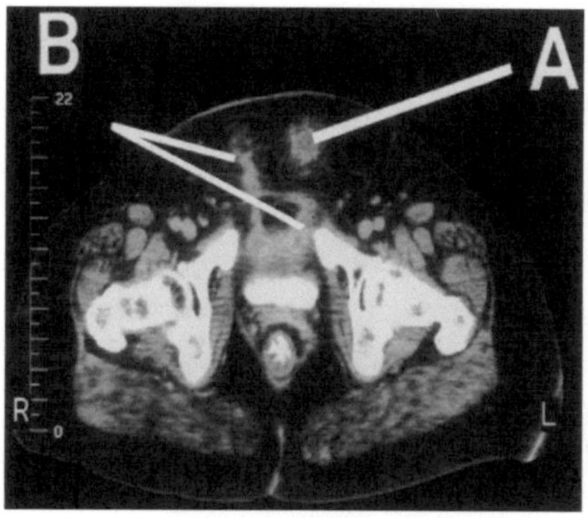

Fig. 10. CT shows inflammation of subcutaneous tissue (*A*) and along arms of the SIS sling **(Ho et al, 2004).**

The SIS graft material is well accepted by the host tissue, and considered safe and effective with lower incidence of erosion and infection than the synthetic midurethral slings. However, Long period of follow up are still required to support the durability of these preliminary results.

4. Stem cell therapy

4.1 Introduction

Stem cells therapy for the regenerative repair of the deficient rhabdosphincter has been the most recent advance in incontinence research. The ultimate goal has been to achieve a permanent cure for SUI by restoration of the intrinsic and extrinsic urethral sphincter and the surrounding connective tissue, including peripheral nerves and blood vessels. Overall, the aim of stem cell therapy is to replace, repair, or enhance the biological function of damaged tissue or organs.

4.2 Cell source

There are two general types of stem cells potentially useful for therapeutic treatment, embryonic stem cells (ESCs) and adult stem cells **(Novara and Artibani, 2007).** The practical use of ESCs has ethical limitations inherent to cell harvesting from fetal tissue and histocompatibility problems. **(Edwards, 2007)**. In contrast, adult stem cells have no significant ethical issues related to their use and have more limited differentiation potential which makes them safer. Tissues engineering therapies are based on autologous multipotent stem cells, of which bone marrow stromal cells are most often used. The bone marrow stromal cells contain mesenchymal stem cells (MSCs) that are capable of differentiating into into adipogenic, osteogenic, chondrogenic and myogenic cells **(Pittenger et al, 1999; Ferrari et al, 1998; Prockop, 1997; Dezawa et al, 2005),** However, bone marrow compartment usage has significant limitations due to its painful nature which usually require general or spinal anesthesia, and low number of (MSCs) are obtained **(Pittenger et al. 1999)**. Muscle derived stem cells (MDCs) and adipose derived stem cells (ADSCs) are advantageous because they can be easily obtained in large quantities under local anesthesia **(Rodríguez et al,. 2006; Strem et al, 2005).**

4.2.1 Bone marrow-derived stem cells (BMSCs)

Bone marrow-derived stem cells (BMSCs) have been most widely studied of all mesenchymal stem cells. BMSCs have been used for the regeneration of cardiac muscle **(Sadek et al, 2009),** bladder detrusor muscle **(Kanematsu et al, 2005),** anal sphincter muscle **(Lorenzi et al, 2008)**, and many other structures **(El Backly and Cancedda, 2010)**. Drost et al. in a pilot study transplanted autologous BMSCs into injured rat urethral sphincter. The cultured BMSCs were injected periurethrally 1 week after the urethral injury. Both histological and immunohistochemistry evaluation showed that transplanted BMSCs survived and differentiated into peripheral nerve cells and striated muscle cells compared to the cell-free group **(Drost et al, 2009).**

4.2.2 Adipose-derived stem cells

Adipose derived stem cells (ADSCs), is a pluripotent cells which have the ability to differentiate into cells of the same and of another germ layer, such as adipogenic, chondrogenic, neurogenic, myogenic and osteogenic cells **(Roche et al, 2010).** In the field of urinary incontinence ADSCs are of special interest for mesodermal and neuronal regeneration and to promote revascularization. Bacou et al, reported that transplantation of ADSCs increases mass and functional capacity of damaged skeletal muscle. They can express specific striated muscle markers (eg, desmin, myod1, myogenin, myosin heavy chain), form multinucleated cells characteristic of myotubules **(Bacou et al, 2004)**. Also, ADSCs can express nerve growth factor at the time of neural differentiation. Zhang et al, reported that neural-differentiated ADSCs present glial characteristics and promote nerve regeneration, after 7 days of transplantation in a rat model in vivo **(Zhang et al, 2010).** Periurethral injection of ADSCs in an immune-competent, incontinent rat model with SUI, exhibited in vivo differentiation into smooth muscle cells and improved urethral resistance **(Lin et al, 2010).** Fu et al. injected predifferentiated ADSCs with 5-azacitidine periurethrally into incontinent rats. A significant difference in bladder capacity and leak point pressure was observed after 3 months of follow-up between the control group and the pretreated group. Also increased number of myoblasts under the mucosa and expression of α-smooth muscle actin was observed 3 months after implantation **(Fu et al, 2010).**

4.2.3 Muscle derived stem cells (MDCs)

Muscle-derived stem cells (MDSCs) can naturally differentiate to multinucleated muscle fibers and display stem cell characteristics **(Seale and Rudnicki, 2000).** MDSCs have also the ability to undergo long-term proliferation, self-renewal, and multipotent differentiation, including differentiation toward endothelial and neuronal lineages **(Lee et al, 2000; Qu-Petersen et al, 2002).** Cannon et al, reported that MDSCs are capable of restoring muscular contraction of the urethral sphincter 2 weeks after injection **(Cannon et al, 2003)**. MDSCs also may improve neurogenic bladder dysfunction in animal models by reconstitution of damaged peripheral nerve cells (eg, Schwann cells, perineum) and vascular cells (eg, vascular smooth muscle cells, pericytes, endothelial cells) **(Nitta et al, 2010)**. For the treatment of SUI myoblasts have been injected to the striated urinary sphincter of a pig model. The animals have shown an increase in urethral pressure profile and muscular myofibrils **(Mitterberger et al, 2008).**

Advantages of MDSCs injection therapy over conventional treatments for SUI:

1. MDSCs that are derived from the incontinent patient (autologous cell transplantation) will not cause an immunogenic or allergic reaction **(Yokoyama et al, 2001a; Lee et al, 2004).**
2. MDSCs are uniquely different from fibroblasts and smooth muscle cells since MDSCs will fuse to form post-mitotic multinucleated myotubes. This limits persistent expansion and risk of obstruction that may occur with other cell sources such as fibroblasts **(Kwon et al, 2006).**
3. MDSCs form contractile myotubes and myofibers that become innervated into the host muscle by activating the intrinsic nerve regeneration and formation of neuromuscular junctions. Therefore, they can not only serve as a bulking agent, but they are also physiologically capable of improving urethral sphincter function **(Chancellor et al, 2000; Yokoyama et al, 2001b; Huard et al, 2002; Hoshi et al, 2008).**

4.3 Isolation of muscle-derived stem cells in humans

Mitterberger M et al. and Strasser H et al. reported biopsy in the right or left upper limb (biceps muscle) to obtain 0.32 to 2 cm3 of muscle tissue (figure 11). At the same time, 250 mL of blood were drawn for autologous serum **(Mitterberger et al, 2008; Strasser et al, 2007b).**

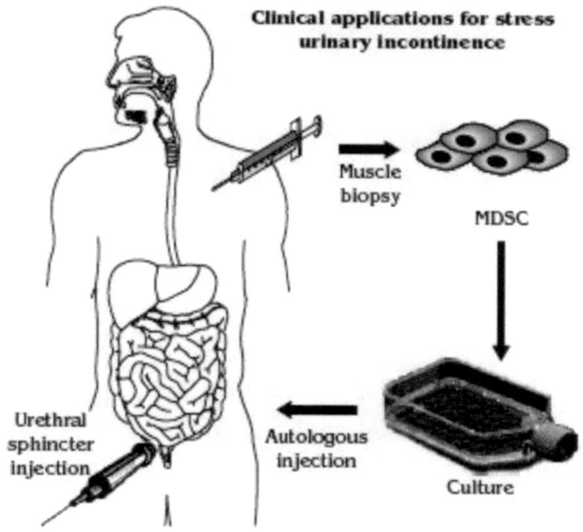

Fig. 11. Diagram showing autologous stem cell injection therapy for SUI. Autologous stem cells are obtained with a biopsy of tissue, the cells are dissociated and expanded in culture, and the expanded cells are implanted into the same host. MDSCs = muscle derived stem cells **(Jankowski et al, 2008)**

Myoblasts and fibroblasts are separated from connective tissue by centrifugation and enzymatic digestion with type I collagenase. Myoblasts are cultured in Ham's F10 medium supplemented with 20% autologous serum, and fibroblasts in DMEM (Dulbecco's modified Eagle medium) and Ham's F12 medium with 10% autologous serum. Cells are accepted when they reach 80% confluence. After 6-8 weeks in culture, fibroblasts and myoblasts are harvested separately by tripsinization and washing with centrifugation. Cell quality is assessed by immunohistochemistry, immunofluorescence, and fluorescence-activated cell sorting. Anti-desmin, vimentin, CD56, CD34 and ASO2 antibodies are used to differentiate myoblasts from fibroblasts. Fusion capacity of myoblasts is measured in differentiation medium without autologous serum to assess their viability, and cells are counted in each culture using the Neubauer chamber (figure 12). Once the cells are "harvested", they are transferred in adequate numbers to sterile syringes, separating myoblasts from fibroblasts. Myoblasts are suspended in 1.4 mL of DMEM/F12 with 20% autologous serum, and fibroblasts in 1 mL of DMEM/F12 with 20% autologous serum mixed with collagen as transport material to prevent cell migration from the injection site, because fibroblasts are mobile following application. Collagen has been shown to stabilize cells so that they remain in place and produce their own extracellular matrix **(Strasser et al, 2007b).**

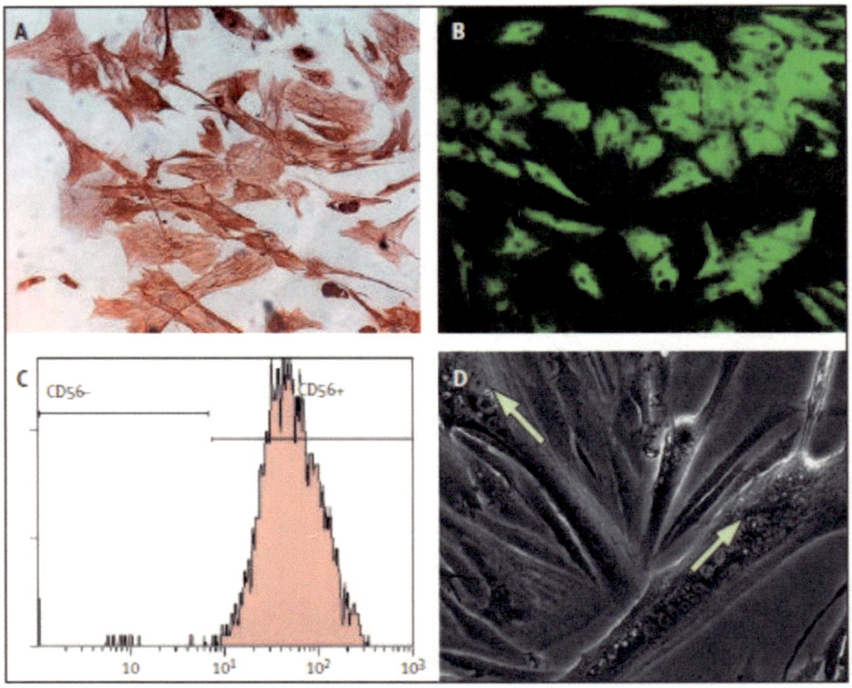

Fig. 12. Characterisation of cells: (A) Immunohistochemical image of human myoblasts stained with antidesmin antibodies. (B) Immunofl uorescence image of human fibroblasts stained with antivimetin antibodies. (C) Fluorescent antibody cell sorter (FACS) analysis of myoblast cell culture showing that 97% of the myoblasts are positive for CD56 antibodies. (D) Phase-contrast microscope image of multinucleated myotubes (marked with arrows) that have formed after fusion of mononucleated myoblasts in diff erentiation medium **(Strasser et al, 2007b).**

4.4 Transurethral ultrasound (TUUS) guided injection of stem cell

At the beginning of the cell injection, the TUUS probe (8 Ch, 15- 20 MHz) was carefully inserted into the urethra. The urethral wall and the rhabdosphincter were visualized. A specially designed patent-pending injection device was used for precisely adjusted injection of several small portions. First, 15-18 portions of the myoblast suspension were injected directly into the omega-shaped rhabdosphincter at two different levels. Then, 25-30 depots of the fibroblast/collagen suspension were injected into the submucosa circumferentially at three levels (Figure 13). After implantation of the cells the patients were instructed to perform PFT and FES for 4 wk postoperatively to support integration of the cells and to improve formation of new muscle tissue **(Strasser et al, 2007).**

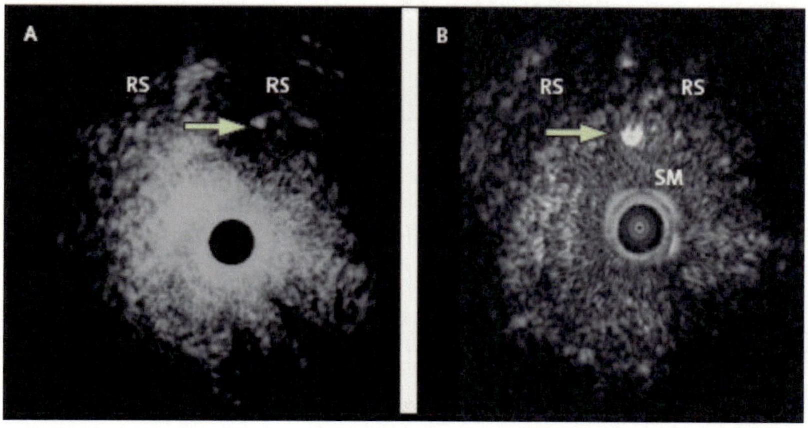

Fig. 13. Cross-sectional ultrasonography images of the urethra and the rhabdosphincter (A) The tip of the needle (marked with an arrow) is positioned at the inner aspect of the rhabdosphincter (RS) for injection of myoblasts. (B) The tip of the needle is placed at the outer aspect of the submucosa (SM) for injection of fibroblasts **(Strasser et al, 2007b).**

4.5 Clinical results of stem cell therapy

Few human trials have been conducted using autologous derived stem cells in the treatment of female SUI, which mainly involved the use of MDSCs. Stem cell therapy, shows an early encouraging results and these results suggest the ability of pure cellular therapy to treat female SUI (Table 8).

Strasser et al. conducted the first clinical experiments in women with SUI. 42 women suffering from SUI were recruited and subsequently treated with transurethral ultrasonography- guided injections of autologous myoblasts and fibroblasts obtained from skeletal muscle biopsies. After a follow-up of 12 months incontinence was cured in 39 women **(Strasser et al, 2007a)**. In another trial 42 women were randomly assigned to receive transurethral ultrasonography guided injections of autologous myoblasts and fibroblasts, at 12-months' follow-up, 38 of the 42 women injected with autologous cells were completely continent **(Strasser et al, 2007b).** Mitterbarger et al. studied 20 female patients suffering from SUI after TUUS guidance injection of autologous myoblasts and fibroblasts. At 1 year follow-up 18 patients were cured and 2 patients improved. At 2 years after therapy 16 of the

18 patients presented as cured, 2 others were improved, and 2 were lost to follow-up **(Mitterbarger et al, 2008a)**. Other studies have been reported early good results for stem cell injection in female with SUI **(Carr et al, 2008; Herschorn et al, 2010).**

Not only stem cell injection therapy is limited to the field of female SUI, however its usage has been extended to treat males with post-prostatectomy incontinence **(Mitterbarger et al, 2008b; Yamamoto et al, 2010).**

Clinical study	Patients (n)	Patient group	Stem cell source	Symptomatic improvement
Strasser et al, 2007a	63 (42) women (21) men	SUI	MDSC, fibroblasts	85%
Strasser et al, 2007b	42 women	SUI	MDSC, fibroblasts	91%
Mitterbarger et al, 2008a	20 women	SUI	MDSC, fibroblasts	90% at 1 yr 89% at 2 yr
Carr et al, 2008	8 women	SUI	MDSCs	63%
Herschorn et al, 2010	29 women	SUI	MDSC	50% cured

Table 8. Results of the first clinical studies have recently become available.

In general, stem cell injection therapy into the middle urethra may restore the contractile response of the striated muscle and rhabdosphincter. Early results were encouraging with no reported serious side effects. Autologous MDSCs and ADSC pure injection therapy may be a promising treatment to restore urethral sphincter function. These promising early clinical results warrant further evaluation to validate results, determine durability and focus on safety and possible adverse reactions.

5. References

Abrams P, Cardozo L, Magnus F, et al. (2002). The standardization of terminology of lower urinary tract function: report from the standardization sub-committee of the International Continence Society. *Neurourol Urodynam*, Vol. 21, pp. 167–178

Abouassaly R, Steinberg JR, Lemieux M, et al. (2004). Complications of tension-free vaginal tape surgery: a multi-institutional review. *BJU Int*, Vol. 94, pp. 110

Aigmueller T, Trutnovsky G, Tamussino K, et al. (2011). Ten-year follow-up after the tension-free vaginal tape procedure. *American Journal of Obstetrics and Gynecology*. Article in Press. doi:10.1016/j.ajog.2011.07.010

Amid P. (1997). Classification of biomaterials and their relative complications in an abdominal wall hernia surgery. *Hernia*, Vol. 1, pp. 15–21

Andonian S, Chen T, St-Denis B, et al. (2005). Randomized clinical trial comparing suprapubic arch sling (SPARC) and tension-free vaginal tape (TVT): one-year results. *Eur Urol*, Vol. 47, pp. 537

Angioli R, Plotti F, Muzii L, et al. (2010). Tension-Free Vaginal Tape Versus Transobturator Suburethral Tape: Five-Year Follow-up Results of a Prospective Randomised Trial. *European Urology*, Vol. 58, pp. 671–677

Atala A, Guzman L, Retik AB. (1999). A novel inert collagen matrix for hypospadias repair. *J Urol*, Vol. 162, pp. 1148–51

Bacou F, el Andalousi RB, Daussin PA, et al. (2004). Transplantation of adipose tissue-derived stromal cells increases mass and functional capacity of damaged skeletal muscle. *Cell Transplant*, Vol. 13, pp. 103–111

Badylak SF. (1993). Small intestinal submucosa (SIS): a biomaterial conducive to smart tissue remodeling. In: Bell E, ed. *Tissue Engineering: Current Perspectives*, 179-189, Cambridge, MA: Burkhauser Pub

Badylak SF, Kokini K, Tullius B, et al. (2001). Strength over time of a resorbable bioscaffold for body wall repair in a dog model. J Surg Res, Vol. 99, pp. 282–287

Badylak SF. (2004). Xenogeneic extracellular matrix as a scaffold for tissue reconstruction. *Transplant Immunology, Vol.* 12, pp. 367-377

Barber MD, Gustilo-Ashby AM, Chen CC, et al. (2006). Perioperative complications and adverse events of the MONARC transobturator tape, compared with the tension-free vaginal tape. *Am J Obstet Gynecol*, Vol. 195, pp. 1820

Barber MD, Kleeman S, Karram MM, et al. (2008). Transobturator tape compared with tension-free vaginal tape for the treatment of stress urinary incontinence: a randomized controlled trial. Obstet Gynecol, Vol. 111, pp. 611

Botlero R, Urquhart DM, Davis SR, et al. (2008). Prevalence and incidence of urinary incontinence in women: review of the literature and investigation of methodological issues. *Int J Urol*, Vol. 15, pp. 230–4

Cannon TW, Lee JY, Somogyi G, et al. (2003). Improved sphincter contractility after allogenic muscle-derived progenitor cell injection into the denervated rat urethra. *Urology*, Vol. 62, pp. 958–963

Carr LK, Steele D, Steele S, et al. (2008). 1-year follow up of autologous muscle-derived stem cell injection pilot study to treat stress urinary incontinence. *Int Urogynecol J Pelvic Floor Dysfunct, Vol.* 19; pp. 881–883.

Chen F, Yoo JJ, Atala A. (1999). Acellular collagen matrix as a possible "off the shelf" biomaterial for urethral repair. *Urology*, Vol. 54, pp. 407–9

Cindolo L, Salzano L, Rota G, et al. (2004). Tension-free transobturator approach for female stress urinary incontinence. *Minerva Urol Nefrol*, Vol. 56, pp. 89–98

Clarke KM, Lantz GC, Salisbury SK, et al. (1996). Intestine submucosa and polypropylene mesh for abdominal wall repair in dogs. *J Surg Res*, Vol. 60, pp. 107–114

Clemens JQ, DeLancey JO, Faerber GJ, et al. (2000). Urinary tract erosions after synthetic pubovaginal slings: diagnosis and management strategy. *Urology*, Vol. 56, pp. 589–94

Chancellor MB, Yokoyama T, Tirney S, et al. (2000). Preliminary results of myoblast injection into the urethra and bladder wall: a possible method for the treatment of stress urinary incontinence and impaired detrusor contractility. *Neurourol Urodyn,* Vol. 19, pp. 279–87

Costa P, Grise P, Droupy S, et al. (2004). Surgical treatment of female stress urinary incontinence with a trans-obturator-tape (T.O.T.) Uratape: short term results of a prospective multicentric study. *Eur Urol,* Vol. 46, pp. 102

Costantini E, Lazzeri M & Porena M. (2007). Managing Complications after Midurethral Sling for Stress Urinary Incontinence. *EAU - EBU update series,* Vol. 5, pp. 232-40

Daneshgari F, Kong W and Swartz M. (2008). Complications of Mid Urethral Slings: Important Outcomes for Future Clinical Trials. *The Journal of Urology,* Vol. 180, pp. 1890-1897

Dedecker F, Grynberg M, Staerman F. (2005). Small intestinal submucosa (SIS): prospects in urogenital surgery. *Prog Urol,* Vol. 15, pp. 405–7

Deffieux X, Donnadieu AC, Porcher R, et al. (2007). Long-term results of tension-free vaginal tape for female urinary incontinence: follow-up over 6 years. *Int J Urol,* Vol. 14, pp. 521–526

DeLancey JO. (1994). Structural support of the urethra as it relates urinary incontinence: the hammock hypothesis. *Am J Obstet Gynaecol,* Vol. 170, No. 20, pp. 1713

De Leval J. (2003). Novel Surgical Technique for the Treatment of Female Stress Urinary Incontinence: Transobturator Vaginal Tape Inside-Out. *European Urology,* Vol. 44, pp. 724–730

DeLorme E. (2001). Transobturator tape urethral suspension: mini-invasive procedure in the treatment of stress urinary incontinence in women. *Prog Urol,* Vol. 11, pp. 1306–1313

Delorme E, Droupy S, de Tayrac R, et al. (2004). Transobturator tape (Uratape): a new minimally-invasive procedure to treat female urinary incontinence. *Eur Urol,* Vol. 45, pp. 203

Deng DY, Rutman M, Raz S, Rodriguez LV. (2007). Presentation and management of major complications of midurethral slings: are complications under-reported? *Neurourol Urodyn,* Vol. 26, pp. 46–52

Deprest J., Zheng F. and Konstantinovic M, et al. (2006). The biology behind fascial defects and the use of implants in pelvic organ prolapse repair. Int Urogynecol J, Vol. 17, pp. S16–S25

Dobson A, Robert M, Swaby C, et al. (2007). Trans-obturator surgery for stress urinary incontinence: 1 year follow-up of a cohort of 52 women. *Int Urogynecol J Pelvic Floor Dysfunct,* Vol. 18, pp. 27–32

Drost AC, Weng S, Feil G, et al. (2009). In vitro myogenic differentiation of human bone marrow-derived mesenchymal stem cells as a potential treatment for urethral sphincter muscle repair. *Ann N Y Acad Sci,* Vol. 1176, pp. 135–143.

Duckett JRA, Constantine G. (2000). Complications of silicone sling insertion for stress urinary incontinence. *J Urol,* Vol. 163, pp. 1835–7

Dwyer PL. (2006). Evolution of biological and synthetic grafts in reconstructive pelvic surgery. *Int Urogynecol J,* Vol. 17, pp. S10–S15

Dezawa M, Ishikawa H, Itokazu Y, et al. (2005). Bone marrow stromal cells generate muscle cells and repair muscle degeneration. *Science, Vol.* 309, pp. 314–7

Edwards RG. (2007). A burgeoning science of embryological genetics demands a modern ethics. *Reprod Biomed Online*, Vol. 15, pp. 34–40

El Backly RM, Cancedda R: (2010). Bone marrow stem cells in clinical application: harnessing paracrine roles and niche mechanisms. *Adv Biochem Eng Biotechnol*, Aug 27 (Epub ahead of print).

Farahat Y, Eltatawy H, Haroun H et al: (2009). The Small Intestinal Submucosa (SIS) as a Suburethral Sling for Correction of Stress Urinary Incontinence: *UroToday International Journal*, Vol. 2/Iss 3/June doi:10.3834/uij.1944-5784.2009.06.02

Fischer A, Fink T, Zachmann S, et al. (2005). Comparison of retropubic and outside-in transoburator sling systems for the cure of female genuine stress urinary incontinence. *Eur Urol*, Vol. 48, pp. 799

Ferrari G, Cusella-De Angelis G, Coletta M, et al. (1998). Muscle regeneration by bone marrow-derived myogenic progenitors. *Science*, 279, pp. 1528–30

Flock F, Reich A, Muche R, et al. (2004). Hemorrhagic complications associated with tension-free vaginal tape procedure. *Obstet Gynecol*, Vol. 104, pp. 989

Fu Q, Song XF, Liao GL, et al. (2010). Myoblasts differentiated from adipose-derived stem cells to treat stress urinary incontinence. *Urology*, Vol. 75, pp. 718–723

Giberti C, Gallo F, Cortese P, et al. (2007). Transobturator tape for treatment of female stress urinary incontinence: objective and subjective results after a mean follow-up of two years. *Urology*, Vol. 69, pp. 703–707

Grise P, Droupy S, Saussine C, et al. (2006). Transobturator tape for stress urinary incontinence with polypropylene tape and outside-in procedure: Prospective study with 1 year of minimal follow-up and review of transobturator tape sling. *Urology*, Vol. 68, 759–763

Hammad FT, Kennedy-Smith A, Robinson RG. (2005). Erosions and urinary retention following polypropylene synthetic sling: Australasian survey. *Eur Urol*, vol. 47, pp. 641–7

Hannestad YS, Rortveit G, Sandvik H, et al. (2000). A community based survey of female urinary incontinnce: the Norwegian EPINCONT study. *J Clin Epidemiol*, Vol. 53, pp. 1150–7

Huard J, Yokoyama T, Pruchnic R, et al. (2002). Muscle-derived cell-mediated *ex vivo* gene therapy for urological dysfunction. *Gene Ther*, Vol. 9, pp. 1617–26

Haylen BT, Freeman RM, Swift SE, et al. (2011). An International Urogynecological Association (IUGA) / International Continence Society (ICS) joint terminology and classification of the complications related directly to the insertion of prostheses (meshes, implants, tapes) & grafts in female pelvic floor surgery. *Int Urogynecol J*, Vol. 22, pp. 3–15

Herschorn S, Carr L, Birch C, et al. (2010). Autologous muscle-derived cells as therapy for stress urinary incontinence: A randomized blinded trial. *Neurourol Urodyn*, Vol. 29, pp. 243–326 [abstract]

Ho KL, Witte MN, Bird ET. (2004). 8-ply small intestinal submucosa tension-free sling: spectrum of postoperative inflammation. *J Urol, Vol.* 171, pp. 268-271

Holmgren C, Nilsson S, Lanner L, et al. (2007). Frequency of de novo urgency in 463 women who had undergone the tension-free vaginal tape (TVT) procedure for genuine stress urinary incontinence - a long-term follow-up. *Eur J Obstet Gynecol*, Vol. 132, pp. 5 - 121

Hoshi A, Tamaki T, Tono K, et al. (2004). Reconstruction of radical prostatectomy-induced urethral damage using skeletal musclederived multipotent stem cells. Transplantation, Vol. 85, pp. 1617–1624

Jankowski R, Pruchnic R, Hiles M, et al. (2004). Advances toward tissue engineering for the treatment of stress urinary incontinence. *Rev Urol*, Vol. 6, pp. 51-57

Jankowski R, Pruchnic R, Wagner D et al. (2008). Regenerative Therapy for Stress Urinary Incontinence. *Tzu Chi Med J*, Vol. 20, pp. 169-176

John TT, Aggarwal N, Single AK, et al. (2008). Intense inflammatory reaction with porcine small intestine submucosa pubovaginal sling or tape for stress urinary incontinence. *Urology*, Vol. 72, pp. 1036-1039

Jones JS, Vasavada SP, Abdelmalak JB, et al. (2005a). Sling may hasten return of continence after radical prostatectomy. *Urology, Vol.* 65, pp. 1163-1167

Jones JS, Rackley RR, Berglund R, et al. (2005b). Porcine small intestinal submucosa as a percutaneous mid-urethral sling: 2-year results. *BJU Int,* 96, pp. 103-106

Juanos JL, Sanchez EB, Soler JP, et al. (2011). De novo urgency after tension-free vaginal tape versus transobturator tape procedure for stress urinary incontinence. *European Journal of Obstetrics & Gynecology and Reproductive Biology*, Vol. 155, pp. 229-32

Kanematsu A, Yamamoto S, Iwai-Kanai E, et al. (2005). Induction of smooth muscle cell-like phenotype in marrow-derived cells among regenerating urinary bladder smooth muscle cells. *Am J Pathol,* Vol. 166, pp. 565–573.

Karram MM, Segal JL, Vassallo BJ, et al. (2003). Complications and untoward effects of the tension-free vaginal tape procedure. *Obstet Gynecol*, Vol. 101, pp. 929

Kassaby EA, Retik AB, Yoo JJ, et al. (2003). Urethral stricture repair with an off-the-shelf collagen matrix. J Urol, Vol. 169, pp. 170–3 Kobashi KC, Govier FE. (2003). Management of vaginal erosion of polypropylene mesh slings. *J Urol*, Vol. 169, pp.2242–3

Kropp BP. (1998a). Small-intestinal submucosa for bladder augmentation: a review of preclinical studies. *World J Urol*, Vol. 16, pp. 262–5

Kropp BP, Ludlow JK, Spicer D, et al. (1998b). Rabbit urethral regeneration using small intestinal submucosa onlay graft. Urology, Vol. 52, pp. 138–42

Kwon D, Kim Y, Pruchnic R, et al: (2006). Periurethral cellular injection: comparison of muscle-derived progenitor cells and fibroblasts with regard to efficacy and tissue contractility in an animal model of stress urinary incontinence. *Urology*, Vol. 68, pp. 449–454

Latthe P, Foon R and Toozs-Hobson P. (2007). Transobturator and retropubic tape procedures in stress urinary incontinence: a systematic review and meta-analysis of effectiveness and complications. *BJOG*, Vol. 114, pp. 522

Laurikainen E, Valpas A, Kivela A, et al. (2007). Retropubic compared with transobturator tape placement in treatment of urinary incontinence: a randomized controlled trial. *Obstet Gynecol*, Vol. 109, pp. 4

Le Roux PJ. (2005). Endoscopic urethroplasty with unseeded small intestinal submucosa collagen matrix grafts: a pilot study. *J Urol*, Vol. 173, pp. 140–3

Liapis A, Bakas P and Creatsas G. (2010). Efficacy of inside-out transobturator vaginal tape (TVTO) at 4 years follow up. *European Journal of Obstetrics & Gynecology and Reproductive Biology*, Vol. 148, pp. 199–201

Liatsikos EN, Dinlec CZ, Kapoor R, et al. (2001). Ureteral reconstruction: small intestine submucosa for the management of strictures and defects of the upper third of the ureter. J Urol, Vol. 165, pp. 1719–23

Lin G, Wang G, Banie L, et al. (2010). Treatment of stress urinary incontinence with adipose tissue-derived stem cells. *Cytotherapy*, Vol. 12, pp. 88–95

Lee JY, Qu-Petersen Z, Cao B, et al. (2000) Clonal isolation of muscle-derived cells capable of enhancing muscle regeneration and bone healing. *J Cell Biol, Vol.* 150, pp. 1085–100

Lee JY, Paik SY, Yuk SH, et al. (2004) Long term effects of muscle-derived stem cells on leak point pressure and closing pressure in rats with transected pudendal nerves. *Mol Cells, Vol.* 18, pp. 309–313

Lorenzi B, Pessina F, Lorenzoni P, et al. (2008). Treatment of experimental injury of anal sphincters with primary surgical repair and injection of bone marrow-derived mesenchymal stem cells. *Dis Colon Rectum*, Vol. 51, pp. 411–420.

Mariappan P, Alhasso A, Ballantyne Z, et al.b(2007). Duloxetine, a Serotonin and Noradrenaline Reuptake Inhibitor (SNRI) for the Treatment of Stress Urinary Incontinence: A Systematic Review. *European urology*, Vol. 51, pp. 67–74

Meschia M, Bertozzi R, Pifarotti P, et al. (2007). Peri-operative morbidity and early results of a randomised trial comparing TVT and TVT-O. *Int Urogynecol J Pelvic Floor Dysfunct, Vol.* 18, pp. 1257–1261

Misseri R, Cain MP, Casale AJ, et al. (2005). Small intestinal submucosa bladder neck slings for incontinence associated with neuropathic bladder. *J Urol, Vol.* 174, pp. 1680-1682

Mitterberger M, Pinggera GM, Marksteiner R, et al. (2007). Functional and histological changes after myoblast injections in the porcine rhabdosphincter. *Eur Urol*, Vol. 52, pp. 1736–1743. (Published erratum appears in Eur Urol 2008, 54:1208

Mitterberger M, Pinggera GM, Marksteiner R, et al. (2008a). Adult Stem Cell Therapy of Female Stress Urinary Incontinence. *European urology*, Vol. 53, pp. 169-175

Mitterberger M, Marksteiner R, Margreiter E, et al. (2008b). Myoblast and fibroblast therapy for post-prostatectomy urinary incontinence: 1-year follow-up of 63 patients. *J Urol*, Vol. 179, pp. 226–231.

Morley R & Nethercliffe J. (2005). Minimally invasive surgical techniques for stress incontinence surgery. *Best Practice & Research Clinical Obstetrics and Gynaecology*, Vol. 19, pp. 925-940

Neuman M & Shaare-Zedek MC. (2007). Training TVT SECUR: the first 150 teaching operations. *Int Urogynecol J*, Vol. 18, S27

Nilsson CG, Falconer C & Rezapour M. (2004). Seven-year follow-up of the tension-free vaginal tape procedure for treatment of urinary incontinence. *Obstet Gynecol*, Vol. 104, pp. 1259–1262

Nilsson CG, Palva K, Rezapour M, et al. (2008). Eleven years prospective follow-up of the tension-free vaginal tape procedure for treatment of stress urinary incontinence. *Int Urogynecol J Pelvic Floor Dysfunct*, Vol. 19, pp. 1043–7

Nitta M, Tamaki T, Tono K, et al. (2010). Reconstitution of experimental neurogenic bladder dysfunction using skeletal muscle-derived multipotent stem cells. *Transplantation,* Vol. 89, pp. 1043–1049

Novara G, Artibani W. (2007). Myoblasts and fibroblasts in stress urinary incontinence. Lancet, Vol. 369, pp. 2139-40

Novara G, Artibani W, Barber MD, et al. (2010). Updated Systematic Review and Meta-Analysis of the Comparative Data on Colposuspensions, Pubovaginal Slings, and Midurethral Tapes in the Surgical Treatment of Female Stress Urinary Incontinence. *European Urology*, Vol. 58, pp. 218 - 238

Nygaard IE and Heit M. (2004). Stress urinary incontinence. *Obstet Gynecol*, Vol. 104, pp. 607

Petros P, Ulmsten U. (1993). An integral theory and its method for the diagnosis and management of female urinary incontinence. *Scand J Urol Nephrol Suppl*, Vol. 153, pp. 1-93

Pittenger MF, Mackay AM, Beck SC, et al. (1999). Multilineage potential of adult human mesenchymal stem cells. *Science,* Vol. 284, pp. 143–7

Prevel CD, Eppley BL, Summerlin DJ, et al. (1995). Small intestinal submucosa: use in repair of rodent abdominal wall defects. *Ann Plast Surg,* Vol. 35, pp. 374–380

Price N, Dawood R and Jackson SR. (2010). Pelvic floor exercise for urinary incontinence: A systematic literature review. *Maturitas,* Vol. 67, pp. 309–315

Prockop DJ. (1997). Marrow stromal cells as stem cells for nonhematopoietic tissues. *Science, Vol.* 276, pp. 71–4

Qu-Petersen Z, Deasy B, Jankowski R, et al. (2002). Identification of a novel population of muscle stem cells in mice: potential for muscle regeneration. *J Cell Biol*, Vol. 157, pp. 851–864

Rezapour M & Ulmsten U. (2001a): Tension-free vaginal tape (TVT) in women with recurrent stress urinary incontinence–a long-term follow-up. *Int Urogynecol J Pelvic Floor Dysfunct*, Vol. 12, pp. S9–S11

Rezapour M & Ulmsten U. (2001b): Tension free vaginal tape (TVT) in women with mixed urinary incontinence–a long-term follow-up. *Int Urogynecol J Pelvic Floor Dysfunct*, Vol. 12, pp. S15–18

Rezapour M, Falconer C & Ulmsten U. (2001c). Tension-free vaginal tape (TVT) in stress incontinent women with intrinsic sphincter deficiency (ISD)–a long-term follow-up. *Int Urogynecol J Pelvic Floor Dysfunct*, Vol. 12, pp. S12–14

Roche R, Festy F, Fritel X. (2010). Stem cells for stress urinary incontinence: The adipose promise. *J Cell Mol Med*, Vol. 14, pp. 135–142

Rodríguez L, Alfonso Z, Zhang R, et al. (2006). Clonogenic multipotent stem cells in human adipose tissue differentiate into functional smooth muscle cells. Proc Natl Acad Sci USA, Vol. 103, pp. 12167-72

Rosch R, Junge K, Hölzl F et al. (2004). How to construct a mesh. In: Schumpelick V, Nyhus LM (eds) Meshes: benefits and risks, 179–184, Springer, Berlin Heidelberg New York.

Roumeguere T, Quackels T, Bollens R, et al. (2005). Trans-obturator vaginal tape (TOT) for female stress incontinence: one year follow-up in 120 patients. *Eur Urol*, Vol. 5, pp. 805–809

Rutner AB, Levine SR, Schmaelzle JF. (2003). Processed porcine small intestine submucosa as a graft material for pubovaginal slings: durability and results. *Urology,* 62, pp. 805-809

Sadek HA, Martin CM, Latif SS, et al. (2009). Bone-marrow-derived side population cells for myocardial regeneration. *J Cardiovasc Transl Res,* Vol. 2, pp. 173–181.

Santucci RA, Barber TD. (2005). Resorbable extracellular matrix grafts in urologic reconstruction. *Int Braz J Urol,* Vol. 31, pp. 192-203

Sharma AK, Secrest CL. (2003). Small intestinal submucosa (SIS) graft reconstruction of urethra. *J Urol,* Vol. 169, pp. 101 (Abstract no. 393)

Stanton SL, Brindley GS, Holmes DM. (1985). Silastic sling for urethral sphincter incompetence in women. *Br J Obstet Gynaecol,* Vol. 92, pp. 747–50

Seale P, Rudnicki MA. (2000). A new look at the origin, function, and "stem-cell" status of muscle satellite cells. *Dev Biol,* Vol. 218, pp. 115–124

Strasser H, Marksteiner R, Margreiter E, et al (2007a). Transurethral ultrasonography-guided injection of adult autologous stem cells versus transurethral endoscopic injection of collagen in treatment of urinary incontinence. *World J Urol, Vol.* 25, pp. 385–92

Strasser H, Marksteiner R, Margreiter E, et al. (2007b). Autologous myoblasts and fibroblasts versus collagen for treatment of stress urinary incontinence in women: a randomized controlled trial. *Lancet,* Vol. 369, pp. 2179-86

Strem B, Hicok K, Zhu M, et al. (2005). Multipotential differentiation of adipose tissue-derived stem cells. *Keio J Med,* Vol. 54, pp. 132-41

Sweat SD, Itano NB, Clemens JQ, et al. (2002). Polypropylene mesh tape for stress urinary incontinence: complications of urethral erosion and outlet obstruction. *J Urol,* Vol. 168, pp. 144–7

Ulmsten U, Henriksson L, Johnson P, et al. (1996). An ambulatory surgical procedure under local anesthesia for treatment of female urinary incontinence. *Int Urogynecol J,* Vol. 7, pp. 81–86

Villet R, Atallah D, Cotelle-Bernede O, et al. (2002). Treatment of stress urinary incontinence with tension-free vaginal tape (TVT). Mid-term results of a prospective study of 124 cases [in French]. *Prog Urol,* Vol. 12, pp. 70–76

Waltregny D, Gaspar Y, Reul O, et al. (2008). for the treatment of female stress urinary incontinence: results of a prospective study after a 3-year minimum follow-up. *Eur Urol,* Vol. 53, pp. 401–408

Ward KL & Hilton P. (2004). The United Kingdom and Ireland Tension- Free Vaginal Tape Trial Group: A prospective multicenter randomized trial of tension-free vaginal tape and colposuspension for primary urodynamic stress incontinence: 2-year follow-up. *Am J Obstet Gynecol,* Vol. 190, pp. 324–331

Ward KL & Hilton P. (2008). The United Kingdom and Ireland Tension- Free Vaginal Tape Trial Group: Tension-free vaginal tape versus colposuspension for primary urodynamic stress incontinence: 5-year follow-up. *BJOG,* Vol. 15, pp. 226-233

Wiedemann A, Otto M. (2004). Small intestinal submucosa for pubourethral sling suspension for the treatment of stress incontinence: first histopathological results in humans. *J Urol,* Vol. 172, pp. 215-218

Winters JC, Fitzgrerald MP and Barber MD. (2006). The use of synthetic mesh in female reconstructive surgery. *BJU International,* Vol. 98 (suppl 1), pp. 70–76

Yamamoto T, Gotoh M, Hattori R, et al. (2010). Periurethral injection of autologous adipose-derived stem cells for the treatment of stress urinary incontinence in patients undergoing radical prostatectomy: report of initial two cases. *Int J Urol*, Vol. 17, pp. 75–82 (Retraction in *Int J Urol*, 2010, Vol. 17, pp. 896)

Yokoyama T, Yoshimura N, Dhir R, et al. (2001a). Persistence and survival of autologous muscle derived cells versus bovine collagen as potential treatment of stress urinary incontinence. *J Urol, Vol.* 165, pp. 271–6

Yokoyama T, Pruchnic R, Lee JY, et al. (2001b). Autologous primary muscle-derived cells transfer into the lower urinary tract. *Tissue Eng,* Vol. 7, pp. 395–404

Zhang Y, Luo H, Zhang Z, et al. (2010). A nerve graft constructed with xenogeneic acellular nerve matrix and autologous adipose-derived mesenchymal stem cells. *Biomaterials,* Vol. 31, pp. 5312–532416.